What Your Doctor Won't Tell You

What Your Doctor Won't Tell You

Jane Heimlich

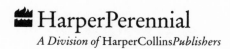

HarperPerennial

A Division of HarperCollins*Publishers*

FIRST EDITION

Designed by Alma Orenstein

Library of Congress Cataloging-in-Publication Data

Heimlich, Jane.
  What your doctor won't tell you/Jane Heimlich. — 1st ed.
    p.   cm.
  Includes bibliographical references.
  ISBN 0-06-055204-2
  ISBN 0-06-096539-8 (pbk.)
  1. Therapeutics—Popular works. I. Title.
  RM122.5.H45   1990
  615.5—dc20   89-46097

90 91 92 93 94 AT/RRD 10 9 8 7 6 5 4 3 2 1
90 91 92 93 94 AT/RRD 10 9 8 7 6 5 4 3 2 1 (pbk.)

To my husband, for encouraging and supporting this venture

Contents

This book is intended to introduce the reader to alternative treatments for chronic and major life-threatening diseases, and to enable the reader to better understand, assess, and decide on the appropriate course of treatment for a given disease or condition. This book should not be substituted for the advice and treatment of a physician but rather should be used in advance of a visit to the doctor in order to assist the reader to better understand the treatment options available. The author and publisher disclaim responsibility for any adverse effects resulting from the information contained herein.

Foreword

I began my medical career as a conventional physician specializing in public health and nutrition. I knew nothing about "alternative" medical treatment until eight years ago when comedian–health writer Dick Gregory checked into the hospital and I was asked to serve as nutrition consultant. Gregory was undergoing one of his extended water fasts and requested medical supervision.

Walking into Gregory's hospital room was like entering a busy office; his phone rang constantly, most often with calls from well-known performers and other notables who wanted his advice about health matters. I wondered, Why is it that these celebrities, who can afford the best medical care, turn to an individual with no medical credentials? Curious, I began investigating some of the treatments that Gregory advocated.

I soon discovered that herbs and other natural remedies, one of Gregory's areas of expertise, are often more effective than drugs and, furthermore, have minimal side effects. I then began to scientifically evaluate traditional diets, such as the macrobiotic diet, and natural remedies, such as evening primrose oil. (Evening primrose oil, a rich source of one of the essential fatty acids, has been shown in clinical trials to lower blood pressure, alleviate eczema, aid in weight loss, and eliminate other health problems.) Before long I became acquainted with numerous "alternative" physicians; some were well trained in the scientific aspects of medicine, and yet they were successfully using diet and centuries-old remedies to treat patients.

I also became aware of efforts on the part of the pharmaceutical industry, allied with some elements of organized medicine and members of the Food and Drug Administration, to discredit nutritional therapies that might compete with costly patented prescription drugs. This powerful medical-drug complex is also engaged in a conspiracy to harass physicians who practice alternative medicine.

In *What Your Doctor Won't Tell You,* Jane Heimlich, a journalist and physician's wife, enlightens you on the ineffectiveness and dangers of medical treatments, operations, and drugs that your doctor may, in good faith, be prescribing for you. (The average doctor is woefully ignorant of alternatives to drug treatment.) The results that Heimlich cites are based on documented evidence that has appeared in leading medical journals. But the focus of her book is on alternative therapies—what they consist of and who provides them. One of these effective and remarkably safe treatments is chelation therapy, a painless procedure performed in a doctor's office. Chelation is not only an alternative to coronary bypass surgery but can help you avoid a heart attack or stroke in the first place. Like other so-called alternative therapies, chelation therapy is based on scientific research that most doctors have ignored.

Congratulations to Heimlich and her publisher for having the courage to produce this much-needed book.

James P. Carter, M.D.
Professor of Nutrition
Tulane University School of Public Health
New Orleans, Louisiana

Acknowledgments

My thanks to the many physicians who took time to describe their work, and to Drs. Michael L. Gerber and George M. Ewing who provided guidance at the beginning of my journey. Another invaluable "compass" was Russell L. Smith, Ph.D., an authority on cholesterol, who generously shared his illuminating research with me.

Grateful thanks to Corinne Capuder and Katherine Mansoor, library sleuths; to Carrie Dlouhy, Information Specialist, Fetzer Foundation; members of the Science Department of the Cincinnati Public Library and Ruth Rosevear, nutritionist, who without benefit of the latest technology could always produce the needed study. Above all, heartfelt thanks to Teresa (Terri) Malloy, superefficient and understanding secretary, friend, and mainstay.

This book would not exist without the ministrations of Lila Karpf, literary agent, who shepherded the project from start to finish. I am most grateful for her expertise and concern. I am also extremely fortunate that this book reflects the skills of Eamon Dolan, editor; Brenda Woodward, copyeditor; and Susan H. Llewellyn, production editor.

Introduction

No one disputes the fact that modern medicine can perform miracles in the case of injury or trauma. An auto accident victim whose lung is crushed and bleeding is rescued from certain death when an emergency medic inserts a tube in his chest that draws off blood and air. New clot-dissolving drugs can save the life of a patient who has suffered a heart attack. A cardiologist using ultrasound can detect a heart attack that has already occurred.

But most Americans experience medical care as chronic disease patients, and my friends who fall into this category are fed up with the medical care they're receiving. (Cincinnati, where I live, is far from being a hotbed of radical thinking; it's an extremely conservative city whose residents are customarily described as "complacent.")

Larry, a middle-aged lawyer who recently married a younger woman, developed joint pains diagnosed as arthritis a few years ago. His doctor prescribed an anti-inflammatory drug that temporarily relieves the pain, but one of its major side effects is sexual impotence.

Beth, a marketing research analyst, recently lost her job and, while unemployed, developed high blood pressure. When she told her doctor that the antihypertensive drug he prescribed has made her chronically constipated, he recommended a laxative and said that she should expect to take the high blood pressure medication indefinitely.

Almost two years ago, six-year-old Susan (her mother is in my aerobics class) developed a low-grade fever, malaise, and stomach pains. Although she underwent a battery of tests (including esophagoscopy, which can puncture the esophagus), her pediatrician admits that he doesn't know what's causing her problem and recommends keeping her on antibiotics.

Mort, who's in his late 50s and until recently was a television producer,

1

suffered a heart attack six months ago and the following day underwent coronary bypass surgery. (His wife, Eleanor, in emotional shock, did not request a second opinion.) Today, Mort's memory, as he describes it, is "shot," and he's unable to work.

Medical consumers aren't the only ones complaining about medical care. The soaring cost of American health care (a projected $650 billion in 1990) appears to be a problem as insoluble as the national debt. Some experts blame the problem on "outrageous medical overkill."[1] According to a Rand Corporation fellow quoted in a recent article in the *Journal of the American Medical Association,* "one-fourth of hospital days, one-fourth of procedures, and two-fifths of medications could be done without."[2]

While medical policymakers debate how to clean up the abuses of the American health care system, there's an alternative to current medical treatment that you may be unaware of — a new world of medical doctors who reserve drugs and surgery as a last resort. (Incidentally, medical drugs have spawned a new crop of pharmaceuticals, a $2-billion-a-year expenditure, whose sole purpose is to treat adverse effects from other drugs.[3]) This "new" breed of doctor,[4] whose methods harken back to Hippocrates, employs diet and nutrients and other nontoxic treatments that encourage the healing process. Nutritional physician Dr. Melvyn R. Werbach describes himself and colleagues as "third line" physicians, who frequently serve as a last resort for patients who have not been helped by either the primary care physician or the specialist.[5]

After interviewing numerous "alternative" physicians (the term I use in this book), and many of their patients, and attending a great many national conferences devoted to new findings in alternative medicine, I have my own ideas as to the basic difference between alternative physicians and their orthodox or "standard" colleagues. The alternative physician, with the zeal of a medical detective, seeks to find the cause of your problem rather than merely treating symptoms with a battery of drugs. Reading the "standard treatment" section for various diseases in this book, you may be struck, as I was, by the number of times you come across the phrase "The cause [of arthritis, heart disease, cancer, cataracts, etc.] is unknown." The alternative physician doesn't subscribe to this thinking. As Dr. Hugh D. Riordan, president of the Olive W. Garvey Center in Wichita, Kansas, expressed it, "If you work hard enough, you can find the cause of the patient's problem." "Working hard" at the Garvey Center entails an initial three-day evaluation that includes analysis of the patient's biochemical makeup — vitamins, minerals, amino acids, blood cells, etc. Alternative physicians have various evaluation techniques, but all employ noninvasive tests that many standard doctors either ignore or are not familiar with. Alternative physicians also devote a great deal of time to discussing the patient's diet and other life-style aspects. To quote Riordan again, "Once you find the cause of the problem, you have the treatment."

The term *alternative* may sound unscientific, but nutritional medicine is based on an enormous body of scientific research. Reflecting on this research, much of it dating from the 1930s and 1940s before the advent of "miracle" drugs, Dr. John A. McDougall, author of *The McDougall Plan,* said, "It took me years to figure why these nutritional studies were gathering dust on library shelves. This research has no economic value." Since a diet or nutritional supplement cannot be patented, which limits its market value, a pharmaceutical company has no interest in funding nutritional research.

If *alternative* still sounds far-out, consider the number of orthodox procedures that were once outside the pale: Louis Pasteur's germ theory of disease; antiseptic surgery, devised by Sir Joseph Lister; Edward Jenner's vaccine against smallpox — when introduced, all were denounced as quackery. In 1948, a time when the radical mastectomy held sway, a Scottish surgeon, Mr. R. McWhirter, who advocated treating breast cancer patients with lumpectomy (partial excision of the breast) and radiation,[6] was denounced by American surgeons. (Surgeons in the United Kingdom are called Mr., not Dr.) Today, this "conservative" approach is one of the options available to the woman who develops breast cancer.

What kind of doctor chooses to practice alternative medicine? These physicians, for the most part, began their medical careers as specialists — internists, pediatricians, ophthalmologists, psychiatrists, cardiologists, surgeons, and the like — practicing standard medicine. But somewhere along the way, as Dr. Fuller Royal of Las Vegas, a former U.S. Air Force flight surgeon, expressed it, "I got tired of doling out pills and never having anyone get well." They "stumbled" on nutritional medicine (some credit a patient who was knowledgeable about vitamins) and, like itinerant scholars in medieval times, set forth to train themselves in the complex subject of nutrition — no mean feat considering that nutrition is a stepchild in medical schools and nonexistent in continuing medical education courses (many of which are sponsored by pharmaceutical companies).

If you've read the book jacket, you know that I'm married to a physician, Dr. Henry Heimlich, who is well known as inventor of the Heimlich Maneuver. People often ask me, "How did you get involved in alternative medicine?" or (a gleam in their eyes) "What does your husband think about what you're doing?" Despite my husband's "establishment" credentials — Cornell Medical School graduate, board-certified thoracic surgeon — he has always been critical of standard medicine. When our four grown children were young — a time when pediatricians were prescribing antibiotics for a simple chest cold — Hank vetoed drugs in favor of the old-fashioned steam kettle and plenty of fluids. We never had an aspirin in the house. (It's now recognized that Reye's syndrome, a serious childhood disorder that is often fatal, is linked with aspirin use.) As a surgeon, Hank was highly critical of unnecessary surgery and ill-chosen operations. Because he was widely recognized as an authority in surgery of the esophagus, many of the patients referred to him were, in plain words, the botched-up cases. I used to dread hearing about another patient who had been subjected to multiple unsuccessful operations, each one an attempt to rectify the original mistake. In a 1975 study of 67 patients who had undergone a procedure he devised called the reversed gastric tube (RGT), one of the patients had previously been subjected to eight major procedures, all of which had failed.[7] (In case you think incompetence and unnecessary surgery are a thing of the past, a recent *New York Times* story describes the current "glut of surgeons [who] may perform too few operations to maintain peak skills."[8])

I had no interest in medicine until the early 1970s when the holistic movement emerged in California and moved eastward. Like medical Marco Polos, health practitioners brought back acupuncture and herbs from the Orient, meditation and imagery from India, and discovered that the First Americans knew a thing or two about health. Fueled by dissatisfaction with the impersonality of medical care and its reliance on drugs and surgery, the holistic revolution called for treating the patient as a whole person, not just a diseased gallbladder or bad heart. Doctors talked about such unlikely subjects as caring and love, and encouraged their patients to take responsibility for their own health by practicing a healthy life-style.

Captivated by this caring approach to health, I sampled the holistic smorgasbord of Eastern practices and folk remedies, then researched a 200-year-old system of medicine called homeopathy and coauthored a book, *Homeopathic Medicine at Home.* For five years I wrote a column, "Helping Yourself," that appeared in the *Cincinnati Enquirer.*

As a columnist, I was deluged with calls from readers, most of whom asked the same question: Did I know a holistic doctor? By *holistic,* they invariably meant a doctor who was knowledgeable about diet and vitamins, who listened, "who doesn't just prescribe a lot of drugs." Most of these callers had been diagnosed with a potentially serious condition—heart disease, high blood pressure, and arthritis topped the list—and were fearful of the drugs their doctor had prescribed. I told each about physicians in neighboring cities who practiced nutritional/preventive medicine, and offered to send them material about these doctors and their work.

Acting as a holistic clearinghouse was enjoyable but time-consuming, and I wished "someone" would write a book about holistic/alternative physicians, the treatments they provide for patients with chronic diseases, who they are, and where you can find them.

In *What Your Doctor Won't Tell You,* you'll meet some of today's leading alternative physicians, and some whose work is little known even to the health-conscious individual. (One of the latter is a Chatham, New Jersey, pediatrician who reports excellent results using ear acupuncture to treat learning-disabled youngsters and those with cerebral palsy.) Although the focus of this book is on alternative treatments for the major life-threatening diseases, I've included information about such disabling conditions as mental illness, autism, chronic constipation, shingles, carpal tunnel syndrome, hypoglycemia, and mono-nucleosis. I've also provided a wealth of self-care information. (In my opinion, one of the most valuable nuggets comes from a scientist, considered the fore-most authority on magnesium, who tells you why you're probably deficient in magnesium, what this means in terms of your health, and what to take as a preventive dose.)

But before you investigate doctor-approved alternative treatments, you need to understand what constitutes mainstream medicine. Reading the section on standard treatment for each disease will enable you to better assess the treatment that your doctors prescribe and to talk their language. Let's say your cholesterol level is high and your doctor recommends a cholesterol-lowering drug. You may recall a newspaper article describing the questionable benefits of one of these drugs, but a vague remark, "I read somewhere in the paper . . . ," will not impress your doctor. Referring to one of several scientific studies that I've provided in the heart chapter will provoke a more satisfying exchange.

During this exchange, don't expect your doctor to be familiar with the alternative treatments I've described, or even be willing to discuss them. A remark in a 1983 *New York Times* editorial about holistic health typifies an attitude that still prevails: "Its emphasis on nutrition, exercise and preventive care are well placed. But with the first twinge of sickness, holism should be quickly forgotten."[9]

As I mention in the chapter on cancer, if possible, don't wait until illness strikes to acquaint yourself with alternative treatments. Listening to a doctor pronounce a dreaded diagnosis, the mind shuts off; reports of patients rushed into major operations or medical procedures are legion. But if you're con-fronted with a serious health problem and smack up against a decision concerning medical treatment, share the appropriate chapter with a close family member or friend, and ask this individual to accompany you on your next visit to the doctor.

Understandably, space does not permit my describing every alternative treatment for every serious disease. But if the condition you're most con-cerned about does not appear in this book, keep in mind that the alternative approach is the same whether the problem is carpal tunnel syndrome (a painful condition of the wrist) or depression. "All disease is biochemical," said Dr. Derrick Lonsdale, former Cleveland Clinic pediatrician. "The trick is to find the biochemical key that fits the lock."

Cancer Treatments Designed to Strengthen the Immune System

Imagine two 747s colliding in midair every day, killing all 862 passengers each time. If this occurred, the public would be up in arms. But every day 1,350 people die of cancer.[1] We are witnessing a cancer epidemic. One in three Americans will develop cancer at some time in their lives and two thirds of these patients will die within five years. This year close to one million people will develop cancer and a half million Americans will die of the disease.

The War on Cancer—Another Vietnam?   In December 1971, President Richard M. Nixon signed the National Cancer Act, officially launching a "war on cancer." Since then, despite the government's expenditure of $1.4 billion every year to the National Cancer Institute (NCI), cancer survival rates have not changed significantly from those of the 1950s.[2] In response to these depressing statistics, the NCI, which must sell its program to Congress, announces at regular intervals that more patients with cancer are surviving more than five years.[3]

But in the early 1980s, members of the cancer establishment began to question the NCI's interpretation of cancer survival statistics. In a 1983 scientific article, a Yale researcher, Dr. Alvan R. Feinstein, stated that cancer survival may be no better today than it was two decades ago. The following year, Dr. Haydn Bush of the London (Ontario) Regional Cancer Center pointed out why the NCI's cancer survival statistics look better than they are. Survival rates are improving not so much because of better treatment, but owing to earlier diagnosis, which simply starts the five-year survival clock sooner, he said.[4]

In 1984 Drs. Robert K. Oye and Martin F. Shapiro from the UCLA School of Medicine in Los Angeles joined the growing number of NCI critics. In a scientific journal, they questioned whether chemotherapy helps people live longer.[5]

The blast came in May 1986 with publication of an article coauthored by a leading cancer researcher from the Harvard School of Public Health, John C. Bailor, in America's most prestigious medical journal, the *New England Journal of Medicine.*[6] The authors concluded that "some 35 years of intense effort focused largely on improving treatment must be judged a qualified failure." Their statement "We are losing the war against cancer" made national headlines.

The following year, a congressional investigation conducted by the General Accounting Office (GAO) concluded that gains in treating cancer over the last three decades had been small and overstated by federal health officials.[7]

If you have been diagnosed with cancer, the information in this chapter will help you assess your doctor's recommendations. If you have cancer and have already embarked on standard treatment, this information will help you assess your original decision.

STANDARD TREATMENT

If a biopsy or another procedure shows that a tumor is malignant, the patient undergoes various tests to determine the extent to which a cancer has spread—that is, the stage to which the disease has progressed. This part of the diagnostic process is called "staging." A localized tumor (or what appears to be one) is classified as Stage I; the most advanced cancer is Stage IV. Based on the stage of a cancer, the oncologist determines what type of treatment is needed. Staging is generally a uniform or standardized procedure, but treatment varies from hospital to hospital. As you'll see, recommendations for treating Stage I breast cancer patients did a 180-degree turn in May 1988.

Standard cancer treatment consists of surgery, radiation, chemotherapy (including hormonal treatment), and immunology. These four types of treatment are used either singly or, more frequently, combined.

Surgery

What It Is.   As described by the American Cancer Society, "Cancer is most often treated by surgery. . . . When dealing with cancer, a surgeon not only removes the malignant tumor or organ, but also a wide margin of normal tissue and, in some cases, the nearby lymph nodes to halt further spread."[8]

Looking Back.   Today, surgeons are aware that by the time a lump in the breast (or another type of tumor) is detected, the cancer may have already spread to other parts of the body. But prior to the 1970s, the prevailing belief was that cancer started as a local disease and was surgically "curable" until that unknown moment when distant metastases occurred.[9] As a result, many surgeons believed that cure could only be achieved by the most "aggressive" surgery. For example, the Halsted radical mastectomy, popularized in the 1890s, involves removal of breast tissue, underlying muscle, and all lymph nodes in the armpit. (Removing nodes in the armpit causes the arm to swell in many patients; removing the muscle gives a sunken look to the chest and makes it difficult to raise the arm.) According to Dr. George Crile, Jr., a former Cleveland Clinic surgeon and early critic of the mastectomy, "[it] seems to have been designed to inflict the maximal possible deformity, disfiguration and disability" on women.[10]

As surgeons in Europe and Canada challenged the rationale for extensive surgery, a more limited form of mastectomy called a *modified* radical mastectomy (removing the breast and lymph nodes) came into use. A ten-year study of women with early breast cancers (*New England Journal of Medicine,* March 14, 1985) showed that the modified mastectomy achieved the same results as the radical in terms of recurrence of tumor and survival.[11] In the same issue of the journal, a national five-year study of women with small tumors detected early showed even more clearly that less may be as good as more in breast surgery. This study compared three treatments: modified mastectomy, lumpectomy plus radiation, and lumpectomy alone. (A lumpectomy is removal of the tumor and a margin of tissue around it.) The five-year results showed no difference in survival between a lumpectomy plus radiation and mastectomy.[12]

Side Effects.   Disfigurement is the most common disadvantage of cancer surgery.

Prostatic cancer has been treated with total prostatectomy (removal of the gland, the capsule, the seminal vesicles, and a portion of the bladder neck) for many years. The procedure, which causes impotence in the vast majority of cases, has been compared to the radical mastectomy.[13] When cancer of the bone occurs in a limb, part or all of it is amputated.

All surgery is traumatic in that it depresses the patient's immune system; in cancer, this may lower resistance to the disease. Two researchers, Drs. Gerald O. McDonald and Warren H. Cole, formerly with the University of Illinois, studied the results of surgical stress in cancer. In a paper delivered at a meeting of the American Medical Association, they wrote, "Most surgeons have encountered the patient whose cancer grows rapidly following operations, resulting in death within a few weeks."[14]

Some scientists have speculated that surgery accelerates the cancerous process. They theorize that cutting into the tumor may spread cancer cells throughout the body.[15] A 1971 textbook, *Clinical Oncology for Medical Students and Physicians* (published jointly by the University of Rochester School of Medicine and the American Cancer Society) warns that surgical biopsy, a procedure to detect cancer in its earliest stages, may contribute to the spread of cancer.[16]

Results.   Surgery is effective in curing early, localized tumors, meaning tumors that have not spread to other parts of the body (metastasized). Of the 1 million people diagnosed with cancer each year, 220,000 are curable by surgery alone.[17]

The problem is, there's no way of determining if a tumor is localized or has metastasized. As Cincinnati surgeon Dr. Harold Pescovitz said in an interview, "Some cancers of the breast at time of detection have already disseminated in the body, even though there's no sign of cancer cells in the lymph nodes. Yet there are other tumors of the same type which remain localized for many years." According to the latest figures from the National Cancer Institute, of the women regarded as having a favorable prognosis after surgery, "30 percent or more have recurrences of their cancer."[18]

Radiation Therapy

What It Is.   Radiation therapy, or radiotherapy, is the use of high-intensity X rays to destroy the ability of cancer cells to reproduce. Radiation can be beamed from outside the body or given by a device called a radioactive implant, known as an interstitial, or "seed," inserted directly into the cancer. Radioactive implants are used in many cancers that are in accessible regions, such as the breast, head and neck area, cervix, and vagina.

Radiation therapy has gained new importance with the advent of the breast-saving lumpectomy, which is almost always followed by radiation. As mentioned in the previous section, lumpectomy followed by radiation has been shown to be as effective as mastectomy (removing the entire breast). According to Dr. Bernard S. Aron, director of radiation, Oncology Division, University of Cincinnati Medical Center, "85 percent of women whose breasts are irradiated suffer no disfigurement from radiation."

Looking Back.   Radiation as an adjunct to breast surgery is nothing new. Prior to the late 1960s, standard treatment for breast cancer was mastectomy followed by radiation until studies showed that mastectomy and radiation offered no survival advantage over mastectomy alone.

Radiation as adjuvant therapy in breast cancer made a comeback with the previously mentioned five-year study published in the *New England Journal of Medicine* in March 1985. This study showed that women treated with lumpectomy and radiation had fewer recurrences than those treated with lumpectomy alone.

Side Effects.   When radiation therapy was introduced at the turn of the century, doctors were unaware of its toxic effects and took few precautions. Several of the early radiologists developed cancer in the fingertips and died from the disease. Patients suffered severe burns.

But radiation therapy is not a "benign procedure," as Mortimer B. Lipsett of the National Institutes of Health points out.[19] Common adverse effects that the patient undergoing radiation must be prepared for are described in the American Cancer Society's *Cancer Book:* "sores or ulcers . . . in the mouth, throat, intestines, genital areas and other parts of the body that are covered with delicate mucous membranes"; mouth sores that make it difficult to eat can be a problem for the weakened malnourished cancer patient; side effects vary according to the area being irradiated; "women undergoing radiation of the pelvic cavity . . . may develop rectal ulcers, fistulas, bladder ulcers, diarrhea and colitis."[20]

The most serious long-term effect of radiation is that the treatment itself can cause cancer. A study of 440,000 cancer patients who received chemotherapy or radiation showed that those treated with radiation had a significantly increased risk of a type of leukemia involving cells other than the lymphocytes.[21] (Lymphocytes are parts of the immune system that attack and destroy cancer cells.) Other long-term effects of radiation are fertility problems and birth defects.

Results.   Like surgery, radiation is only effective in treating localized tumors, such as Hodgkin's disease, lymphoma, and tumors of the head, neck, and cervix. Some of these cancers are treated with radiation alone and some with radiation and surgery or chemotherapy.[22] In breast cancer treatment, lumpectomy and radiation appear to be more effective than lumpectomy alone. In the 1985 five-year study already mentioned, only 8 percent of women who received both lumpectomy and radiation had a recurrence of their tumors, as compared with almost one-third of women who were treated with lumpectomy alone.[23] Roberto Lipsztein of Mount Sinai Medical Center in New York warned about long-term effects of radiation: "An increase in breast cancer attributed to radiation is generally not observed until ten years after exposure."

Chemotherapy

What It Is. Chemotherapy in cancer treatment is use of toxic drugs, or chemicals, to kill cancer cells. "Chemo" drugs are taken by mouth or given as an injection in the muscle or vein, and thus carried by the bloodstream throughout the body. Since chemotherapy drugs kill normal cells as well as cancer cells, they cause a wide spectrum of adverse effects.

Looking Back. Chemotherapy, a stepchild of the chemical weapons and forms of biological warfare developed during World War II, was introduced in the 1950s. The discovery that mustard gas and other poisonous chemicals had tumor-inhibiting effects came at a time when cancer treatment had reached a standstill. Another weapon besides surgery was needed to control cancers that had spread beyond the primary site.

Chemotherapy was originally used as a primary treatment to shrink and destroy cancer cells that were known to exist in the body. In the early 1970s, oncologists began to give chemotherapy immediately after surgery or radiation to the patient with a high risk of developing a recurrence. This use of chemotherapy is called "adjuvant" chemotherapy. It is intended to wipe out cancer cells that may remain hidden in the body after the visible tumor has been removed.

Since the advent of adjuvant chemotherapy, this treatment has been given to patients with a high risk of developing a recurrence, meaning women whose cancer has spread to the lymph nodes. On May 21, 1988, the National Cancer Institute changed the rules about adjuvant chemotherapy. At that time the NCI issued a "clinical alert" in the form of a letter sent to 13,000 cancer specialists recommending that *all* women with breast cancer have chemotherapy or hormonal treatment after their initial surgery. (This news was considered too urgent to wait for publication in a medical journal.) The NCI recommendation was based on the findings of three then unpublished studies, which show that 30 percent of all women with early breast cancer will have a recurrence.[24]

Another recent change in breast cancer treatment concerns postmenopausal women. From the early 1970s to 1986, adjuvant chemotherapy was given to patients of all ages who were found to have one or more positive underarm lymph nodes (Stage II), and thus considered to be at high risk of recurrence. Since the majority (75 to 80 percent) of breast cancer patients are postmenopausal, this meant that older women, who are least able to withstand the rigors of chemotherapy, underwent this treatment along with their younger sisters.

This policy changed when an analysis of more than a hundred clinical trials showed that there was no scientific basis for giving chemotherapy to postmenopausal women.[25] Toxic drugs not only failed to extend their lives, but harmed them. Studies showed that a hormone-blocking drug called tamoxifen, which has minimal side effects, gives older women two or more additional years of life.[26]

This change to a more humane and effective treatment for the older woman was aided by the efforts of a feisty breast cancer advocate, the late Rose Kushner, member of the National Cancer Advisory Board. In a 1984 article that appeared in an American Cancer Society journal, Kushner charged that doctors are "literally making healthy people sick" by administering toxic drugs that are "of only marginal benefit to the vast majority of women who develop breast cancer."[27]

Other issues in breast cancer treatment remain unresolved. One is dosage of chemo drugs. Bruce Chabner, director of cancer treatment at the National Cancer Institute, urges doctors treating breast cancer patients to raise the doses of chemotherapy "as high as the patients can tolerate."[28] Other experts argue that too high a dosage will suppress the bone marrow's production of blood cells, which can cause multiple harmful effects including death through infection.

As there is no "best" dosage, so there is no "best" drug or combination of drugs, as Kushner observed in 1984. Dr. Orlando J. Martelo, director of the Division of Hematology/Oncology at the University of Cincinnati Medical Center, explained why oncologists are in the habit of trying one "toxic cocktail" after another: "The disease becomes resistant to the combination of chemo drugs. We try another regimen, but at some point we run out of drugs and have nothing else to offer." Commenting on the practice of chemotherapy, Dr. Petr Skrabanek of the University of Dublin's Trinity College, wrote in a 1985 issue of *The Lancet,* "Fashions in chemotherapy change too fast for allowing a reasonable time to assess them, but rapid changes are themselves indicative of unfulfilled promise."[29]

Side Effects.   According to a psychologist whose article appeared in the American Cancer Society journal, "the side effects of cancer chemotherapy can cause more anxiety and distress than the disease itself."[30]

A major adverse effect is suppression of bone marrow. As one of the authors of the American Cancer Society's *Cancer Book* explains, "The bone marrow produces the white blood cells that fight infections, the red blood cells . . . that carry life-sustaining oxygen to the body's organs, and the platelets, which help the blood to clot. When the bone marrow is suppressed, fewer blood cells are produced and the patient becomes more vulnerable to infection, anemia and at risk for serious bleeding."[31] Infection is a major cause of death in cancer patients, as in AIDS patients.[32]

Each chemotherapy drug produces its own set of side effects, as described in the product "insert." Methotrexate, one of the most widely used of the thirty chemo drugs, in addition to producing marked depression of bone marrow, "may be hepatotoxic" (damaging to the liver). Warnings for Adriamycin, one of the most powerful chemo drugs, include "serious irreversible myocardial toxicity [damage to the muscle of the heart] with delayed congestive failure [heart failure] often unresponsive to any cardiac supportive therapy." Another chemo drug, Cytoxan, can cause "secondary malignancies."

Common side effects of chemo drugs are loss of appetite, diarrhea, fatigue, nausea and vomiting, and mouth and lip sores. In addition, "25 to 65 percent of cancer patients develop phobia-like reactions," most commonly, anticipatory nausea and vomiting provoked by stimuli associated with treatment, such as the sound of the doctor's voice or a particular smell.[33] The need to cope with nausea and vomiting in the chemotherapy patient has spawned a line of antiemetic agents, which in turn cause side effects. For some patients, the most devastating effect of chemo drugs is hair loss, which affects 85 percent of patients.[34]

Long-term effects of chemotherapy include damage to the heart,[35] loss of fertility, and an increased risk of developing a second cancer.[36] Patients with breast cancer, ovarian cancer, and multiple myeloma who were treated with chemotherapy had a significantly higher incidence of acute nonlymphocytic leukemia.[37] As early as 1983, cancer experts warned nurses and other health professionals to follow strict safety precautions in preparing anticancer drugs because the substances have caused malignancies and birth defects in laboratory animals.[38]

Results.   According to the National Cancer Institute's 1977 Cancer Data, of the 1 million new cases a year, 11,000 with advanced disease can be cured with chemotherapy.[39] These 11,000 patients who can benefit from chemotherapy are afflicted with one of twelve rare cancers. These rare cancers, which make up less than 10 percent of all cancers, include Hodgkin's disease, which used to be fatal; Burkitt's lymphoma, found primarily in certain parts of Africa; choriocarcinoma, a rare tumor that occurs in pregnancy; and a type of testicular cancer. Before chemotherapy, few children with leukemia survived. Now most can be cured, or at least live longer. The treatment, however, exacts a price: survivors of childhood cancer have an increased risk of developing bone cancer later in life as a result of radiation therapy and chemotherapy.[40]

Apart from these successes, no sudden change in death rates from any of the major cancers can be credited to chemotherapy. Dr. Orlando J. Martelo, Hematologist/Oncologist of the University of Cincinnati Medical Center, calls the results of cures with present chemotherapy drugs "unacceptably low." In breast cancer, he says, "We cannot cure patients with metastatic cancer, but with chemotherapy we can extend their lives three or four years." In a 1980 article in *Lancet,* six British cancer researchers disputed the claim that chemotherapy prolongs survival, contending that "survival may even have been shortened in some patients given chemotherapy."[41]

Immunotherapy

What It Is. Cancer immunotherapy is based on the theory that if the immune system recognizes tumor cells as foreign invaders, it will destroy them.[42] The immune system substances that do this are naturally manufactured by the body and called biological response modifiers (BRMs). Some BRMs with familiar names are interferon, interleukin-2, and tumor necrosis factor (TNF). Another type of biological regulator is called a monoclonal antibody. These are used to detect cancer cells as well as to destroy them.

Looking Back. The founder of immunology was a New York surgeon, Dr. William B. Coley, who practiced almost a century ago.[43] Coley, disheartened by the number of patients who died soon after undergoing cancer surgery, puzzled over why these patients died while others appeared to be cured after removal of a tumor. Searching hospital records, Coley found that the common denominator among cancer survivors was that each had suffered a severe infection at the time of surgery. To induce a similar infectious response, Coley began giving cancer patients a bacterial "cocktail," with some notable successes.

    Present-day immunology began in the 1960s, but it was major technological advances in the 1980s that ushered in the present era. These advances, namely genetic engineering, make it possible to produce large quantities of proteins, such as interferon and interleukin-2, which occur only in small amounts in the body.[44]

Side Effects. Using cancer drugs that consist of substances produced naturally by the body's immune system sounds natural and homespun compared to existing "cut, burn, and poison" treatments, but BRMs have proved to be as toxic as chemotherapy and radiation therapy. Treatment with interleukin-2 requires weeks of hospitalization, primarily in an intensive care unit, "to survive the devastating toxic reactions," which include anemia requiring multiple transfusions, severe bleeding, shock, and confusion.[45] Interferon causes rapid onset of fever, chills, and severe muscle contractions that may require morphine.[46]

Results. Are these biologicals, originally hailed by the press as a "cancer breakthrough,"[47] likely to fulfill this promise? Mayo clinic oncologist Dr. Charles G. Moertel finds "no evidence that unacceptably severe toxicity and

astronomical costs of interleukin-2 are balanced by evidence of true therapeutic gain."[48] At present, excitement about biotechnology for cancer appears to have shifted to products that are designed to help doctors detect and
diagnose disease. The newest of these are called monoclonal imaging
products.[49]

Why the Changes?

You may be wondering why the constant changes? These are most
apparent in breast cancer treatment, but extend to all areas of treatment. As
the American Cancer Society's *Cancer Manual* states, "New drugs and new
combinations of drugs appear frequently, and surgical techniques and radio-
therapeutic strategies change almost year by year."[50]

One opinion about the reason for these changes comes from an expert in
artificial intelligence, Edward A. Patrick, M.D., Ph.D., professor of electrical engineering and computer science at the University of Cincinnati Medical
Center and author of *Decision Analysis in Medicine* (Boca Raton, Fla.:
C.R.C. Press, 1978). According to Patrick, "The outcome of existing cancer
therapies is unknown because the data has never been looked at properly. The
most important reason for this failure is politics. Researchers at various
university medical centers who control the data have also influenced funding."
In a 1975 article in *Science,* Patrick emphasized the need for expert statisticians to interpret results of cancer studies.[51] In 1988 he noted, "Thirteen
years later, almost nothing has been done to correct the situation."

Criticism of cancer treatment on the part of mainstream physicians
continues. According to Allan Oseroff, associate professor of dermatology at
the New England Medical Center in Boston, existing cancer treatments "are
all different and they're all lousy, so you pick the one with the least side
effects."[52]

FREEDOM OF CHOICE IN CANCER
TREATMENT

Imagine that the scenario you dread is unfolding. Your doctor tells you that
you have cancer—say, a malignant tumor in one of your kidneys. After a
surgeon removes the kidney, your doctor tells you that the cancer has
metastasized to your liver and lungs and then tells you your options: you can
have chemotherapy (here you are told about the results and side effects of
chemotherapy) or you can try one of the alternative cancer therapies. "I can't
guarantee any results," your doctor says, "but I've had some success treating
cancer patients with high doses of vitamin C given intravenously."

Of the two options, which would you choose: a course of chemotherapy that might take months—even a year—during which you can expect to lose your hair, become debilitated, and all the rest, or a vitamin C "drip" given every few days whose only side effect is an energy boost?

If this improbable choice were routinely offered in doctors' offices, the cancer industry, estimated at $80 billion a year, would be out of business. Those who work in the industry—a greater number than have cancer—would lose their jobs. But the economic factor is just one of many reasons why your doctor doesn't tell you about alternative cancer treatments. In fact most doctors know nothing about these treatments since reports about them never appear in medical journals except under the heading of "cancer quackery." This is also one of the reasons why you never read about alternative cancer treatments in the medical section of your newspaper, and why it's so difficult to obtain any information about the subject. When I called the National Cancer Institute's information service, (1/800) 4–CANCER, the young woman who answered told me, without missing a beat, "Alternative treatments have been tested in the lab and found to have no tumor-inhibiting effect." (At that time, an investigation of alternative cancer treatments was still in the works.)

To understand why a "cancer blackout" exists (the term is the title of a book published in 1959[53]), a brief lesson in cancer politics is in order.

The Elephant and the Mouse

On one side is the gargantuan cancer establishment, dubbed Cancer, Inc., by some of its critics. The kingpin of Cancer, Inc., is the National Cancer Institute (NCI). The NCI is part of the National Institutes of Health and has a yearly budget of $1.4 billion. (As in all areas of standard medicine, Cancer, Inc., is aligned with the American Medical Association, pharmaceutical companies, and insurance companies.) Also affiliated with the NCI are medical centers (called Comprehensive Cancer Care Centers), private hospitals, university research facilities, and the American Cancer Society (ACS), "the world's richest private charity."[54] The ACS's yearly budget of $150 million comes largely from public contributions. Like the NCI, the ACS derives much of its power from its ability to dispense grants to major research institutions.[55]

On the other side is a group of physicians, allied health practitioners, and their patients (let's call them Alt, Inc.) who endorse nontoxic therapies for cancer.

Cancer, Inc., maintains that proponents of "unproven" methods of cancer management deceive patients and their families with "false promises and exaggerated claims."[56] For this reason, they say, consumer protection laws are necessary to restrict the sale of "worthless" health products and services to a "vulnerable" public.[57] These products and services are lumped together as "cancer quackery."

Alt, Inc., maintains that patients have the right to choose whatever form of treatment they wish. This right was articulated by Supreme Court Justice Benjamin Cardozo in 1914: "Every human being of adult years and sound mind has a right to determine what shall be done with his own body. . . ."[58] Cardozo's statement also established that an individual has a "right to privacy." This "right," and its subsequent interpretations, serves as the basis for freedom-of-choice arguments.

To control cancer quackery, the American Cancer Society formed a Committee on Unproven Methods of Cancer Management in 1954.[59] One of the committee's functions is to maintain an official blacklist, a list called Unproven Methods of Cancer Management. Inclusion on the list leads to loss of grants and other punitive measures.[60] Occasionally a blacklisted method is rediscovered by scientists and inspires a new approved treatment. Coley's "cocktail," mentioned previously, was such a method. More often, "unproven methods" are lost to the medical community. This was the case with Krebiozen.

In the early 1950s, Dr. Andrew C. Ivy, a distinguished medical scientist, began treating terminal cancer patients with a drug called Krebiozen. Many of these "hopeless" cases recovered. (This anticancer agent was discovered by a Yugoslavian cancer researcher, Stevan Durovic, who brought it to Ivy's attention.) Despite Ivy's impeccable credentials, the AMA refused to test Krebiozen. Ivy was expelled from the Chicago Medical Society[61] and eventually indicted by a federal grand jury for conspiracy, mail fraud, and violations of the Food, Drug and Cosmetic Act.[62] He was later acquitted, but the National Cancer Institute showed no interest in testing Krebiozen.[63]

To protect the public from cancer quackery, Cancer, Inc., has at its disposal a "complex web of federal and state laws and regulations designed to restrict the availability of these [alternative] treatments and direct consumers towards so-called 'proven' methods."[64] One of the federal agencies primarily responsible for enforcing these laws is the Food and Drug Administration (FDA). The FDA has the responsibility for determining whether a 7product intended to treat or prevent cancer is safe and effective before it enters the marketplace. In order to test a medical treatment, the researcher must apply to the FDA for investigational new drug (IND) status. Over the years, the FDA has spurned a long line of IND applications for unorthodox cancer treatments, beginning with Krebiozen in 1963.[65]

Substances that are promoted as medical treatments also come under the FDA's jurisdiction. During the 1960s and 1970s, laetrile was the chief target of the FDA, "but today we're more concerned about cancer treatments than products," said Kenneth Durham, the FDA's director of consumer affairs.

One of the cancer treatments of concern to the FDA is a form of immunotherapy administered by Dr. Stanislaw R. Burzynski, president of the Burzynski Research Institute, Inc., in Houston. This Polish-born physician, who is also a Ph.D., is the author of 110 scientific papers and holds fifteen medical patents. Burzynski's treatment, which he calls Antineoplaston Therapy, is a means of activating a natural defense system in the cancer patient.[66] On July 17, 1985, FDA agents raided Burzynski's office and confiscated patient medical records. The agency charged Burzynski with violating interstate commerce laws by furnishing out-of-state patients with his antineoplaston serums. Burzynski patients filed a class action suit, but the appeal is still pending.

Several states have enacted laws to prohibit or severely curtail unorthodox cancer treatment. According to Michael T. Bugumill, program coordinator of California's Department of Health Services, Food and Drug Branch, in 1959 California became the first state to institute a law prohibiting the sale of products for cancer "either unproven, worthless or judged not safe and effective." Those found guilty of "prescribing, administering, or dispensing drugs or devices that have not received prior approval for cancer treatment are committing quackery," said Bugumill. According to legislation enacted in 1974, a first conviction on a quackery charge is a felony, "with jail terms of up to five years and fines as high at $10,000."[67]

One of the half-dozen California physicians who have been charged with quackery is Dr. Bruce Halstead, a marine biologist who has published more than two hundred scientific papers and served as consultant for the World Health Organization and the United Nations, among others. Halstead was prosecuted under California's Health and Safety Code for prescribing a Japanese herbal tea to twenty cancer patients. In 1985, a jury found him guilty on twenty counts. In addition to losing his medical license, he was fined $10,000 and sentenced to four years in state prison.[68]

Some states, on the other hand, have passed laws that protect unorthodox methods of treating cancer. Based on laetrile statutes passed in the 1970s, laetrile is legal in nineteen states.

The conflict between Cancer, Inc., and Alt, Inc., is only one aspect of the struggle going on in other areas of medicine, but as we've seen, suppression of alternative cancer treatments has a particularly virulent quality. Assuredly there are unprincipled cancer quacks who exploit the fears of cancer patients, and here we welcome protection. But is the government, in its zeal to stamp out quackery, suppressing treatments that could improve your odds of surviving cancer? For the past four decades, we've allowed Cancer, Inc., to make that decision. Today, in view of the failure of the war on cancer, a growing number of Americans want to make that decision themselves. They also contend that cancer quackery laws have diminished our chances of finding a cure for cancer. "We have lost more courageous, innovative practitioners in cancer treatment than in any other area of medicine," said Michael S. Evers, attorney and executive director of Project Cure, a political action organization.

An individual who has experienced this loss personally is medical writer John Maxwell Desgrey, coauthor of *Beyond Pritikin*. At age 63, Desgrey's father, a corporate vice president, decided to retire early. Although pronounced "sound as a dollar" at his recent annual medical checkup he wasn't feeling well. An X ray taken at a mobile X-ray unit told the story: cancer of the lungs had metastasized to the brain. He was given six months to live.

Having no knowledge about alternative treatments, his son began searching for answers. "My aunt suggested that I investigate Krebiozen— 'That's what saved your grandfather's life.'" (His grandfather had prostate cancer.) Desgrey called Dr. Ivy, the scientist who had introduced Krebiozen, and went to Chicago to meet him.

> I was appalled to find a broken man. He warned me that I'd be under surveillance—it was against the law to transport Krebiozen to a patient. But Dr. Ivy couldn't turn down a cry for help and, after looking at my father's medical records, prepared a serum and specified the dosage. 'You'll have trouble getting a nurse to administer this,' he said. So I asked him to teach me how to give an injection, which he did— bringing out an orange for demonstration purposes!
>
> My father was deteriorating fast—his sight, speech, motor functions were shutting down. But I gave him the injections, as Dr. Ivy specified, and, within a month, his symptoms had begun to reverse. By then his doctor was convinced that something was happening, and agreed to have a nurse give the injections.

Desgrey went home. His father continued to improve. Then one day a call came from his mother who informed him that an FDA agent from Washington, D.C., had come to their home with an affidavit and warned her that her son could be put in jail for transporting Krebiozen across state lines. Frightened, she turned over her entire supply of Krebiozen. "My father died a few months later." His father's case is not an isolated example, Desgrey said. "I've talked to a great many cancer patients who were given Krebiozen and recovered."

Cancer Patients Search for a Better Way

Despite the cancer blackout and cancer quackery laws and regulations, thousands of cancer patients, disillusioned with the results of standard cancer treatment and fearful of its harsh treatments, turn to alternative or nontoxic therapies.[69] Estimates of the numbers range from 15 to 40 percent of those diagnosed. In Ohio, which is distinguished by extremely conservative attitudes, a cancer official estimates that nearly one third of diagnosed cancer patients "seek some form of treatment outside the proven methods of radiation therapy, chemotherapy and surgery."[70] A 1985 Associated Press/Media General public opinion poll, projecting to an estimated 161 million adults, showed that one half of the respondents believed that alternative cancer clinics should be allowed to operate in the United States.

One patient who chose alternative treatment is June Pruitt, of Miami, Florida, a 59-year-old homemaker and mother of four. In August of 1973, Pruitt was diagnosed with multiple myeloma, as shown by medical records from two university hospitals. This form of cancer, according to the *Merck Manual,* is an "ultimately fatal disease," which is associated with lesions that can destroy the bone, cause kidney damage, and increase susceptibility to bacterial infections.[71] Pruitt, a patient at the University of Miami Hospital, was given chemotherapy for one year. "My weight dropped to ninety; I was sick and nauseated all the time." Learning that the University of Arizona was conducting research in bone marrow disease, she went there "hoping for a miracle." After two weeks of grueling diagnostic tests, "They rolled me into the radiology department where the technician proceeded to draw black marks on my ribs. 'What are you doing?' I asked. 'We're going to radiate your ribs.' At that point, I was fed up being a guinea pig, and insisted on going home."

Returning for treatment at the hospital in Miami, "They gave me stronger chemo drugs along with Compazine (to counteract nausea and vomiting caused by chemotherapy) and Valium. Finally my body couldn't take it any longer. I developed pneumonia, my lung collapsed, and they sent me home to die.

"I started praying in earnest—'Please Lord, I'm not ready to die.' My youngest was only seven. At this time, a friend called, 'Ever hear of laetrile?'"

Learning that laetrile was not a drug but a food substance made from apricot seeds that could then be purchased at a health food store, Pruitt read about laetrile as well as the laetrile diet (fresh fruits and vegetables and raw vegetable juices), and incorporated both in her regime. "I kept a diary. At first I had one good day now and then, but gradually the 'good days' increased."

When she had regained some of her strength, she spent two weeks at a clinic in Jamaica that offered "metabolic" treatment (nutrition and enzymes). "It was such a peaceful environment, caring doctors and nurses—I could feel myself healing." (This clinic no longer exists.)

Pruitt continues to take laetrile (one 500-milligram tablet each day) supplemented by an infusion of laetrile every week or two, which her husband administers. ("I have a friend who's an R.N. as backup.") Every six months she spends a week to ten days at the American Biologics Hospital in Tijuana where she receives chelation therapy (see chapter 4); a "slow drip" that includes laetrile, vitamin C, calcium, magnesium, and zinc; and live cell therapy. (More about these therapies later in this chapter.)

"I regard my cancer as if it were diabetes; I follow a certain regime to keep it under control. Putting good things in my body is no hardship. I feel much healthier than I did before I had cancer."

Interviewing June and other cancer patients you'll meet in this chapter, I found intelligent, resourceful, spunky individuals—very much like the subjects of Judith Glassman's book, *The Cancer Survivors*. Glassman describes these survivors as individuals who "despite the worst prognosis . . . are thriving, full of energy and enthusiasm for life."[72] These individuals also resemble Bernie Siegel's "exceptional patients who refuse to be victims." They are the patients that physicians consider "difficult or uncooperative."[73]

Shades of the Old-Fashioned Family Doctor.   One moving account of a caring physician came from 36-year-old William Rosenberg of Brooklyn, a social worker. Rosenberg's mother had undergone major thoracic surgery and six weeks of radiation, but her lung cancer had metastasized to the liver, and the doctors gave her two months to live. At this point, listening to Gary Null's radio show, Rosenberg heard about Dr. Emanuel Revici, a 91-year-old Romanian-born New York physician who had devised a complex theory of "biological dualism" to explain the nature of disease and correct the underlying imbalance in the patient's chemistry.[74] Rosenberg called Revici and made an appointment for his mother and other family members to see him.

"With a waiting room full of patients, he spent almost two hours with us. 'I can't cure your mother, but I can affect the quality of her life,' he said. For three months, she gradually improved—some days she sounded like her old self. Then she went downhill."

On several occasions, Revici visited Rosenberg's mother at home, but would never accept payment beyond his regular fee of $65, Rosenberg said. The last visit occurred the night she was dying. "He gave her an injection, and she regained consciousness. I held her hand. 'Can you hear me?' She squeezed my hand. Dr. Revici stayed with us till the very end. The man is another Albert Schweitzer."

Profile of a Cancer Patient.   I was pleased to have my impression of these cancer patients and their doctors confirmed by a study conducted by University of Pennsylvania researcher Barrie Cassileth, Ph.D., based on 660 cancer patients receiving alternative care. Cassileth reported that they "do not conform to the traditional stereotype of poorly educated, terminally ill patients who have exhausted conventional treatment." On the contrary, "Patients who use unorthodox therapies are well educated . . . in the early stages of disease" and frequently without symptoms. Furthermore, the unorthodox practitioners they consulted were not the unscrupulous quacks we are warned about "who play upon patients and others to use their unproven methods." Instead, the study shows that "many are well trained, few charge high fees, and most sincerely believe in the efficacy and rationality of their work. . . . The cost of unorthodox regimes was relatively modest with most patients spending under $1,000 for the first year of treatment."[75]

The Bottom Line

The big question is, What are the results of alternative treatment? How effective is a particular therapy for a particular type of cancer? Regrettably, there are no reliable statistics that can provide an answer. As journalist Gary Null, who conducted a two-year survey of alternative centers in North America, discovered, "Many of the clinics . . . are understaffed or don't have the funds to do important statistical analysis and follow-up of patients that would provide the general public, as well as the scientific community, with some idea of the results they're getting."[76] Michael Lerner, Ph.D., author of *Integral Cancer Therapies,* who visited thirty alternative cancer centers in the early 1980s, also noted "absence of funds for careful inquiry" and the need for "careful scientific research."[77]

To add to the confusion, some clinics in Tijuana, Mexico, give survival statistics while emphasizing that the majority of their patients come to them as a last resort. The late Harold Manner, Ph.D., director of the Manner Metabolic Clinic, told me that case studies from his clinic show a survival rate of 68 to 74 percent. Dr. Ernesto Contreras, medical director of the hospital that bears his name, claims 90 to 95 percent survival for patients with prostate cancer. The American Biologics (A-B) Research Hospital claims that the clinic has achieved 80 percent survival rates for patients with breast and colon cancer.[78]

One of the Tijuana clinics, the Gerson Institute, is making an effort to supply reliable statistics. "We're compiling a 'best case retrospective review,' with help from the University of California in Los Angeles," said the clinic's spokesperson.

In 1987, when I first began investigating alternative cancer treatment, I was hopeful that statistics concerning the results of such treatment would be forthcoming. At that time, the first major evaluation of an alternative cancer therapy was underway. A congressional agency, the Office of Technology Assessment (OTA), was developing a protocol for a clinical trial of "Immuno-Augmentative Therapy," an immunology treatment devised by Dr. Lawrence Burton, whose clinic is located in the Bahamas. (More about Burton later in this chapter.) "This trial," according to the OTA, "would be the first step towards finding out whether the IAT is an effective treatment for cancer."[79] Optimism about the study was premature. In the spring of 1989, one of the agencies that had originally lobbied Congress to request the study reported that the OTA project on unorthodox cancer treatments "appears headed for trouble as evidence mounts that the agency has not handled its assignment in an objective and evenhanded manner."[80] For further information about the OTA project, call Project Cure, (1/800) 552–CURE.

So, for the time being, we have to depend on anecdotal evidence; that is, case histories of recovered cancer patients. Assessing the treatments that her cancer survivors received, Judith Glassman concludes, "These methods were far from cure-alls, but they gave life to a percentage of 'terminal' cases.[81]

ADJUNCTIVE CANCER THERAPIES

Bridging the Gap between Standard and Alternative Cancer Therapies

According to the University of Pennsylvania study that I mentioned, more than half of the patients who choose "unorthodox" cancer treatments use these treatments simultaneously with conventional treatment.[82] Anne, a Cincinnati housewife in her mid-40s, who has breast cancer, follows that route. She's undergoing radiation treatment as her doctor has advised, but to sustain her during this period, she has a weekly session with a psychotherapist, who helps "quiet my mind," and meditates several times a day. Meanwhile, "lying on the table while my breast is heating up, I hold my crystal in my hand and pray that I won't be burned."

Albert Marchetti, M.D., author of *Beating the Odds; Alternative Treatments That Have Worked Miracles Against Cancer,* teaches patients how to use these treatments as adjuncts to surgery, chemotherapy, and radiation. Therapies include diet and nutritional supplements, exercise, meditation, visualization, and hypnosis. Marchetti advises obtaining professional help in learning any of these self-treatments.[83]

Psychotherapy.   Since the advent of modern medicine, doctors have resisted the idea of a psychosomatic basis for cancer. A professor of radiology at the University of Cincinnati Medical College, whom I interviewed in 1978, said flatly, "No one has demonstrated a link between stress and cancer." A Cincinnati psychologist, who specializes in counseling cancer patients, had her office in a suite occupied by nine oncologists. Despite the proximity, "I never received a single referral from a member of this oncology group," she said.

The debate goes on. A recent (1989) *Science News* article reported a study that concludes, "Chronic feelings of depression do not affect a person's likelihood of developing cancer."[84]

Dr. Lawrence LeShan, humanistic psychologist and researcher and author of *You Can Fight for Your Life,* published in 1977, was one of the first contemporary practitioners to claim that emotional factors play a role in causing cancer. LeShan describes the cancer personality as being unable to express anger or resentment, disliking oneself, having no respect for one's own accomplishments, feeling absolutely alone in one's despair, and seeking "no way out of the emotional box . . . short of death itself." LeShan's goal, he says, is to try to help these patients "develop or regain their will to live."[85]

O. Carl Simonton, M.D., in *Getting Well Again,* added his voice to the argument that stress is linked to cancer. "Effects of emotional stress can suppress the immune system, thus lowering our resistance to cancer, and other diseases." But it isn't the external event—an unlucky roll of the dice— that does us in, he says. "The amount of emotional stress depends on how the individual interprets or copes with that event." In other words, you get cancer "when your coping techniques are faulty."[86] Simonton was bitterly criticized for giving the cancer patient a guilt trip.

Bernie Siegel, M.D., says more or less the same thing: "Most illnesses do have a psychological component and a realization of one's participation and responsibility in the disease process is entirely different from blame or guilt. . . ."[87] Somehow the verbal hug that accompanies his teaching takes away the sting.

Visualization.   Visualization, or mental imagery, as a tool to influence the immune system in cancer, was pioneered by radiation oncologist O. Carl Simonton and Stephanie Matthews Simonton, a psychotherapist, who was then his wife. One of their self-help methods, described in *Getting Well Again,* involves combining deep relaxation with mental imagery to reinforce the goals of medical treatment. The Simontons emphasize that these psychologi- cal techniques "do not replace standard medical procedures, but are used in conjunction with them."[88] The authors suggest images to use: "Depict your cancer cells as anything soft that can be broken down . . . like hamburger meat or fish eggs." Visualize your white blood cells "as aggressive, eager for a battle. . . ."[89]

Virginia Veach, Ph.D., a psychotherapist in the San Francisco Bay area who specializes in counseling cancer patients, rejects the Simonton method "as coming from the outside." (Veach is associated with Commonweal, de- scribed below.) Veach does not give her patients ready-made images but encourages them to create their own. "One woman with breast cancer visualized sheep grazing all over her body, as if she were a meadow. This image gave her a sense of being healthy and nourishing others, but obviously was one I could never have come up with." This "inner" approach also enables patients to get in touch with their own bodies, Veach says. "One patient told her doctor that the tumor in her left breast had receded, but there was another emerging in her right breast. Tests showed that she was right."

In addition to the Simontons' book, two other excellent accounts of visualization are *Imagery in Healing* by Jeanne Achtenberg (Boston: New Science Library, 1985) and *Healing Yourself: A Step-by-Step Program for Better Health Through Imagery* by Martin L. Rossman, M.D. (New York: Pocket Books, 1989).

Although mental imagery is by its nature a self-help technique, Veach and other therapists emphasize that for the cancer patient who is under stress, using the mind as a healing tool can be achieved more easily by working with a therapist, at least as a starter.

Joining a Group.   Some organizations teach cancer patients how to use alternative methods in conjunction with standard treatment. One is Commonweal, a health research institute just north of San Francisco, founded in 1976. Commonweal holds the Commonweal Cancer Help Program, a week-long retreat, at regular times throughout the year. At this retreat, cancer patients experience visualization, massage, a vegetarian diet, and yoga, and become informed about cancer therapies, both orthodox and "complementary." ("Complementary" refers to either alternative or adjunctive cancer therapies.)

Commonweal's founder and president, Michael Lerner, Ph.D., a Mac-Arthur Award winner, depicts his organization as bridging the gap between orthodox and alternative therapies. Lerner, who has been both a Yale professor and a yoga teacher, recommends that the cancer patient explore both orthodox and complementary therapies and then "make a choice that the person feels good about." It is the patient's sense of participating in this decision, rather than the treatment itself, that defines what Lerner calls "integral cancer therapy."[90] For further information about Commonweal and its services, write to Commonweal, P.O. Box 316, Bolinas, CA 94924.

The Wellness Community, a self-help group for people with cancer, in Santa Monica, California, has become well known as a result of Gilda Radner's deeply moving book, *It's Always Something.* Radner, a comedian of "Saturday Night Live" fame, who developed ovarian cancer, describes the Wellness Community as "an oasis in the desert."[91] It was there that she connected with herself again, regaining her humor and her skills as a comedian and adjusting to being in the "well world." (Radner died of cancer May 20, 1989.)

According to its founder, ex-lawyer Harold H. Benjamin, author of *From Victim to Victor,* "The Wellness Community is a place where cancer patients can learn whatever they need to know to fight for their recovery."[92] The Wellness Community teaches relaxation, visualization, nutrition, cancer education, and, above all, the benefits of group support and laughter. All services are free of charge. For further information about the Wellness Community, see Benjamin's *From Victim to Victor* (Los Angeles: Jeremy P. Tarcher, 1987) or contact the Wellness Community, 1235 5th Street, Santa Monica, CA 90401, (213) 393–1415.

Comparing Standard and Alternative Treatments

Standard treatment, according to German physician Dr. Josef Issels, "the grand old man of alternative cancer treatment,"[93] is based on the belief that cancer starts as a localized tumor and, if not detected in time, spreads throughout the body.[94] Based on this belief, standard treatment has focused on eradicating the tumor—cutting it out, or burning it, and, if that fails, flooding the body with poisonous chemicals to search out and kill cancer cells wherever they may be hiding. (As you've probably noticed, standard physicians use military terms to describe the "war" on cancer.)

The alternative view, says Issels, is that "a healthy body has an immune system that can destroy cancer cells and prevent them from multiplying."[95] But when the body's immune system is weakened below a certain threshold, it can no longer do so, and eventually, the disease culminates in formation of a tumor. Alternative cancer treatment, like most alternative treatments, consists of stimulating the body's own natural defenses to heal itself.

Differences between standard and alternative medicine are becoming less clear-cut as standard medicine revises its thinking about cancer. According to a 1985 standard text, "Use of the body's own defense system, the immune system, is gaining momentum as an alternative to traditional cancer treatments."[96] According to medical writer Robert G. Houston, immunotherapy, the new excitement in standard medicine, is based on approaches that were pioneered decades ago by Lawrence Burton and other "alternative" immunologists.[97]

ALTERNATIVE TREATMENT

Although there is considerable overlap, alternative therapies fall into four categories: diet, metabolic (diet plus related treatments), immunotherapy, and eclectic (a combination of therapies).

Diet

Of the three well-known therapeutic diets—Pritikin, McDougall, and macrobiotic—only the macrobiotic, meaning "way of life," claims to both prevent and treat cancer. (These three therapeutic diets are described in chapter 7.)

After several decades in which the cancer establishment maintained that diet had no effect on cancer, the National Academy of Sciences reversed its stand in 1982 and announced that a host of dietary factors reduce cancer risks.[98] Today the American Cancer Society says that nutrition can help prevent cancer[99] but does not recognize nutrition as a treatment for cancer. Dr. Robert A. Good, former president and director of the Sloan-Kettering Institute for Cancer Research, has devoted most of his working life to researching the influence of nutrition in preventing cancer and other diseases. When I asked Good, now a professor in the Department of Pediatrics at the University of South Florida, if he treated cancer patients with diet, he said, "We don't know enough at this time. Maybe ten or fifteen years from now we'll have the data."

But Michio Kushi, leading proponent of macrobiotics, has no hesitation about wading into this controversial area. In his book *The Cancer Prevention Diet,* he cites numerous cases of recovered cancer patients as proof that the macrobiotic diet can cure cancer as well as prevent it.[100]

The macrobiotic diet, Japanese in origin, is not an exotic creation but the traditional diet that has sustained the human race throughout recorded history, Kushi says. Individuals who follow this time-tested diet are "immune" to cancer, heart disease, and even tooth decay, a few of the conditions common among "civilized" peoples. This "perfectly balanced" diet consists of 50 percent whole cereal grains, 20 to 30 percent local vegetables (preferably organically grown), and smaller amounts of soups and beans and sea vegetables; white meat, fish, and fruit are permitted occasionally. There is no need for vitamin and mineral supplements in a balanced diet, Kushi says.

Yin and Yang.   The relation of diet and disease in macrobiotics is expressed in terms of yin and yang. Yin and yang have been described as "convenient labels used to describe how things function in relation to each other and to the universe [and] to explain the continuous process of natural change."[101] According to Kushi, cancer results from an imbalance of dietary factors. The type of cancer, whether more yin or yang, depends on its location in the body. Yang cancers are found in the deeper parts of the body and are caused by overconsumption of animal foods such as eggs, meat, fish, poultry, and cheese, which are yang foods. Yin cancers appear nearer the outside of the body and result from an excess of soft drinks, sugar, milk, ice cream, and foods containing artificial additives (yin foods).

To prevent cancer, one must avoid foods that are extremely yin or yang, Kushi says. You can do this by following the standard macrobiotic diet, which is suitable for any healthy person. But treating cancer requires a stricter diet, one that takes into account the patient's type of cancer and individual needs. Prescribing a cancer diet is a complex undertaking that requires the services of a trained macrobiotic counselor.

A macrobiotic success story was related by a 74-year-old physician in Miami, Florida, whom I'll call Dr. P since he requested that his name be withheld. Eight years ago, Dr. P was diagnosed with widespread prostatic cancer, Stage IV. After treating him with surgery and radiation, his doctors told him that he had at most three months to live. They also told him, "Chemo will give you a 30 percent increase in life expectancy, but you'll be in bed during most of the treatment." Dr. P rejected that option. "I looked at myself in the mirror and said, They've given up on you—it's time to try something else."

Dr. P was familiar with macrobiotics and other dietary approaches. Years ago, as head of a committee to fight health fraud, he had investigated a number of so-called quack treatments and had ended up convinced of their merit. But although he gave lip service to the importance of nutrition, he indulged his sweet tooth and, before his illness, the five-foot eight-inch physician weighed 175 pounds. Now, too ill to travel to macrobiotics head-quarters in Brookline, Massachusetts, he located a macrobiotic counselor in his area who taught him the rudiments of the diet.

"When I started the diet, the cancer had spread to the bone—I was in terrible pain. Seven months later, all tests were negative. I showed before and after bone scans to my doctors; nobody believed it." Today, a trim 140 pounds, Dr. P does "fast dancing," which he considers good aerobic exercise, several times a week. He says, "I've turned down requests from macrobiotic organizations to talk to groups about my recovery. I don't want to give false hope. I've seen people on the macrobiotic diet who developed cancer, and I've seen people on the diet die of cancer."

For information about View of Life seminars, the three-day program conducted by Michio Kushi, contact the East/West Foundation, 17 Station Street, P.O. Box 850, Brookline, MA 02146, (617) 738–0045. These semi-nars, which mainly attract cancer patients, are held twice a month and cost $450 ($350 for a support person).

Testing Needed. Scientists dismiss case histories like Dr. P's as "anecdotal," but the catch is that research organizations show little interest in testing the effect of diet on cancer. Dr. James P. Carter, professor at Tulane School of Public Health, Nutrition Program, has proposed the following study: Take a group of patients with advanced (Stage IV) cancer of the prostate and instruct them in the macrobiotic diet. Then at a later date, compare survival rates with a control group of patients who eat a standard American diet. Carter first submitted this project to research organizations in the early 1980s, but thus far, no takers.

Meanwhile, Carter has conducted what is called a retrospective study. He compared survival rates of 29 patients with cancer of the pancreas, who were practicing macrobiotics, with those of a control group that included the longest living survivors with pancreatic cancer according to National Cancer Institute statistics. (Average life expectancy for cancer of the pancreas is six months.) Carter found that 55 percent of the macrobiotic patients survived one year as compared to 10 percent of the control group. "At least two macrobiotic patients are still living eight years later," he said.

Carter has a theory that may explain the success of the macrobiotic diet, and other vegetarian diets, in treating cancer. "Cancer of the prostate tops the list of cancers in which patients with widespread cancers, who change their diet, experience a dramatic turnabout," he says. The significant fact, he continues, is that prostate is one of the endocrine-dependent or hormone-sensitive tumors (a type that responds to hormonal treatment). Other cancers of this type include cancer of the breast, pancreas, uterus, ovary, and colon. Carter speculates that these endocrine-dependent tumors are the ones that respond best to a macrobiotic diet.

But the patient must follow the diet very strictly, Carter emphasized. Patients can never consider themselves "cured"; remnants of cancer cells remain. Says Carter, "A low-fat diet enables the immune system to keep the cancer in check, but once the individual increases the amount of fat in his diet, the cancer comes back."

Metabolic

Metabolic therapy is twofold: it consists of flushing out the body's toxins and supplying a well-balanced diet plus various vitamins and enzymes. The diet is vegetarian, with emphasis on raw "live" foods and fresh vegetable juices. Sugar, white flour products, processed foods of any kind, coffee, and alcoholic beverages are not permitted.

Gerson Therapy. Gerson therapy, offered at the Gerson Institute, located just over the California border in Tijuana, Mexico, is the granddaddy of nutritional metabolic programs and the model for many nutritional physicians who work with cancer patients. The program was devised by the late Dr. Max Gerson, a German-born physician whom Albert Schweitzer described as "one of the most eminent geniuses in medical history."[102] Gerson cured Schweitzer's wife of advanced lung tuberculosis and, with the same diet, enabled Schweitzer, at the age of 75, to control his diabetes. Fleeing the Nazis, Gerson established a practice in New York, and in 1946 he was invited to appear before a Senate committee investigating cancer treatment to discuss his methods. Gerson's premise that diet can both prevent and treat cancer was swiftly attacked by the medical establishment.

The Gerson program, supervised by Gerson's daughter, Charlotte Gerson (a commanding presence at cancer conventions), aims to rid the body of a lifetime's accumulation of toxins and to flood the body's cells with the nutrients they need. The diet, the centerpiece of Gerson therapy, consists of organically grown fresh vegetables and fruits, thirteen glasses of freshly squeezed juices daily, including raw liver juice, plus "biologicals" (substances that occur naturally in the body), such as thyroid, iodine, potassium, and liver extract. The diet also includes linseed oil, a rich source of omega-3 fatty acids. Gerson recommended one tablespoon of cold-pressed linseed oil each morning and evening for four weeks, then one tablespoon per day.[103]

The key detoxification measure is the coffee enema, which the patient self-administers several times a day. Caffeine taken rectally is believed to have a twofold effect: it dilates the bile ducts so the liver can more easily excrete cancer toxins, and it cleanses the blood of toxins by way of the intestines. Gerson stressed that the liver plays a major role in overcoming cancer.[104]

Years before standard medical doctors were aware of vitamin A's tumor-inhibiting effect, Gerson prescribed quantities of carrot juice and liver juice; both contain large amounts of beta-carotene, a substance the body converts to vitamin A. Gerson's use of linseed oil jibes with new understanding of the function of essential fatty acids. Despite scientific thinking edging closer to Gerson's principles, the Gerson method "is not considered an effective means of cancer treatment," according to the National Cancer Institute, and Gerson therapy remains on the American Cancer Society's list of unproven methods of cancer management.[105]

A major disadvantage of Gerson therapy is that adhering to it strictly, as patients are advised to do, is practically a full-time job. (One former Gerson patient told me that she got so fed up with the program, "I threw my glass of carrot juice across the room!") But among patients who stick to the demanding regimen, success stories abound.

One of many Gerson success stories is Donald Lindseth, former Pan American pilot and flight engineer. In 1978 Lindseth began having grand mal seizures and was diagnosed with a brain tumor. "The tumor was as big as your fist," Lindseth said. "The doctors told me I needed radiation treatment. I asked them, 'Will I be OK after that?' They gave me three years at most."

Since conventional treatment didn't sound like a bargain to Lindseth, he began searching for other methods. Learning about the Gerson program, Lindseth read Gerson's book, *A Cancer Therapy: Results of Fifty Cases* (New York: Whittier Books, 1959) and was encouraged to find that several of the patients described in the book had been cured of brain cancer. Lindseth spent a month at La Gloria Clinic, then followed the Gerson regime of diet, juices, and coffee enemas at home. Within two to three weeks, the seizures had stopped, and two months later, the tumor had shrunk. Elated, Lindseth went back to work as a ground officer for the airline, but after two years the seizures returned, and he resigned himself to following the Gerson program for life.

Today Lindseth grows his own vegetables and continues the juice and enema routine — "Sure, it's time-consuming, but I'd be dead without it." Recently, he had an MRI (magnetic resonance imaging), which showed that the tumor was continuing to recede. "The doctors don't know what to make of me," he says.

For information about Gerson therapy, contact the Gerson Institute, P.O. Box 430, Bonita, CA 92002, (619) 267–1150.

Laetrile. Detoxification measures and diet are the mainstays of a metabolic program, but most of these programs include laetrile, high doses of emulsified vitamin A, and proteolytic enzymes. These three nutrients attracted media attention in September 1977 when the late Dr. Harold W. Manner, then a biology professor at Loyola University, reported that the three caused an 89 percent regression of breast tumors in laboratory mice.[106]

Although laetrile remains a symbol of alternative cancer treatment, it is not used alone but as part of a metabolic program that includes megadoses of vitamins, minerals, and enzymes. Manner and others who prescribe it say that it helps relieve pain, increases appetite, and promotes a feeling of well-being. A surprising tribute to laetrile appeared in *American Medical News,* a publication of the American Medical Association, in a 1982 letter to the editor. A San Antonio physician, Dr. Eva Lee Sneak, wrote, "Laetrile, properly used, has had, in my hands at least, as good a success as chemotherapy, with far less side effects."[107]

Laetrile, also known as vitamin B17, is derived from a chemical compound called amygdalin. Amygdalin is found in the seeds of all common fruits, most abundantly in apricot pits, as well as in twelve hundred plants including buckwheat and millet. Like so many healing substances, laetrile was known to the ancient Egyptians, Chinese, Greeks, and Romans, all of whom described the "sacred seeds" as anticancer agents.[108]

Laetrile was introduced to the United States in the early 1950s by a San Francisco physician, Ernst T. Krebs, and immediately attracted media attention. The Food and Drug Administration's vendetta against laetrile, which began in the early 1960s, reached its height in 1977 when the FDA issued a Laetrile Warning claiming that laetrile was "worthless in the prevention, treatment or cure of cancer [and] can cause poisoning and death when taken by mouth." Although at that time an estimated 50,000 to 100,000 cancer patients were taking laetrile, at most three deaths had been reported from accidental overdoses of the substance.[109]

Ignored in the hysteria was a series of experiments performed by a well-respected researcher, Dr. Kanematsu Sugiura, at the Sloan-Kettering Cancer Center in New York between 1972 and 1976. Sugiura found that while amygdalin did not destroy primary tumors, it inhibited the growth of tumors and significantly retarded growth of lung metastases.[110]

A surprise finding emerged from a 1980 study at Rutgers University. Investigators studying the effect of amygdalin in diabetes found that the substance helps protect the body from a dangerous free radical, the hydroxyl radical. (Free radicals are unstable oxygen molecules that play a harmful role in a variety of degenerative diseases. Cancer, for example, cannot spread without production of free radicals, the most virulent of which is hydroxyl radical.)

A 1982 National Cancer Institute study of laetrile, conducted by Dr. Charles G. Moertel of the Mayo Clinic, appeared to sound the death knell for laetrile in the scientific community. Investigators concluded that "laetrile was ineffective as a treatment for cancer and did not substantially improve symptoms of the disease in study patients."[111] Laetrilists charged that Mayo Clinic investigators did not administer pure laetrile or give it in conjunction with a laetrile diet and appropriate nutrients.[112]

Vitamin C.   A key nutrient in metabolic therapy is vitamin C, or ascorbic acid.

In the late 1960s when Linus Pauling, Nobel laureate, turned his attention to the subject of nutrients and disease, he theorized that megadoses of vitamin C would increase the resistance of the cancer patient. A Scottish surgeon, Dr. Ewan Cameron, with thirty years' experience in cancer treatment, had independently hit on the same idea, and for some time had been giving vitamin C along with conventional treatment to patients at his hospital in Glasgow. In the early 1970s, the eminent scientist and the cancer specialist teamed up to test the efficacy of vitamin C in cancer.

After publishing several preliminary clinical reports, the two investigators studied Cameron's first 100 cancer patients, all terminally ill, who had been given 10 grams of vitamin C a day. These 100 patients were compared with a control group of 1,000 patients who were also considered untreatable. (The control group was selected from case records of cancer patients who had received identical treatment at the Vale of Leven Hospital except that they were not given vitamin C.)

Results looked promising. Cameron and Pauling found that ascorbate-treated patients, on the average, survived ten months longer than matched controls. Of the 100 ascorbate-treated patients, 22 lived longer than one year; only 4 of the 1,000 patients in the control group lived this long.[113] The two researchers reported these results in 1976.

Extended survival time was not the only criterion in judging vitamin C's performance. As Cameron had observed since he first began giving vitamin C, ascorbate-treated patients felt better, gained weight, and experienced less pain. (Although criticized later for not conducting a double-blind randomized clinical trial, Cameron was unwilling to deprive any patient of the benefits of vitamin C.)

Placebo or Anticancer Agent?   Cameron and Pauling's claims that a vitamin powder costing pennies could accomplish what drugs failed to do inevitably raised hackles in the scientific establishment. After repeated requests were made to the National Cancer Institute for a controlled trial of vitamin C in

advanced cancer patients, the Mayo Clinic finally ran two double-blind studies, the first reported in 1979, the second in 1985. In both studies, the
investigators concluded that in treating advanced cancer patients, vitamin C
was no better than a placebo.[114, 115] Pauling criticized the first study on the
grounds that the patients had been treated with chemotherapy. (Only 4 of the
100 patients in the Vale of Leven study had received chemotherapy.) His
objection to the second study, in which the participants had not been treated
with chemotherapy, was that the patients were only given vitamin C for an
average of ten weeks. (Pauling and Cameron kept advanced cancer patients
on vitamin C indefinitely.)

Alternative to Chemotherapy.   One of the physicians who is treating cancer
patients with megadoses of vitamin C is Dr. Hugh D. Riordan, president of
the Olive W. Garvey Center for the Improvement of Human Functioning, Inc.,
in Wichita, Kansas. (The Center's clinical services are available to the patient
who has been seen by one or more physicians "without adequate results.")
     One of Riordan's patients, George Williams, a retired Wichita business-
man, was diagnosed with a tumor in the right kidney in November 1985. "The
kidney was removed and the urologist thought he got it all," Williams said. But
in March of 1986, a CAT scan showed multiple pulmonary lesions in his lungs
and several areas in his liver. He said, "I didn't want chemo; I've never known
anyone who had that treatment and recovered."
     Williams went to the Garvey Center—his wife had been a patient
there—and conferred with Riordan, who suggested vitamin C therapy. That
March, Williams embarked on a course of intravenous infusions of vitamin C
(starting with 15 grams and increasing to 30 grams) three times a week.
Riordan also advised him to drink one glass of fresh carrot juice every other
day, and recommended beta-carotene. In April, an X ray taken at the hospital
showed no evidence of cancer in his lungs and only two lesions in the liver. As
Williams continued to improve (he was back to playing golf), vitamin C
treatments were tapered off to twice a week, then once a week. By July there
was no evidence of cancer in the liver, lungs, or lymph nodes. He has a vitamin
C drip every six weeks "as a preventive."

Vitamin A.   According to Henry Dreher, author of *Your Defense Against
Cancer,* "no other single nutrient has excited cancer scientists quite as much"
as vitamin A and its precursors. (A vitamin A precursor, the best known of
which is beta-carotene, is a substance the body converts to vitamin A.)
There's good reason for the recent excitement: large-scale studies (one
involved 2,000 men who were followed for nineteen years) showed that
people who ate foods rich in vitamin A or beta-carotene had a lower than
expected incidence of lung, stomach, and other cancers. Although treating a
cancer patient with vitamin A is "unproven" (and considered a felony in

California), Dreher says that vitamin A "appears to have such powerful anticancer effects that the cancer establishment is starting clinical trials for its use in the treatment of cancer as well as for its prevention."[116]

Vitamin A is a fat-soluble nutrient; that is, it does not dissolve in water. For this reason, fat-soluble vitamins (others of this type are vitamins E, D, and K) are prepared by dissolving in oil. Metabolic practitioners recommend high doses of emulsified vitamin A taken orally. (*Emulsification* means breaking down the oil into particles small enough to mix well with water, thus enabling the intestinal tract to absorb most of the nutrients.) When I asked Dr. Harold W. Manner why emulsified vitamin A is not toxic, he said, "When an ordinary source of vitamin A—cod liver oil or fish oil—or its synthetic form leaves the small intestine, it enters the liver through the portal vein where it can damage membranes. Instead, emulsified vitamin A enters the blood and lymph system bypassing the liver."

Luke R. Bucci, Ph.D., lab director for Biotics Research in Houston, a nutritional supplement manufacturer that sells only to health care practitioners, further clarified why it's safe to take large doses of emulsified vitamin A:

> Emulsified vitamin A gets into the lymph system faster than a standard form of vitamin A because it's absorbed faster by the intestinal tract. The lymph system then carries the vitamins along with dietary fats into the bloodstream, which in turn distributes the vitamin throughout the body. Since the vitamin is disseminated in the bloodstream rather than flooding the portal system (direct gateway to the liver), the liver can handle a larger amount of vitamin A without any damage to membranes.

Proteolytic Enzymes.   Enzymes help us digest our food. The function of proteolytic enzymes is to digest protein. Here's how Manner relates this to cancer: "The cancer cell shields itself from anticancer agents by forming a fibrin coating around each individual cell; this fibrous coating is made of protein. Proteolytic enzymes digest this protein coating, which allows the body's white cells to attack the cancer cells and destroy them." Manner traces the use of proteolytic enzymes to research by two German scientists, Drs. Max Wolf and Karl Ransberger, in the 1930s. The enzyme product they devised, called Wobe-Mugos, is widely used in West Germany and Austria.[117] According to Manner, "Proteolytic enzymes are well accepted in all parts of the world except this country."

The Hoxsey Treatment.   The Hoxsey treatment, as described by Judith Glassman in *The Cancer Survivors,* is "absurdly simple." It consists mainly of an herbal tonic for internal cancers and a powder, salve, or clear solution for external cancers. Patients who use the external treatment also take the tonic.

It's understandable why Glassman describes the Hoxsey program as "the hardest to accept . . . of all the alternative therapies." Harry Hoxsey, who devised the program, seems the prototype of a snake oil salesman—a charismatic, self-taught healer. Furthermore, the herbal tonic, centerpiece of the program, was originally concocted by one of Hoxsey's forebears, he said, as a tonic for horses, and the formula had been handed down through the generations. Despite these inauspicious origins, the tonic reportedly worked miracles, and a series of Hoxsey Clinics, first established in the 1920s, attracted patients from all over the country. Hoxsey's dream was to have his treatment accepted by the medical establishment, and over the years he made valiant efforts to persuade the AMA and NCI to investigate his methods. But early in his career Hoxsey incurred the wrath of the AMA, and after countless legal skirmishes, the FDA banned the sale of all Hoxsey medications in 1960.

The Hoxsey story is the subject of a much-acclaimed 1988 film, *The Quack Who Cured Cancer?* To obtain a video, contact Project Cure, (1/800) 552–CURE.

Today the Hoxsey treatment is available at the Bio-Medical Center in Tijuana. The Center, directed by Hoxsey's long-time chief nurse, Mildred Nelson, was opened in 1963. One of the Hoxsey patients I've met, all eager to describe their "cures," was 62-year-old Shirley McCray of Alliance, Ohio. McCray, tall, slim, wearing a blue silk blouse that matched her eyes, looked the picture of how to age gracefully.

McCray's story began when she read in a magazine that a "dimpling" in your breast can be a sign of cancer. Examining her breasts, she found a lump in one and, alarmed, went to her doctor. He ordered a mammogram, which was inconclusive, then referred her to a surgeon who performed a lumpectomy and removed lymph nodes in the axilla (armpit). "He said the tumor was malignant and five nodes were cancerous." McCray then underwent a course of thirty radiation treatments, but nine months later, a CAT scan showed that the cancer had metastasized to the liver, and the oncologist recommended chemotherapy.

"It felt like a death sentence," she said. "I was terrified of chemo, but I didn't know anything about alternative treatments, so I followed my doctor's advice and began chemotherapy. I lost my hair, had terrible pains in my stomach, felt so weak it took me twenty minutes to make my bed." During chemotherapy, she had two bouts of bronchitis and colitis. Five months later, a CAT scan showed that the cancer had increased by one third. "The doctor told me, 'This isn't working—we'll have to give you stronger chemo drugs.'"

On her way home from the doctor's office, McCray stopped at the library to look up the side effects of methotrexate, one of the drugs she was to be given. Consulting the *Physicians' Desk Reference,* she read "Methotrexate can cause liver or kidney failure, and continued use weakens the heart muscles." She thought, "This will wipe me out before the cancer does." Standing there, she saw another book on the shelf that seemed to be saying

"Take me, take me." The book was Judith Glassman's *The Cancer Survivors,* and it fell open to the section about Harry Hoxsey and his cancer treatment. There she read about the Bio-Medical Center in Tijuana.

Despite McCray's qualms about methotrexate, she began chemotherapy and experienced the same side effects as before—mouth blisters, weakness, and stomach pain. But this time, she also had double vision. Frightened, McCray told her doctor she wanted to stop chemotherapy and try the Hoxsey treatment at a clinic in Mexico. To her surprise, he encouraged her and agreed to monitor her condition. (According to the University of Pennsylvania study I mentioned, 75 percent of the patients told their physicians about their use of alternative care, and 30 percent of these physicians were supportive.)[118]

"A patient spends only one day at the Bio-Medical Center," McCray said, recalling her visit in March of 1986. "You take your medical records; the doctor examines you; you have all the lab tests." When the results are in, the doctors and Mildred Nelson, R.N., confer on your case and decide on dosage of the tonic and other matters, she said. "I began with one teaspoon of the tonic in water four times a day and gradually increased the dosage to one tablespoon. It has a faint licorice taste."

She described the center as "Spanish-style, very attractive and clean. I couldn't believe all the people there were cancer patients. The oncologist's office was so depressing—all those sick-looking frightened people waiting for their chemotherapy treatment. Here, the atmosphere was upbeat; people were talking and laughing, some were swapping recipes."

McCray was instructed to eat a diet of fresh foods, with no salt, sugar, or alcohol. Also forbidden were carbonated beverages, pork, tomatoes, vinegar, and highly seasoned foods, which are claimed to interfere with the action of the tonic. "I drink at least a quart of unsweetened grape juice and water (half and half) a day. It's a wonderful body cleanser."

After five months on the program, McCray asked her oncologist to order a CAT scan. According to the radiologist's report, dated August 18, 1986: "Although metastatic disease is still present in the liver, the previously described lesions are smaller, no new lesions have appeared and some lesions are no longer identifiable. Overall appearance of the liver shows considerable improvement."

Is McCray a "spontaneous remission" (medical term for unexplained recovery) or was she misdiagnosed? Or is it possible that the tonic has some value? James Duke, Ph.D., former chief botanist at the U.S. Department of Agriculture's Medicinal Plants Laboratory, has analyzed the tonic, which consists of potassium iodide combined with such familiar North American herbs as licorice, red clover, burdock root, poke root, and buckthorn bark.[119] All of the Hoxsey herbs have known anticancer properties, he said.[120]

Immunotherapy

The Burton Treatment.   One of the best-known alternative cancer treatments is the Immuno-Augmentative Therapy (IAT) devised by Lawrence Burton, Ph.D. The Immunology Research Center, an outpatient facility directed by Dr. Burton, is located in the Rand Memorial Hospital in Freeport, Grand Bahama Island. (Before his "exile" to the Bahamas, Burton was an oncologist for fifteen years at St. Vincent's Hospital in New York City.)

Like all immunology treatments, the IAT uses substances produced naturally by the patient's body to bolster the patient's immune system. The unique aspect of IAT is Burton's finding that certain components of the blood must be present to enable the immune system to ward off cancer. These components—four blood proteins—are deficient in the cancer patient. IAT patients receive injections of these four blood proteins twice a day in amounts based on daily measurements of their blood. Unlike standard immunologic treatments, IAT is nontoxic and produces minimal side effects.

Among Burton's enormous coterie of devoted patients is Cornell Medical College graduate Dr. Philip J. Kunderman of North Brunswick, New Jersey. In 1978 Kunderman, a thoracic surgeon, was diagnosed with cancer of the prostate. A bone scan and biopsy both showed that the disease had spread to the breastbone and right shoulder.

Soon after that, Kunderman retired, and he and his wife acquired a second home in the Bahamas. (Mrs. Kunderman firmly believes that they were "led" there.) As a newcomer to the island, Kunderman learned about Burton's cancer clinic, a short drive from their condominium. Kunderman had a long talk with Dr. Burton and was impressed. Back in New Jersey, Kunderman checked on Burton's scientific papers in the medical library and was again impressed. A month later, Kunderman returned to the Bahamas and enrolled for treatment at the IAT clinic.

Today, seven years later, Kunderman, age 77, says he's feeling fine: "My last bone scan showed complete clearing of the metastases in sternum and shoulder, indicating repression of my disease."

Kunderman, who has observed a great many Burton patients, says he is "astounded" by results in advanced cancer patients who failed to respond to conventional therapies. Having practiced in an industrial area, Kunderman has treated a large number of factory workers with mesothelioma, a type of cancer caused by exposure to asbestos that is invariably fatal. "At the IAT clinic, I've seen patients with mesothelioma whose disease either regressed or was controlled," he says.

As a thoracic surgeon, Kunderman was particularly impressed by the case of a man with a large malignant tumor of the left lower lobe of the lung with invasion of the mediastinum: "After several months of IAT, this mass had disappeared and his chest X ray appeared normal."

Kunderman has observed other apparent cures of cancers considered incurable, including metastatic carcinoma of the pancreas, cancer of the pharynx, cancer of the colon with liver metastases, malignant melanoma of the skin, and lesions of the brain. "I've seen patients arrive in wheelchairs and stretchers, who appeared to be terminal, respond to IAT. A month later, they're free of pain and walking about."

The Livingston Treatment.   Unlike IAT, which is primarily a vaccine, the Livingston treatment, another well-respected immunotherapy for cancer, involves diet and psychotherapy.

This holistic form of immunotherapy was devised by a physician, Dr. Virginia Livingston, whose long, illustrious career includes a professorship at Rutgers University. Treatment takes place at the Livingston-Wheeler Medical Clinic in San Diego, California, an outpatient facility established in 1969.

The basis of Livingston's treatment is an autogenous vaccine (a vaccine prepared from a culture of the patient's own bacteria) given in conjunction with the BCG (tuberculosis) vaccine. Use of these vaccines reflects Livingston's belief that cancer is caused by a microbe. (This explanation of cancer was accepted thinking in the early nineteenth and twentieth centuries.[121]) Livingston also believes that the cancer virus is pleomorphic, or capable of changing form at different stages of its development. This theory may account for the difficulty in identifying the cancer microorganism, since each researcher, like the blind men and the elephant, sees it a little differently. The cancer microbe, which Livingston calls *Progenitor Cryptocides,* exists in all of us, but only causes disease when the immune system is in a weakened state, she says.

Nutrition is an important aspect of treatment at the Livingston-Wheeler Medical Clinic. Livingston recommends a "live food" vegetarian diet (similar to the McDougall diet described in chapter 7), which she describes in *Food Alive.*[122] Livingston forbids all poultry, which she says is contaminated with the *Cryptocides* microbe.

The day I visited the Livingston-Wheeler Clinic, I heard a lively and frequently humorous talk by a clinical psychologist. "The typical cancer patient is a Mr. Nice Guy who never thinks about his own needs," he said. "Learn to say no, even though your family may fight it." Members of the audience, visibly tense at the start of his talk, soon relaxed and at times roared with laughter.

For a copy of *The Patient's Handbook* and other materials about Livingston's treatment, contact the Livingston-Wheeler Medical Clinic, 3232 Duke Street, San Diego, CA 92110, (619) 224–3515.

Eclectic

The term *eclectic* denotes a smorgasbord of treatments. Eclectic cancer treatment includes metabolic therapies (diet and a wide range of immune system–enhancing nutritional substances) plus "anything that works," as one practitioner described it.

The American Biologics (A-B) Hospital in Tijuana, according to spokesperson Michael L. Culbert, offers eclectic treatment. Therapies given at the A-B Hospital include a Japanese vaccine, ozone therapy developed in Germany, live cell tissues from Germany, Chinese herbs, and biomagnetism. In the early 1980s, Michael Lerner, considered an unbiased observer, described the A-B Hospital program as "the most ambitious and comprehensive program integrating alternative cancer modalities currently available in North America."[123] For information, contact the A-B Hospital, 1180 Walnut Avenue, Chula Vista, CA 92011-2622, (1/800) 227–4458.

A newly founded clinic that offers eclectic cancer treatment is the International Medical Center in Juarez, Mexico (ten minutes from El Paso, Texas). The center, designed to treat all types of chronic degenerative disease, is directed by Dr. H. Ray Evers, pioneer in chelation therapy and long-time proponent of holistic care. Cancer therapies available at the center include live cell, Koch vaccine, Dr. Virginia Livingston's vaccine, and hydrazine sulfate. For further information, contact the International Medical Center, 424 Executive Center Blvd., Suite 100, El Paso, TX 79902, (1/800) 621–8924.

An example of what eclectic treatment can achieve, at least in the hands of a master, was demonstrated by Dr. Josef Issels of Germany. For forty years, Issels, director of the Ringberg-Klinik in Baden-Baden, treated cancer patients with a combination of therapies designed to shrink the tumor and restore the body's defense mechanisms. Issel's "whole body therapy" included hyperthermia (fever therapy), ozone infusion, enzymes and organ extracts, and various types of immunotherapy, along with nutrition, exercise, and psychotherapy. When necessary, he gave short-term chemotherapy and radiation. In a speech delivered in New York City in May 1987, Issels emphasized the importance of removing sources of infection, which he said contribute to the development of cancer, such as infected teeth, teeth whose dead pulp has been removed by root canal treatment, amalgam fillings, and infected tonsils. Issels' results in treating cancer patients, almost all of whom had progressive metastases, were impressive. Two independent studies, one at the University of Leiden in Holland, the other at King's College Hospital in London, showed a five-year "cure" rate in terminal patients of 16.6 to 17 percent.[124]

If you consult a physician who offers eclectic cancer treatment, here are some of the therapies you can expect to find.

Live Cell.   Live cell therapy involves injecting animal fetal cells, most often cells taken from an unborn calf, into the muscle. One of the advantages of using embryo cells of an animal instead of adult tissue is that the fetus has not yet developed an immune system and, consequently, the patient's immune system will not reject the cells as a foreign substance.

A Swiss surgeon, Paul Niehans, developed cell therapy in the 1930s and treated patients with it for the entire spectrum of degenerative diseases. The treatment is unlicensed in the United States, but there's a growing interest among scientists in using human fetal tissue to treat incurable diseases.[125]

According to Michael L. Culbert, spokesperson, American Biologics (A-B) Hospital in Tijuana, live cell therapy diminishes symptoms in patients who receive it within one to three months; they have greater energy and improved appetite. In the ten years that cell therapy has been used at A-B, "We've seen no adverse side effects."

In cancer treatment, endocrinologist Wolfram Kuhnau, M.D., the A-B Hospital's live cell expert, injects the thymus, "the key gland of the immune system," along with fibrous tissue from the umbilical cord. After a weekly treatment for three weeks, the cancer patient returns for live cell injections at three months, six months, and finally one year. One way to test whether live cell therapy is working is to give an HLB blood test a few days after treatment, Kuhnau said. (This is a test using dried blood to indicate the activity of toxic oxygen in the body.) The newest innovation in live cell treatment at A-B Hospital is the use of shark embryo cells. "The shark has a perfect immune system, never gets cancer, and has a placenta that resembles a human one," said Kuhnau. Researchers say the mystery substance found in shark cartilage that may be responsible for the shark's perfect health also inhibits tumor growth in other mammals. In an article published in *Science,* Dr. Robert Langer of the Massachusetts Institute of Technology writes, "Shark cartilage contains a substance that strongly inhibits the growth of new blood vessels toward solid tumors, thereby restricting tumor growth."[126]

To obtain *Live Cell Therapy* by Dr. Wolfram Kuhnau, contact Cancer Book House, 2043 N. Berendo Street, Los Angeles, CA 90027, (213) 663–7801.

Oxidative Therapies.   Ozone and hydrogen peroxide are oxidative therapies, which means that each supplies oxygen to the body. Both are used in alternative cancer treatment.

The use of oxidative treatment in cancer is primarily based on the research of Otto H. Warburg, a two-time Nobel Prize winner. In the mid-1950s Warburg showed that cancer cells are anaerobic (live without oxygen) and will die in the presence of a high oxygen concentration.[127] A newer theory given to explain the effectiveness of oxidative treatment in various diseases involves free radicals (reactive chemicals that form continuously in the body and have been shown to damage cells). Supposedly, oxidative treatment creates "good" free radicals that quench dangerous free radicals.

Ozone.   Ozone therapy is the use of a mixture of ozone and oxygen to treat a wide variety of diseases and conditions, including cancer and AIDS. Ozone gas kills viruses, bacteria, and fungus; hence its commercial use, which is to purify water. (Los Angeles uses ozone rather than chlorine in its water system.) Medically pure ozone, which is created by a device called an ozone generator, is administered by injection, subcutaneous and intramuscular, or enema.

Used in Germany since World War I, ozone therapy has been shown to shrink tumors. One authority, Dr. Renate Viebahn, coauthor of *The Use of Ozone in Medicine,* lists twenty-two scientific papers that show the effects of ozone in cancer treatment.[128] Viebahn, whose clinic is in Iffezheim, Germany, gives daily intramuscular injections of ozone to cancer patients. Ozone is also used in conjunction with radiation treatment.

Gerard V. Sunnen, M.D., biological psychiatrist and associate professor at New York University, became interested in ozone therapy several years ago when a friend developed cancer and the friend's family asked him to investigate the treatment on a trip to Germany. There, Sunnen visited Dr. Viebahn's clinic. "I observed a number of patients with different types of cancers — lung, gynecological, skin cancer — who had been treated for some time. Judging from their charts, the tumors had not increased; some had regressed, and others appeared to have disappeared." Sunnen has since written an article that provides the first bibliography of scientific papers about ozone therapy that has appeared in the world medical literature.[129]

Despite the wealth of clinical reports and animal studies using ozone therapy (Sunnen gives fifty-nine references) ozone therapy in this country has ground to a halt. Medizone International, Inc., the New York–based company that holds the patent to the Hansler ozone generator, applied to the FDA for permission to treat AIDS patients with ozone in December 1985 but has been on "clinical hold" since then.

At present, the cancer patient who wants to be treated with ozone must travel to Europe or to one of the Mexican clinics that offers this treatment. In 1983 the Gerson Institute in Tijuana introduced ozone therapy as an adjunct to its metabolic program. "We're pleased with the results," said spokesperson Gar Hildebrand.

Hydrogen Peroxide.   Hydrogen peroxide is administered by intravenous injection for therapeutic purposes, although the director of a laboratory in St. Clair Shores, Michigan, considers therapeutic use of hydrogen peroxide to be "extremely dangerous" (more about this below). This use of hydrogen peroxide is being pioneered by Oklahoma physician and researcher Charles H. Farr, M.D., Ph.D., who says that internal use of hydrogen peroxide destroys microorganisms. He reports good results giving hydrogen peroxide infusions to patients with influenza, asthma, emphysema, sinusitis, and chronic obstructive pulmonary disease.[130] When I asked him about treating patients with cancer, he said, "We're working with oncologists and seeing some interesting results, but it's too soon to make recommendations."

One of these oncologists is Dr. V. J. Speckhart of Virginia Beach. Among his patients is a 60-year-old woman with chronic lymphocytic leukemia whose chemotherapy was discontinued when she developed suppression of the bone marrow and a dangerously low white blood cell count. At this time Speckhart began hydrogen peroxide treatment. "Almost immediately she felt better, appeared more alert," he told me. "Lymph nodes grew alternately smaller and larger but ultimately decreased markedly in size. A mass in her armpit shrank so much she told me that she now wears a bra two sizes smaller than before."

If peroxide treatment were given in the early stages of disease, results would be more dramatic, Speckhart believes. "But even when used in advanced cancer, patients are more energetic, less depressed, lose that sallow, pasty look. I've observed no serious complications with hydrogen peroxide and feel increasingly confident using it."

Hydrogen peroxide is also given in conjunction with radiation therapy in cancer treatment. A study conducted by investigators at Dallas's Baylor University Medical Center in the 1960s (one of a series undertaken by this group) shows that oxidizing patients while they are receiving radiation increases the cancer-killing effect of radiation.[131] Speckhart would like to use peroxide as an adjunct to radiation, "but there's a lot of resistance to overcome," he said.

For further information about hydrogen peroxide clinical studies and research, contact International Bio-Oxidative Medicine Foundation (IBOM), P.O. Box 61767, Dallas/Ft. Worth, TX 75261.

Philip Hoekstra III, Ph.D., who is highly critical of the use of hydrogen peroxide infusions, is director of ThermaScan, a laboratory that performs thermography (heat) studies in St. Clair Shores, Michigan. Hoekstra said that he first became aware of the danger of hydrogen peroxide treatment while studying films of patients being treated for atherosclerosis. Noticing that these patients were not improving but getting worse, he contacted their physicians and discovered that they were being treated with hydrogen peroxide infusions.

Hoekstra contends that administering hydrogen peroxide according to Farr's protocol damages the lining of arteries. Unlike cells in other parts of the body, cells that line arteries are not protected by enzymes against the toxic effects of hydrogen peroxide. H_2O_2 acts like Drano on these cells, he said. According to Hoekstra, hundreds of scientific articles published in the last twenty years support his position on the damaging effects of hydrogen peroxide. (Note: These researchers are describing hydrogen peroxide produced in the body in the form of free radicals, not that given therapeutically.)

All this talk about hydrogen peroxide causing free radical damage isn't true, said Ed McCabe, author of *Oxygen Therapies* (Morrisville, N.Y.: Energy Publications, 1988). McCabe says that scientists don't understand how hydrogen peroxide given therapeutically works in the body. "When a physician infuses a patient with hydrogen peroxide, the peroxide selectively kills weak diseased cells. Once the process, called a cleansing reaction, is completed (it can take days or even weeks during which the patient may feel sick), the body begins to produce brand new spanking clean cells." The misunderstanding stems from the fact that scientists study hydrogen peroxide's cell-killing action and are not aware of its restorative effects on the body, he said.

Farr points out that close to 5,000 articles describing beneficial effects of hydrogen peroxide treatment appear in the medical literature. Researchers in the 1960s treated several hundred patients with hydrogen peroxide infusions, "with no reported serious side effects."[132]

Hydrogen peroxide is also being used as a self-help remedy. Diluted amounts of food-grade 35-percent hydrogen peroxide are drunk to relieve arthritic pains and other ailments. For information about these self-help uses, write ECHO, Box 126, Delano, MN 55328.

For further information about these two oxidative therapies and others, see *Oxygen Therapies* by Ed McCabe (Morrisville, N.Y.: Energy Publications, 1988), available at health food stores.

DMSO Therapy.   DMSO (dimethyl sulfoxide) was introduced to the scientific community in 1963 by a research team at the University of Oregon Medical School. Since that time, almost 6,000 articles about it have appeared in the scientific literature. Although DMSO, a cheap industrial solvent, is used as a medical drug in fifty-five countries, in this country it is approved by the FDA only for treatment of a rare bladder inflammation.

But according to Dr. Stanley Jacob of the University of Oregon, pioneer in DMSO research, DMSO is an antitumor agent. Research appears to support his statement. Animal studies show that DMSO delays the development of breast cancer[133] and colon cancer in rats,[134] retards the growth of leukemia[135] and slows the growth of one type of bladder cancer cell.[136] DMSO has also been shown to increase the effectiveness of cytotoxic chemotherapy drugs when tested in mice.[137] For further information, see *DMSO* by Barry Tarshis (New York: William Morrow, 1981).

Hydrazine Sulfate Therapy.   One of the most devastating aspects of cancer is the way the patient with advanced disease wastes away, becoming "skin and bones." This condition, called cachexia (ka-KEK-sia), causes 70 percent of cancer deaths.

Hydrazine sulfate, a drug that costs pennies, reverses weight loss in the emaciated patient. Furthermore, clinical trials, both in this country and the Soviet Union, have shown that hydrazine is not only capable of inducing weight gain but also extends survival time and causes tumors to stabilize or regress.

This cancer wonder-worker is derived from a cheap industrial chemical used as rocket fuel in World War II. It was introduced as a medical therapy by Dr. Joseph Gold, director of the Syracuse Cancer Institute, in 1969. Used in minuscule amounts in cancer treatment, hydrazine prevents cachexia by inhibiting an enzyme used by the tumor to "steal" energy from the host body, Gold explained in a phone conversation.

With such a lifesaving drug available, why are two million cancer patients starving to death each year? Blame it on cancer politics. From 1976 to 1979 hydrazine sulfate languished on the American Cancer Society's list of un-proven methods, the agency's blacklist. Inclusion on the list was based on a clinical trial of the drug at New York's Memorial Sloan-Kettering Cancer Center in 1976. The trial, which involved 29 patients there, concluded that hydrazine sulfate was not beneficial. ("The study was so poorly done it would never be published today," Gold says.) Appearing on the ACS's "quack list" scared away other researchers and cut off Gold's funding.

The tide has turned. In 1987 three double-blind studies conducted at the University of California Medical Center in Los Angeles were reported in the ACS journal *Cancer,* and the following year Gold was one of the presenters at the ACS's Science Writers' Seminar. At that time he said that hydrazine sulfate was being investigated as a possible treatment for AIDS patients.

But it's still premature to talk about a happy ending for hydrazine sulfate, says Gold. The drug, which now has investigational new drug (IND) status, can only be used in a clinical trial, and thus far no major drug house is marketing hydrazine. The stumbling block, says Gold, has been Dr. Vincent T. DeVita, former director of the National Cancer Institute (NCI), who has described hydrazine as a "ho-hum idea." Says Gold, "We're a small institute with a tiny budget. It's an embarrassment to the NCI when we come up with a major finding."

Black and Yellow Salves. Many of the alternative treatments we've discussed so far in this section have been tested in literally thousands of scientific studies and are standard treatment in other parts of the world. Black and yellow salves are a notable exception. According to Kenneth Michaelis of A & O Supply Company in Millersport, Ohio, who sells these two products, "Black and yellow salves, used alternately, open a hole in the flesh and draw out the tumor." Michaelis doesn't know how it works but says the salves are derived from an herbal formula used by American Indians.

H. Ray Evers, M.D., a well-respected pioneer in alternative medicine and director of the International Medical Center in Juarez, Mexico, says that black and yellow salves are beneficial for skin cancers and breast tumors. Here's how one of his patients, who was cured of breast cancer, described her experience with these salves:

> Dr. Evers told me, "The tumor has to come out on its own." He first applied the black salve, then on the third day, the yellow salve. It burned very badly and was an angry red. I could feel a drawing sensation in my neck, stomach, under the arm, and, after one and a half weeks, little tumors began to emerge. The malignant tumor in my breast looked as if it were festering but it finally came through taking some of my nipple. The entire process took one month. It was very painful but by the time I left the clinic, I was well.

Dowsing. With growing awareness that spending extended periods of time in a geopathic zone is detrimental to health, the dowser, who uses a forked stick to search for water, is playing a new role. (A geopathic zone contains underground water, mineral veins, fault lines, and underground caverns, all of which emit harmful electromagnetic vibrations.) Dr. Hans Nieper of Hanover, Germany, estimates that 93 percent of all cancer patients have been exposed to geopathic zones. Geopathic exposure is also a factor in multiple sclerosis, he says. Nieper recommends that all cancer and MS patients have their home, bed, and favorite chair dowsed for geopathic radiations.

Dr. Emil Levin, a Russian-born Beverly Hills physician, related the case history of a patient, a lawyer in his 40s, whom I'll call Paul, who was exposed to geopathic stress. Some years ago, Paul (while under another doctor's care) was diagnosed with lymphoma, a malignant tumor of the lymph glands. Treated with chemotherapy, the tumor receded. But two years later, Paul (now a patient of Levin's) had a recurrence of his cancer. Despite receiving similar treatment, Paul failed to improve and became progressively weaker and more emaciated. Levin, trained in Europe, was aware of research that associated this particular type of lymphoma with geopathic stress, and advised his patient to have a dowser check his house in Malibu. The dowser found that Paul's house was situated over buried water veins and advised him to move as soon as possible. "Paul complied, and his health improved immediately," Levin said. "Today, four years later, he is alive and well."

Abandoning your house when "noxious emanations" are present is obviously a last resort. In most cases, there are a number of ways to counteract the damage. For information about dowsing and how to locate a dowser in your area, write to the American Society of Dowsers, Inc., Danville, VT 05828-0024.

Mind and Spirit. Psychotherapy figures in almost all alternative cancer programs. Michael L. Culbert of American Biologics Hospital, in a weekly talk to incoming patients, asks the group, "Is anybody here dying of cancer?" Surveying the show of hands, he says, "Correction. You are not dying of cancer—you are living with cancer. Others are living with diabetes, arthritis, acne."

The spiritual element in healing often goes hand in hand with psychotherapy. Dr. Ernesto Contreras, medical director of the hospital in Tijuana that bears his name, says that mind, emotions, and spirit are more important than any other factor in cancer. A weekly church service is held at the hospital, and patients can also attend Sunday services at a nondenominational church adjoining the hospital.

One of Contreras's "miracle" patients is Beatrice Super, who recovered from advanced stomach cancer. Recalling her darkest days, when the cancer had metastasized to her pancreas, gall bladder, and liver, she said, "Dr. Contreras taught me if I wanted to live, I must get well spiritually and call on the power of God."

Some of the most effective psycho-spiritual therapy undoubtedly takes place informally among patients. Wanda Black, a 52-year-old bookkeeper, told me that she accompanied her father to the Contreras Hospital some years ago when he was dying of cancer. "No one stayed despondent for long," she said. "We kept each other's spirits high."

How to Locate Nontoxic Cancer Treatments

Considering that two out of three cancer patients will die of the disease within five years, there's good reason to prepare for this medical emergency. After all, we're accustomed to doing so in other areas. If you're the parent of a toddler, you post the telephone number of the Poison Control Center on the bulletin board. If your spouse has a heart condition, you may have learned cardiopulmonary resuscitation. Even small children have been taught to perform the Heimlich Maneuver to prevent choking to death on food. But we fear cancer, and we avoid thinking about it. When cancer has struck, however, is not the best time to research alternative cancer treatments. Not long ago I received a phone call from a young man whose wife had been diagnosed with breast cancer. "The doctor recommends that she start chemotherapy right away, but is there a diet that could help her?" I told him about various diets—the Gerson diet, Dr. Ruth Long's, and others that have helped cancer patients. But he sounded so distraught that I doubt he took in all this new information, let alone summoned the energy to follow up the leads.

In some instances, cancer patients stumble on an alternative treatment that feels right to them. (Remember McCray at the public library?) Others embark on a search for the right treatment, as Grace Aldworth did.

Aldworth, 54, a Chicago cultural arts leader and a tall, striking brunette who looks as if she belongs on the pages of a fashion magazine, developed breast cancer in 1982. Despite misgivings about chemotherapy — "As a volunteer at a cancer hospital, I had seen what these chemo drugs did to people" — Aldworth followed her doctor's advice and began chemotherapy. "At that time, I knew nothing about alternative treatment, but was interested in nutrition." Three months later, when her white blood count dropped dangerously low ("I was so weak I could barely walk") and she experienced heart palpitations among other symptoms, she called a halt to chemotherapy. Searching for a direction, she discovered that certain diets were said to cure cancer. She visited Ann Wigmore's Hippocrates Institute, now in Boston, which recommends the use of sprouted foods, particularly wheatgrass. Aldworth tried this diet, and also investigated macrobiotics at the East-West Center in Brookline, Massachusetts. Feeling the need for a more complete and supervised medical program, she then embarked on a tour of cancer clinics and eventually became a patient at the Livingston-Wheeler Clinic in San Diego. Recalling her arduous search, "I was fortunate to have the energy and the means to do all that traveling," she said.

At the time that Aldworth was making her solo journey (1982), Michael Lerner, director of Commonweal, was engaged in the same pursuit on a larger scale. Lerner's account of his tour of thirty alternative cancer centers, plus other valuable material pertaining to alternative treatment, appears in *Integral Cancer Therapies* (available from Commonweal, P.O. Box 316, Bolinas, CA 94924).

In your search for direction, a certain amount of legwork is necessary, but you don't want to reinvent the wheel. Another guide to alternative cancer centers, this one more limited in scope, is Sally Wolper's *16 Year Analysis of Tijuana Clinics, Where and How to Go* (Wolper Publications, 14134 Gladeside Drive, La Mirada, CA 90638), which includes a description of metabolic cancer therapies.

A comprehensive and highly professional guidebook is John M. Fink's *Third Opinion: An International Directory to Alternative Therapy Centers for the Treatment and Prevention of Cancer* (Garden City Park, N.Y.: Avry Publishing Group, 1988). Fink is an actor whose involvement in alternative health care began when his daughter, Phoebe, developed a rare form of cancer at age 2. When conventional treatment failed to help her, the Finks discovered nontoxic therapies. Although at this late date alternative treatment could do no more than relieve their daughter's pain and suffering, the Finks' investigation of these therapies inspired them to make this information available to others.

After reading one of these guidebooks, you may feel overwhelmed by the sheer number of alternative treatment centers (Fink's directory contains about seventy-five entries). What you need is a travel guide — someone who is familiar with these centers and can fill you in on the nitty-gritty.

Filling this need are a dozen or more "information resources" that have sprung up in the past decade to provide information about alternative cancer therapies and where to find them. These resources fall into two categories: (1) organizations that focus on specific needs of the cancer patient and (2) those that are primarily political action organizations. Most are nonprofit educational organizations supported by memberships, with minimum fees of, on the average, $25.

What these resources have in common is that, with few exceptions, each was founded by a recovered cancer patient or someone whose child, parent, spouse, or loved one had cancer. So in addition to obtaining up-to-date information about alternative treatment, you're plugging into a support system of individuals who have traveled the same road and are eager to listen, advise, and put you in touch with other cancer patients.

Information Resources

The Arlin J. Brown Information Center, Inc.
P.O. Box 251
Fort Belvoir, VA 22060
(703) 451–8638

What It Is.   A clearinghouse for information on nontoxic cancer treatment.

Services.   Refers patients to cancer clinics that offer metabolic treatment in this country and Europe; publishes a monthly newsletter, *Health Victory Bulletin* (sample subjects: our deadly water supply, danger of vaccines, healing power of herbs); dispenses books and brochures about nontoxic treatments, including Brown's handbook, *March of Truth on Cancer;* holds an annual conference in Belvoir, Virginia.

Background.   Brown, a retired physicist with the U.S. Army, is a veteran crusader for freedom of choice in medicine. His information center, founded in 1963, was the first organization in the United States devoted to nontoxic cancer therapies.

Cancer Control Society
2043 N. Berendo Street
Los Angeles, CA 90027
(213) 663–7801

What It Is.   With a membership of 5,500, it's probably the largest information resource.

Services.   Provides a directory of alternative health care practitioners here and in Europe; has a 24-hour hot line; publishes a bimonthly journal; offers a large selection of mail-order books; holds an annual cancer convention over the July 4th weekend in Los Angeles, which features leading alternative practitioners (the 1989 convention, its seventeenth, attracted one thousand attendees); sponsors a tour of Tijuana clinics four times a year.

Background.   The society was originally a chapter of the International Association of Cancer Victors and Friends, and became independent in 1973. The contact person is Lorraine Rosenthal, cofounder.

CanHelp
111 Paradise Bay Road
Port Ludlow, WA 98365-9771
(206) 437–2291

What It Is.   A unique cancer patient advisory service operated by a well-known medical writer, Patrick M. McGrady, Jr., coauthor of *The Pritikin Program for Diet and Exercise*. Using a computer linkup with MEDLARS (the National Library of Medicine computer data bank) and other systems, McGrady provides up-to-date information about cancer treatments here and overseas.

Services.   One week after McGrady receives information from a patient (specifics on what to send are contained in a brochure), the patient receives a computer printout telling what cancer specialists or centers achieve the best results treating patients with cancer of the patient's type. There's a fee for the computer search but no charge for telephone consultations.

Background.   McGrady, former Moscow bureau chief for *Newsweek* magazine, launched CanHelp after his father's death from cancer in 1980. (Ironically, his father was science editor for the American Cancer Society.) "My father's experience as a cancer patient showed me how difficult it is to get information about cancer treatment, and how 'the Cancer Church' operates," McGrady says.

Foundation for Advancement in Cancer Therapies
P.O. Box 1242, Old Chelsea Station
New York, NY 10013
(212) 741–2790

What It Is.   FACT distributes literature and tapes about nontoxic therapies for cancer and supports scientific investigation of nutrition and biologicals (substances that occur naturally in the body). In addition to its New York office, there are FACT chapters in Philadelphia, Boston, and Detroit.

Services.   This resource's distinctive asset is counseling provided by its founder-director, Ruth Sackman. Sackman, 73, with twenty years of experience in cancer counseling, spends unlimited time with the cancer patient and family, in person, by phone, or by mail. There's no fee involved. After determining the patient's condition and needs, Sackman makes referrals to one or more doctors or clinics that provide appropriate treatment. She also arranges support groups led by professionals for cancer patients.

Background.   When Sackman's daughter, after undergoing chemotherapy, was dying of leukemia, Sackman in desperation investigated alternative therapies. Her faith in nontoxic therapies has never dimmed.

The International Association of Cancer Victors and Friends, Inc.
7740 West Manchester Avenue, Suite 110
P.O. Box 5400, Playa del Rey, CA 90293
(213) 822–5032, 5132

What It Is.   IACVF is a clearinghouse for information about cancer research and treatment and acts as a consumer advocate on behalf of patients and of family physicians and oncologists who provide nontoxic therapies. There are IACVF chapters throughout the United States, Canada, and Australia and a worldwide membership.

Services.   Emphasizes benefits of networking; provides updated list of alternative practitioners plus names of recovered patients and their type of cancer; publishes the *Cancer Victors Journal* (news about cancer treatment and research, case histories of Cancer Victors); operates a cancer hot line; holds regional seminars and conventions; distributes books and periodicals.

Background.   IACVF was founded in 1963 by Cecile Hoffman, a cancer patient who credited her recovery to a laetrile program. Its president, Marie Steinmeyer of Atlanta, a feisty recovered cancer patient, is founder-director of the Georgia Womens' Coalition for Medical Freedom, emcees a weekly radio show, and counsels cancer patients.

The following are political action groups that can also provide information about alternative centers and support groups.

The Alliance for Alternative Medicine
P.O. Box 59
Liberty Lake, WA 99019
(509) 255-9246

What It Is.   A lobby that advocates testing promising alternative therapies and making them available.

Services.   Networking among cancer patients and alternative practitioners.

Background.   The Alliance was founded in 1987 by Marge Jacob, a Washington C.P.A. whose son, San, was diagnosed with metastasized melanoma at age 11. After San failed to improve with chemotherapy, the Jacobs investigated alternative treatment, and San became a patient of Dr. Lawrence Burton (see page 38). After one year of treatment, the Jacobs' son was doing well. Then Burton's clinic was closed by the Bahamian government (charges leveled against Burton were later dismissed). During the nine months the clinic was closed, the boy's condition deteriorated rapidly and he died.

Coalition for Alternatives in Nutrition and Healthcare, Inc.
P.O. Box B-12
Richlandtown, PA 18955
(215) 346-8461

What It Is.   A grass roots coalition to educate the public about alternative health care and lobby legislative agencies on behalf of freedom of choice in medicine.

Services.   Dispenses publications and free brochures largely pertaining to abuses in standard medicine.

Background.   CANAH's founder-director, Catherine J. Frompovich, Ph.D., developed a life-threatening disease (Legionnaire's) as a young adult. When standard medicine failed to help her, she discovered alternative treatment and, with the help of naturopathic physicians, regained her health.

Immuno-Augmentative Therapy Patients' Association, Inc.
P.O. Box 10
Otho, IA 50569-0010
(515) 972-4444

What It Is.   IATPA protects the rights of patients who have been treated at the IAT clinic in Freeport, the Bahamas, and works closely with other political action groups on behalf of freedom of choice in medicine.

Services.   Disseminates information about IAT and provides cancer patients with names of IAT patients who have similar types of cancer.

Background.   IATPA was formed in July 1985, shortly after the IAT clinic in Freeport was closed by Bahamian health authorities. (The charge by U.S. health authorities that serum being used at the clinic was contaminated with the AIDS virus was later retracted.)

One of IATPA's three founding members is Jack Link, 59, of Kalamazoo, Michigan, retired company president. (All three are ex-captains of industry.) Link was diagnosed with advanced prostate cancer at the Cleveland Clinic in 1984. After refusing castration and chemotherapy, Link was treated at the IAT clinic and today is in excellent health. IATPA president since 1985 is Frank Wiewel, whose father-in-law was a patient at the IAT clinic.

Project CURE
2020 K Street, Suite 350
Washington, DC 20069
(202) 293–3479 or (1/800) 552–CURE

What It Is.   The nation's second largest health-related lobby.

Services.   Provides information on alternative therapies, clinics, and practitioners as well as on the politics of cancer; refers patients to other support groups.

Background.   Project CURE was founded in 1979 by a cancer patient, Robert DeBragga, who had been diagnosed with terminal lung cancer the previous year. DeBragga's exhaustive search of alternative cancer treatments led him to Emanuel Revici, M.D., of New York City (see page 22). Current Project CURE executive director, attorney Michael S. Evers (not a cancer patient), was instrumental in the decision of a congressional agency, the Office of Technology Assessment (OTA), to evaluate Immuno-Augmentative Therapy.

LOOKING AHEAD

Chemotherapy drugs are not the first poisons that doctors have employed to combat disease. Beginning in the early nineteenth century and continuing for most of it, a mercury preparation called calomel was prescribed for almost every disease. Given in large doses and for an extended period, it was a treatment only the strongest patient survived. *Gunns' New Family Physician,* 1872, recommended calomel doses of 5 to 10 grains (320 to 640 milligrams) taken at night. In 1984 the smallest amount of mercury chloride reported to cause death was 500 milligrams. As a physician at the time described the effects of calomel, "The blood itself is altered in character . . . recently healed wounds open afresh; the body becomes emaciated, the face pallid, the whole system becomes peculiarly susceptible to irritating or depressing influences . . ." Another physician recalling the abuse of calomel wrote, "Look at the poor wretch . . . unable to swallow even liquids without torture and with his tongue swollen to three or four times its usual size, protruded far beyond the lips . . . discharging [stinking mucus] into a spittoon. . . ."[138]

Earlier in the century, physicians who practiced "botanical medicine" and other unorthodox therapies protested the use of mercurial medicines along with bloodletting and other "heroic" measures. As time went on, large segments of the public, always distrustful of these torturous treatments, deserted orthodox medicine.

2

Treating High Blood Pressure Without Drugs

High blood pressure, which accounts for more doctor visits and prescriptions than any other ailment, affects more than 60 million Americans, or 30 percent of adults in this country. These patients with high blood pressure spend a total of $11.1 billion each year on health care relating to their disease. High blood pressure, or hypertension, is known as the "silent killer" because it doesn't produce any symptoms until the condition becomes advanced, but, at the same time, may be damaging your heart and blood vessels. Uncontrolled hypertension is "the leading cause of the 500,000 strokes that occur each year, and is a major contributor to the 1.25 million heart attacks that occur each year."[1]

How can high blood pressure create such havoc? Dr. Norman M. Kaplan, head of the hypertension section at the University of Texas, Southwestern Medical School, explains it this way: "As blood pressure rises, the heart must pump harder and the blood vessels are pounded harder with every heartbeat. After many years, the heart may enlarge and finally weaken, the blood-vessel walls roughen or rupture. . . ."[2]

Doctors don't know what causes 90 percent of high blood pressure. This type of high blood pressure is called *essential hypertension.* In the remaining 10 percent of cases, high blood pressure is caused by kidney disease, a tumor of the adrenal gland, or a congenital defect of the aorta (the large blood vessel leading from the heart to the body). This type of high blood pressure is called *secondary hypertension.*[3]

55

Blood pressure readings are expressed in two numbers: an upper one, called the *systolic* pressure, and a lower one, called the *diastolic* pressure. A reading of 120 systolic over 80 diastolic is considered normal blood pressure. Systolic blood pressure represents the pressure in the arteries when the heart is pumping blood; diastolic pressure is the pressure in the arteries when the heart is resting and filling with blood for the next beat. Because the earliest method of measuring blood pressure involved the use of a mercury-filled glass column, blood pressure is usually expressed as millimeters of mercury, or mm Hg.

If your blood pressure is 140/90 mm Hg or higher, your doctor will tell you that you have high blood pressure. An elevated reading should be confirmed on at least two subsequent visits since some people are "office hypertensives": their blood pressure goes up just from being in a medical setting. According to a recent study conducted at New York Hospital–Cornell Medical Center in New York City, if you're a woman under age 40 and of normal weight, you're the most susceptible to "white coat hypertension," particularly when a male physician rather than a female technician takes your blood pressure.[4]

An individual whose blood pressure is 85 to 89 diastolic is classified as "high normal," or at risk of developing high blood pressure, and needs to be closely monitored. The majority of hypertensive patients (estimates vary from 75 to 90 percent) have "mild" hypertension (90 to 104 diastolic). Others are classified as "moderate" (105 to 114 diastolic) and "severe" (115 diastolic and above). Black Americans have almost a 33 percent greater chance of having high blood pressure than whites. Men are more likely to have high blood pressure than women, and there's a tendency for the condition to increase with age.

STANDARD TREATMENT

Since 1977 the Joint National Committee (JNC) on Detection, Evaluation, and Treatment of High Blood Pressure has issued a report every four years advising physicians as to the best way to treat hypertension. These JNC recommendations, issued through the federal National High Blood Pressure Education Program, are based on the latest scientific studies.

If you have high blood pressure, here's how doctors will treat you if they follow the recommendations contained in the 1988 report of the JNC.[5]

Nondrug Treatment

If you are classified as having mild hypertension (by the above definition) and if you are *not* at risk for heart disease (meaning that you don't smoke or have signs of heart damage, are not diabetic, and have normal levels of cholesterol and triglycerides), then your doctor will treat you with "nonphar-macologic approaches." Since there's no scientific evidence, the report says, that a low-fat diet has any effect on hypertension, if you are not obese this nondrug treatment boils down to restricting salt. According to Kaplan, "About 50 percent of the people who cut their sodium in half will have a significant fall in blood pressure."[6] But if you are obese, weight reduction is essential since studies show that "obesity and blood pressure are closely associated." What constitutes a weight-reduction diet is not mentioned.

Drug Treatment

If these nondrug measures, mainly salt and alcohol restriction and a weight-reduction diet left to the doctor's discretion, don't enable you to maintain a blood pressure below 140/90 mm Hg, then the next step is drug treatment. Since the report says that in mild hypertensive patients, clinical trials have shown that drug treatment keeps blood pressure down and protects against stroke, congestive failure, and death, it's not likely that your doctor will spend much time advising you about life-style changes, which carry no such guarantee. Your doctor can choose among four classes of antihypertensive drugs: diuretics, beta blockers, angiotensin-converting en-zyme inhibitors, and calcium channel blockers. If, after one to three months, the drug does not reduce your blood pressure sufficiently, your doctor has three options: to increase the dose of the first drug, add a second drug from another class (the "stepped-care" approach), or discontinue the first drug and substitute a drug from another class. "The goal of therapy is to control blood pressure with the fewest drugs at their lowest dose," says the 1988 JNC report.

If you have moderate hypertension (105 to 114 diastolic) or severe hypertension (115 diastolic or above), your doctor will prescribe a high blood pressure drug but will also recommend nondrug measures (diet, salt restric-tion, and limited alcohol consumption).

Stepped-Care Approach—the More the Merrier

If you think that doctors treating high blood pressure are drug-happy now, consider treatment prior to 1988. At that time, standard drug treatment for high blood pressure was limited to the stepped-care approach. As de-scribed in the 1977 JNC report, "A stepped-care program . . . calls for initiating therapy with a small dose of an antihypertensive drug, increasing the dose of that drug, and then adding, one after another, other drugs as needed."[7] The stepped-care approach is responsible for the familiar plight of the patient who's taking three or four different high blood pressure drugs. As a pharmacist based at a university hospital explained, "One tablet may cause the vessels to dilate and thus lower pressure, but dilating causes the heart to speed up, which requires a second agent to slow the heart down. In addition, one of these two drugs may cause fluid retention, which calls for a diuretic, known as a water pill." Each of these drugs can cause numerous side effects such as impotence or increasing weakness of the heart muscle that can be life-threatening.

Looking Back

Today, criticism of standard treatment for high blood pressure focuses on abuse of antihypertensive drugs. But surprisingly enough, twenty years ago physicians were reluctant to treat mild hypertensives with medication. This conservative attitude took a 180-degree turn when studies conducted in the 1960s and 1970s were interpreted as indicating that hypertensive patients treated with drugs lived longer than untreated hypertensive patients. (I've said *interpreted* because subsequent studies showed different results.) One of these studies, the 1979 Hypertension Detection and Follow-up Program (HDFP) conducted by the National Heart, Lung, and Blood Institute (NHLBI), found that mortality in people with high blood pressure, including those with mild hypertension, could be reduced by almost 20 percent with antihypertensive drug treatment.[8] Studies showing the efficacy of antihypertensive drug treatment ushered in mass blood pressure screening programs. Such programs have led to the present situation, in which at least 20 million Americans take pills every day to lower their blood pressure and spend close to $3 billion a year on these medications.

Growing Concern Over Water Pills

On the heels of the National Heart, Lung, and Blood Institute finding, another NHLBI study, the Multiple Risk Factor Intervention Trial (known by the jaunty title of MRFIT) presented some contradictory evidence. One disturbing finding that emerged from the one-year MRFIT study, the largest clinical trial on the prevention of coronary heart disease, was that patients who were treated "intensively" with thiazide diuretics (the most widely used class of drugs against high blood pressure) had higher death rates than those taking other drugs or no drugs at all.[9] This finding caused speculation that high doses of diuretics, which rid the body of excess fluids and salts, may be toxic. Some doctors began to question whether mild hypertensives—who constitute close to 90 percent of patients with high blood pressure—should be treated with such potentially harmful medications.

At present, 15 to 25 million Americans take diuretics, which have been the mainstay of hypertensive drug treatment for almost fifty years. Meanwhile, studies have shown that lowering blood pressure with diuretics reduces the risk of stroke but does not prevent heart attacks. In addition, diuretics can cause biochemical changes that increase susceptibility to heart attacks. These recent findings are nothing new. Studies published in the early 1980s showed that diuretics deplete potassium levels, increasing the risk of heart irregularities and sudden death, and raise blood cholesterol and triglycerides, which are associated with an increase in coronary heart disease. [10, 11] Diuretics have long been known to cause elevations of blood sugar and uric acid, which exacerbate or cause diabetes, gout, or both.

Discovering Diet

Starting in the mid-1980s, a few investigators began to look at diet as a treatment for mild hypertensives. A University of Mississippi researcher conducted a one-year study in which obese hypertensives lost weight and ate a low-salt diet. At the end of the year, 78 percent of the patients, who had previously been on antihypertensive medication for at least five years, were drug-free and were maintaining normal blood pressure. [12]

A husband-and wife team, Rose and Jeremiah Stamler, from Northwestern University Medical Center, also set out to prove that diet alone can control hypertension. In a four-year trial reported in *JAMA* on March 20, 1987, they showed that many people can stop taking drugs to lower their blood pressure if they change their diets. For those who still need drugs, a healthy diet can lessen some side effects of these drugs. [13]

The Mineral Brigade

It's agreed that minerals, such as sodium, calcium, potassium, and magnesium, play a role in regulating blood pressure. But since each researcher appears to have a pet mineral, it's hard to get an objective assessment of the general role minerals play in high blood pressure. Even salt, long acknowledged as the "heavy" in hypertension, is now regarded by some experts as only one of many culprits. Confusing the issue is the theory that those with high blood pressure can safely ingest a certain amount of salt if they include certain protective nutrients in their diet. [14]

Calcium. Dr. David A. McCarron, of the Oregon Health Sciences University in Portland, believes that calcium may be the key to reducing or preventing hypertension. McCarron's own studies, beginning in 1984, show that adding 1,000 milligrams of calcium per day to the diet lowers blood pressure a "modest" amount (3.8 to 6 mm Hg) in patients with mild to moderate hypertension. [15] Interestingly enough, men are more responsive to calcium than women, he says. McCarron suggests that adding calcium is more important as a cause of hypertension than reducing sodium.[16] (One of his critics, Dr. Norman Kaplan, who recommends that *everyone* cut down on salt, points out that McCarron's research is heavily supported by the National Dairy Council.)

Potassium.   Potassium supplements may lower blood pressure in patients treated with diuretics, according to a study conducted at the University of Texas Health Science Center at Dallas.[17] Potassium appears to have a see-saw relationship with salt because "whenever sodium is deleted from the diet . . . (as happens when you replace processed products with natural foods) potassium intake increases."[18] Kaplan, who conducted the potassium study, recommends that you get your potassium from food, not potassium tablets. (Good sources of potassium are low-fat, high-fiber fruits, vegetables, and beans.) Researchers at the Hadassah Hospital in Tel Aviv suggest that the lower blood pressure of vegetarians relates to their large intake of potassium.[19]

Magnesium.   Dr. Lawrence Resnick, endocrinologist and cardiologist at Cornell University Medical Center in New York, has discovered that "everybody with high blood pressure has lower than normal levels of magnesium inside their cells." (This intracellular magnesium, called free magnesium, differs from magnesium in the bloodstream, which is known as circulating magnesium.) Furthermore, this low level of magnesium inside the cells occurs not only in hypertensives but in people who are obese and in diabetics. Resnick's discovery may help explain why these three conditions are so often found in the same individual.

Does this mean that all hypertensives will benefit from additional magnesium? No, said Resnick, "You can't lump all hypertensives together. We believe that those people with high blood pressure who need extra amounts of magnesium are the ones with lower than average levels of magnesium in the bloodstream." (Your doctor can administer a simple test to determine your level of circulating magnesium.) Resnick has also found that hypertensives with low magnesium values have unusually high renin activity. (Renin is an enzyme released by the kidneys that produces a hormone, angiotensin, that causes constriction of blood vessels and thus an increase in blood pressure.) These two measurements indicate which people with high blood pressure need magnesium supplementation, Resnick said.

Despite this intriguing research about potassium, calcium, and magnesium, don't expect your doctor to treat you with any of these minerals. As Resnick explained, "We're trying to establish criteria that the average doctor can use in treating hypertension." According to the 1988 JNC report, data concerning potassium, calcium, magnesium, and other minerals are "still developing, . . . inadequate, [and] too meager to justify any recommendations."[20]

High Blood Pressure Drugs— Decisions, Decisions

Until recently, physicians treating patients with high blood pressure relied on diuretics and beta blockers. But now that two new types of drugs are available (the newcomers are angiotensin-converting enzyme or ACE inhibitors and calcium channel blockers), high blood pressure specialists are taking sides as to which drug is best. Some contend that the newer drugs will prevent heart attacks. For example, a group of Swedish researchers found that a new drug, metoprolol, a beta blocker with the brand name Lopressor, can reduce the heart attack death rate as well as the death rate from strokes in patients with high blood pressure.[21] But the real attraction of these new drugs is that they cause fewer side effects than the old standbys. Captopril, one of the new ACE inhibitors, is being touted as a "quality of life" drug based on a 1986 study in which patients gave it high marks in terms of "general well-being."[22] Doctors hope that these new drugs will solve the problem of noncompliance—patients who stop taking their high blood pressure pills because the medication makes them feel worse than they did before. In a British study, 40 percent of the subjects discontinued taking their medication because of its side effects.[23]

Other physicians criticize the rush to treat patients with ACE inhibitors and calcium channel blockers, saying these new drugs have never been scientifically tested and furthermore are extremely costly.

Whatever drug your doctor chooses (and according to a November 5, 1989, *New York Times Magazine* article, that choice may depend on which drug company sales representative is most ingratiating), keep in mind some differences between the sexes.

If you're a man, high blood pressure increases your risk of having a stroke or heart attack, but there is no evidence that lowering blood pressure with drugs will prevent you from having a heart attack. Drug therapy may protect you from a stroke, however.

If you're a woman and have high blood pressure, drug therapy may not confer the same benefits, said Dr. Thomas G. Pickering, professor of medicine at the Cardiac Center of New York Hospital-Cornell Medical Center. "You have less risk of heart attack and stroke than a man, and there is no documented evidence that drug therapy benefits women with any degree of hypertension."

Pickering came to these conclusions by analyzing the scientific studies we've discussed, whose subjects, for the most part, are all male. In treating both men and women, "the important thing is to look at high blood pressure as one of many risk factors."[24]

Diet vs. Drugs

What's happening in the real world of the doctor's office? If you have mild hypertension (and three-quarters of all people with high blood pressure do), will your doctor reach for a prescription pad or recommend a diet? Said Dr. E. Paul MacCarthy, director of the hypertension clinic at the University of Cincinnati Medical Center, "In a university setting, we have dieticians available and utilize them extensively. Dietary counseling is particularly important for a hypertensive patient, who is likely to have elevated cholesterol levels and to be overweight."

According to Dr. Herbert Benson of the Division of Behavioral Medicine, New England Deaconess Hospital, Boston, doctors are more likely to give lip service to diet. "Your doctor will tell you to lose weight, stop smoking, exercise more, and relax, but he doesn't have the time or the know-how to give you the tools to make these changes. So you continue the same unhealthy life-style as before and, naturally, when you return for your next doctor's visit, your blood pressure hasn't come down. So the doctor has no choice but to start drug treatment or increase medication."[25]

ALTERNATIVE TREATMENT

The Pritikin Promise

Diet, not drugs, is the cornerstone of alternative treatment for hypertension. This approach isn't new; in the late 1940s, Dr. Walter Kempner of Durham, North Carolina, treated hypertensive patients and others with his rice and fruit diet and reported that diet alone normalized blood pressure.

But it was Nathan Pritikin, a self-styled medical expert, who, appearing on the scene in the mid-1970s, popularized the revolutionary notion that a program of diet and aerobic exercise could transform sick people into active healthy ones. (Aerobic exercise, such as walking, jogging, swimming, and bicycling, generates heat in the body and speeds up the heart rate.) In a four-week period at Pritikin's Longevity Center in Santa Monica, California, more than 83 percent of hypertensive patients who entered the program on medication lowered their blood pressures and left drug-free.[26] (I've described the Pritikin program in considerable detail in chapter 7.)

The Pritikin program isn't confined to Longevity Centers. Pritikin, a gifted teacher, attracted a group of outstanding young physicians and researchers. These individuals, who were disillusioned with standard medicine, absorbed the master's philosophy of health care, learned his methods, and set forth to preach the Pritikin gospel in their own fashion.

Hans A. Diehl, M.D. One of the Pritikin disciples you'll meet in this chapter is Dr. Hans A. Diehl, director of the Lifestyle Medicine Institute in Loma Linda, California, and author of *To Your Health* (Redlands, Calif.: The Quiet Hour, 1987). Diehl was formerly director of research and education at the Pritikin Longevity Center. Today, he conducts workshops in different parts of the world. Like Pritikin, in one instance he took on an entire community.

In March 1988, Diehl, with two dieticians and a minister in tow, arrived in the town of Creston, British Columbia (population 4,000), and conducted a four-week health improvement program. The program, Live with All Your Heart, is designed to reduce the risk of cardiovascular disease. "Over 400 people enrolled," Diehl said. Each day participants attended a two-hour lecture dealing primarily with nutrition. Before and after the program, participants had the option of enrolling in the Heartscreen, a coronary workup that includes testing cholesterol, triglycerides, and glucose, blood pressure, and heart rate. (Of the 400 participants, 332 people took part in the Heartscreen.)

Diehl's approach is to ease participants gently into making life-style changes, good advice to heed if you're trying to influence family members. Said Diehl, "Instead of eliminating meat from the diet, I suggest one meatless day, and after people become acquainted with the endless variety of vegetarian meals, they're ready to try two or three meatless days."

Diehl's message had an immediate impact on sales patterns in Creston food markets. "We showed them how to make frozen banana ice cream. [The recipe for this ice cream sans milk or cream appears on page 155 of *To Your Health*.] That week, the merchants sold three tons of bananas. During the program, the two supermarkets ran out of fresh produce."

After one month of diet and exercise, "400 people lost one ton of excess fat—that's 2,000 pounds, or the equivalent of 13 people. (Average weight loss for each participant was five pounds.) Cholesterol levels dropped an average of 35 points. [This drop is half of what the Pritikin program achieves, but as Diehl pointed out, Crestonites were living on their own, not in a controlled environment.] In addition, 13 people discovered they were diabetic and 12 of the 13 were no longer diabetic after four weeks on the diet."

Diehl invited Creston's nine physicians to the health improvement program, but only two attended a lecture, he said. "Participants were shocked that their doctors did not support the program."

Diehl's successful effort to help participants lose weight, reduce cholesterol levels, and control diabetes was immensely important to people with high blood pressure, since obesity, elevated cholesterol levels, and diabetes are all considered risk factors for high blood pressure.

Diehl was co-investigator of a study in California to show that people taking antihypertensive medication can become drug-free.[27] In this study,

186 high blood pressure patients (85 percent of the study group) had taken anti-hypertensive drugs for several years. With diet, which included reducing salt intake to one teaspoon or less a day, and exercise, they were able to gradually reduce and finally discontinue their medications after only four weeks.

Diehl doesn't question the fact that excessive salt is harmful, as some researchers have done lately. "When we eat more salt than our kidneys can cope with, it accumulates like a toxic waste that must be diluted before the body can get rid of it. To keep the salt diluted, the body begins to retain water, pounds of it. In an attempt to drive that extra salt water through the kidney filters, the body begins to raise the blood pressure, eventually leading to permanent kidney damage.

For more information about Diehl's program to reverse high blood pressure and other cardiovascular conditions naturally, see his lively, readable book, *To Your Health* (available from the Quiet Hour, 630 Brookside Avenue, Redlands, CA 92373-4699). To subscribe to his newsletter, *Lifeline,* write to the same address.

Cleaves M. Bennett, M.D.   Another Pritikin protégé who has a special interest in high blood pressure is Dr. Cleaves M. Bennett, director of the Innerhealth Center in Los Angeles. Bennett, author of *How to Control Your High Blood Pressure without Drugs* (New York: Doubleday & Co., 1988) has devised a twelve-week program that demands a high degree of commitment on the patient's part. The program includes taking your own blood pressure, changing your diet, practicing stress reduction techniques, doing aerobic exercises, and enlisting your doctor as a partner in this endeavor.

True to the Pritikin tradition, "teaching good nutrition is the biggest gun in my arsenal," Bennett says. But he does not go the Pritikin route and provide a list of "approved" and "forbidden" foods. "You've got to discover your own diet," Bennett says. To do this, he suggests that you keep a food diary. By listing everything that you eat, you'll become aware of how salty some of these foods are and how much oil and fat they contain, he says. The diet that Bennett recommends is the basic Pritikin Diet, consisting of whole grains, vegetables, and fruits. No meat, dairy foods, or processed foods permitted. In a casual, unthreatening way, Bennett recommends that you follow this diet for one week to see how your body responds to it.

As Bennett explains, he was once a member of the academic establishment. "I have done research in the best labs, taught in the finest schools, and worked in the most advanced medical clinics. . . ." But at some point Bennett realized that all this publish or perish research was only helping the researchers—not the patients. So he quit the academic rat race.

As you'll discover reading the section on older drugs (the two new classes of drugs were not in use at the time he wrote his book), Bennett is well acquainted with antihypertensive drugs and their side effects. "For years and years I have sat across the desk from patients with high blood pressure. While making out their prescriptions, I've glanced up and caught a look in their eyes. I've seen a very special kind of sadness."

Bennett discovered the world of alternative health when he was searching to improve his own health. "I wasn't exercising, my diet was abominable, and with my insatiable sweet tooth I was looking more and more like a Hostess Twinkie." During this period he spent two years at the Pritikin Longevity Center. "It turned my life around to see what happened to people who got on an excellent diet, started exercising, lost their stress, and gave up smoking and coffee habits."

One of the thousands of people who has benefited from Bennett's home study program for hypertension is David Bleich, owner of a high-tech metals company. Three years ago Bleich went to his doctor for a routine examination and was told he had high blood pressure. Bleich was considerably overweight at the time. His doctor started him on Diazide (a diuretic). "Then every time I changed doctors [Bleich was a patient at a health maintenance clinic] the new one added another drug." Within two years, Bleich was taking three high blood pressure drugs—a diuretic, Lopressor (a beta blocker), and Clonidine (a centrally acting alpha blocker).

"Before I started the pills, I was running eight, nine miles a day. Now I could barely walk. I was falling into bed after dinner—I had no interest in sex. My business slowed down; I lost my competitive edge."

Learning about Innerhealth from a business acquaintance whose company sent its executives there, Bleich made an appointment. Enrolling at the center, he was given a complete workup (blood tests, EKG, treadmill stress test, etc.) and then conferred with Dr. Bennett. "I told him my symptoms—the tiredness, all the rest. He looked at me, 'Do you want to spend the rest of your life living like this?' I saw a copy of his book on his desk, and bought it. I read it two, three times." Bleich then embarked on the twelve-week program described in Bennett's book. Following the vegetarian diet that Bennett recommends, he soon felt energetic enough to resume exercising three hours a day. Convinced that the diuretic wasn't doing him any good, "I stopped taking Diazide but let Dr. Bennett wean me off Lopressor and Clonidine." (In his book, Bennett strongly advises readers *not* to stop taking their blood pressure pills without their doctor's supervision.)

Today, Bleich thrives on his largely vegetarian diet. "I eat lots of fish, vegetables, brown rice, fruit. I've lost thirty pounds. My blood pressure stays around 120/65 (considerably below "normal"). Last Sunday I ran ten miles in one and a half hours. My sex life is fine—business is good. I would never go back to living that way with pills again."

Julian M. Whitaker, M.D.   Dr. Julian M. Whitaker, medical director of the Whitaker Wellness Institute, Inc., in Newport Beach, California, and the Whitaker Wellness Institute, Inc., in Newport Beach, California, and author of *Reversing Heart Disease* (New York: Warner Books, 1985) offers another variation on the Pritikin theme. The institute's low-fat, high-carbohydrate vegetarian diet is classic Pritikin. This diet is ideal for hypertension, Whitaker says. It's extremely low in salt (2 to 4 grams per day) and high in potassium, a ratio that lowers blood pressure. Restricting dietary fat and eliminating all animal products also has a pressure-lowering effect.

But on the issue of nutritional supplements, which Pritikin said were unnecessary if one followed his diet, Whitaker parts company with his mentor. He prescribes for all his patients substantial amounts of vitamins C, B6, and other nontoxic water-soluble vitamins, and smaller amounts of the fat-soluble vitamins E, A, and D, which have a higher potential for toxicity. One of the minerals he gives is magnesium (500 milligrams daily by mouth). Other minerals are calcium and potassium, in the form of potassium salt substitutes, and certain amino acids, such as tyrosine. All these nutrients are provided in a single high-potency multivitamin. For information about this "therapeutic supplement" and how to obtain it, write to Whitaker Wellness Institute, Inc., 4400 MacArthur Blvd., Suite 630, Newport Beach, California 92660.

In addition to the multivitamin, patients at the institute take a fish oil supplement (MaxEpa) and Coenzyme Q10 "to increase overall health." (More about these two nutrients in chapter 3.)

Whitaker, 44, was trained as a surgeon, but after meeting a doctor (a supporter of Pritikin's) who treated patients with nutrition and exercise, began investigating this natural form of treatment. Since opening his institute in 1979, Whitaker has treated around 3,500 patients with diet and exercise. At any one time, 16 people, on the average, are enrolled in the program. Participants in the twelve-day program (a five-day program is also available) can expect a drop of 10 to 20 points in systolic blood pressure and a decrease of 5 to 10 points in diastolic pressure, Whitaker said, and "75 to 85 percent of high blood pressure patients are able to control their blood pressure without medication."

Matt, a 51-year-old pastry chef, recently consulted Whitaker. Matt, who weighed 287 pounds, loved to sample his wares; he also ate a lot of cheese and drank a quantity of whole milk. Laboratory findings showed that he was at high risk of having a heart attack. His blood pressure was 212/108 (approaching the crisis range); blood cholesterol level was 264 (normal is below 200); triglycerides were 519 (normal is below 160). His legs were swollen with edema and his feet were a dark reddish blue, indicating poor circulation, pooled blood, and inadequate oxygenation of the blood to the feet.

First Whitaker prescribed an extremely low-fat diet with additional fiber in the form of two apples a day. He also told Matt to drink a glass of fresh, unsalted vegetable juice each day, an excellent source of potassium and magnesium. Matt was given multiple vitamins and minerals, twelve capsules of fish oil daily, and daily injections of magnesium to lower his blood pressure as fast as possible.

Matt followed instructions and his condition improved rapidly. Over a period of nine days, his blood pressure dropped to 146/80. Both blood cholesterol levels and triglycerides also dropped dramatically. He lost eleven pounds, mostly the excess fluid that had caused swelling in his legs.

Six months later, he had lost fifty-five pounds and felt great. He takes a thermos of freshly squeezed juices—carrot, apple, or celery—to work. Yes, his job requires that he taste his pastry creations, but "I take very small bites."

The Pritikin Credo. As we've seen, each of these Pritikin disciples interprets the Pritikin program a little differently, but all agree on a few basic points.

- The doctor is primarily a teacher whose job is to educate patients about nutrition and other life-style matters.

- Antihypertensive drugs can artificially lower high blood pressure, but they cannot improve or cure the condition. All these drugs have harmful side effects, which range from unpleasant to life-threatening.

- The best way to lower blood pressure is by natural methods such as diet, exercise, and stress management. A healthy diet is a starch-based vegetarian diet that is low in fats, salt, and sugar. Aerobic exercise, which burns up oxygen, should be done on a regular basis. Ways to cope with chronic stress included imagery, relaxation techniques, and psychological counseling.

The Atkins Diet

In my experience, most physicians who practice nutritional medicine recommend the Pritikin, starch-based diet for hypertension. A notable exception is Robert C. Atkins, M.D., whose well-known Atkins diet, introduced in 1972, is low in starch (complex carbohydrates). The diet that Atkins recommends as a weight-loss diet for hypertensives consists of animal foods (meat, fish, fowl, shellfish), eggs, cheese, salad vegetables, and other selected vegetables. Items not permitted on the Atkins diet include bread, flour, fruits, skimmed milk, yogurt, and canned soups. Following this low-carbohydrate diet, people quickly lose weight as well as excess fluids, he says.[28]

For hypertensives who don't need to lose weight, Atkins recommends a low-sugar (meat and millet) diet, which primarily restricts sweets of any kind. In his latest book, *Dr. Atkins' Health Revolution* (Boston: Houghton Mifflin Co., 1988) he emphasizes nutritional supplements rather than diet in his program for hypertensives. Supplements that Atkins prescribes for all patients with high blood pressure include fish oil, evening primrose oil, taurine (a sulfur-containing amino acid), magnesium, calcium, potassium, and Co-enzyme Q10.

Diet and Megadoses

Eric R. Braverman, M.D., director of the Princeton Total Health Center in Skillman, New Jersey, treats hypertensives with a two-part program of diet and nutrients. The first part he describes as "the best of Pritikin and Atkins." The second part, which involves nutrients, reflects Braverman's expertise as an orthomolecular physician—using megadoses of nutrients to treat disease. Braverman, at 30, qualifies as a genuine *wunderkind;* he's author of dozens of scientific articles on what he calls "biochemicals of the brain" and coauthor of *The Healing Nutrients Within* (New Canaan, Conn.: Keats Publishing, 1987).

To lower your blood pressure, Braverman says, first stop smoking: "Tobacco smoke contains harmful cadmium that can harden arteries and damage your heart. Next, eliminate caffeine. Drinking two cups of coffee a day can raise your blood pressure 5 or 10 points. But the key factor in lowering blood pressure is weight loss. Anyone who wants to control his blood pressure and increase his life span must lose weight. If you lose thirty pounds you can expect to lower your blood pressure at least 4 points."

The best way to lose weight initially, Braverman says, is to eat a low-carbohydrate diet, but *not* the Pritikin diet, which is around 85 percent complex carbohydrates (vegetables, starches, and fruit). "Carbohydrates cause fluid retention. High protein, on the other hand, acts as a diuretic—it removes fluids. So if you eat plenty of protein, you don't need a diuretic."

The diet that Braverman recommends as a starter to his hypertensive patients, most of whom are overweight, consists of fish, fresh vegetables (not the starchy variety such as potatoes, corn, peas, and carrots), a small amount of cheese, and salads.

> Fish (not shellfish) has a tremendous blood pressure–lowering effect, as do vegetables. This high-protein diet that restricts salt and fried foods I call Plan A. Once a person has lost weight, then he switches to Plan B—your standard complex carbohydrate Pritikin-type diet, which is fish, chicken, whole grains (such as brown rice), salads, vegetables, and fruit. I advise my patients to increase their intake of polyunsaturated oils, such as safflower and sunflower, as well as monounsaturated oils, and eliminate saturated fats, such as butter. (Polyunsaturated oils have a diuretic effect and lower cholesterol.)
>
> I appreciate the merits of a complex carbohydrate (starch-based) diet, but this diet doesn't work for everybody. Even though I restrict the Plan B diet to 1,500 to 1,800 calories, many obese hypertensives have biochemical imbalances and once they follow a diet high in complex carbohydrates gain weight. In this case, I design a tailormade diet.

Part two of Braverman's program for hypertension consists of mega-doses of nutrients to treat biochemicals of the brain.

High on Braverman's list of essential nutrients is fish oil, which contains a fatty acid called omega-3. "I've used fish oil in over two thousand cases in which hypertensives had elevated triglycerides and low HDL levels, factors which greatly increase the risk of an individual having a stroke or heart attack. In five years using fish oil, I haven't had a single patient who suffered such an event." Dosage of fish oil supplements depends on the individual. "A patient with extremely elevated triglycerides and reduced HDL might need twelve to fifteen capsules of fish oil a day."

But to effectively lower blood pressure, fish oil must be part of a total program of nutrients. Nutrients Braverman finds particularly beneficial are linoleic acid (5 to 15 grams), magnesium (500 to 1,500 milligrams), vitamin B6 (200 to 1,000 milligrams), taurine (1 to 3 grams), and zinc (15 to 60 milligrams). Other nutrients that he gives for high blood pressure include Coenzyme Q10, calcium, and potassium (as a salt substitute or in fruit). Ginger, garlic, and onions also lower blood pressure and are valuable for their anticlotting properties.

Many of these nutrients are contained in a multivitamin and mineral supplement that Braverman devised for hypertension and heart problems. To obtain this product, write to Total Health Nutrients, P.O. Box 334, Skillman, NJ 08558.

Braverman claims excellent results treating hypertensive patients with this diet and nutrient program. "I can't think of a single patient who has come to me taking one or two drugs who was unable to control his blood pressure with diet and nutrients. Once the number of drugs exceeds two, it's harder to get rid of all medication, but it can be done."

Biofeedback—Learning to Be a Yogi

During the first half of this century, standard physiology textbooks taught that our biological processes are governed by two separate nervous systems. To stand, you control the skeletal muscles of the voluntary nervous system. The other system, the involuntary autonomic nervous system, governs functions over which we have no conscious control such as heart rate, blood pressure, and body temperature.

But biofeedback training, which was first reported in 1960,[29] blasted this concept that the mind and body are separate entities. Biofeedback practitioners showed that there is no such thing as an involuntary process, one that is "out of bounds" to the conscious mind. With proper training, ordinary people can perform some of the feats once thought to be the province of yogis—change their heart rate, lower their blood pressure, raise their body temperature, and more.

"Biofeedback," as its name implies, "is any instrumentation to give a person immediate and continuing signs of change in a bodily function of which he is usually unaware."[30]

In the 1950s, psychologist Elmer Green, Ph.D., at the Menninger Foundation in Topeka, Kansas, was training people to "self-regulate" various parts of the body. This training involved first quieting the mind using a relaxation technique called autonomic training (developed in the 1920s by a German psychiatrist, Johannes Schultz), then visualizing the physiological change the individual wished to effect. Green emphasized that the equipment was only a tool. "When a person watches a temperature feedback meter, it is not the movement of the needle that brings about self-regulation of blood flow." The movement merely reveals what works to the person.[31] Tapping into the unconscious mind, almost anything seemed possible. Persons afflicted with tension headaches and migraines, whose hands were icy cold, eliminated their pain by learning to warm their hands, as much as 25 degrees. (Warmth coupled with a feeling of heaviness indicates that the body is relaxed and ready to accept suggestion.[32]) A musician who played a woodwind instrument learned to relax the muscles of his face and throat and thus improve his performance. A middle-aged woman, paralyzed from the waist down and confined to a wheelchair for ten years, regained the ability to stand. A stroke patient was able to walk without her leg brace.[33]

Using this same self-regulating process, patients with high blood pressure learned to control it. One of the case histories that Green reports is a 38-year-old woman who had been on hypertensive medication for sixteen years but was still unable to control her blood pressure. In five months her blood pressure was normal and she was off all medication.[34] Learning to "un-stress," which is the art of the self-regulation process, has rewards beyond controlling one's blood pressure, Green says. "A Type A person [aggressive, impatient, hard driving, governed by a sense of urgency about time] often turns into a Type B [a calm, relaxed individual]." One of Green's hypertensive patients, a psychiatrist, who had taken antihypertensive medication for ten years, recognized this change in himself. "Instead of racing to make the light, I welcome pausing at a red light so I can practice my relaxation exercises. I've learned to smell the roses. I notice the trees, the sky; I'm taking a new pleasure in life."[35]

Another benefit of biofeedback training that Green points out is a sense of mastery, of being in control of one's body. I had a taste of this when I asked a psychiatrist who uses biofeedback in his practice if I could experience the technique. Reclining on a couch, a sensor strapped to my fingers, I was told to imagine I was warming my hands at a campfire. "Your hands are growing warmer and warmer—you can feel the warmth." As my hand temperature went up, he called out the numbers—"85 degrees, 88 degrees, 91 degrees." I felt as if I had superhuman control.

If you're taking medication for high blood pressure, can biofeedback training help you get off those drugs? Steven Fahrion and colleagues at the Menninger Foundation conducted a study of 77 hypertensive patients who were trained to warm their hands and feet, a standard self-regulation technique. Of the 54 patients taking antihypertensive drugs, 58 percent were able to eliminate their drugs while at the same time significantly reducing their blood pressure. An additional 35 percent were able to cut their dosage in half while reducing their blood pressure. The remaining 7 percent showed no improvement in either blood pressure or medication required.[36]

To locate a biofeedback practitioner in your area, contact Applied Psychophysiology and Biofeedback, 10200 West 44th Avenue, #304, Wheat Ridge, CO 80023, (303) 422–8436.

How do you judge the capabilities of a biofeedback practitioner? Fahrion advises, "Question the person about his own experiences with biofeedback. Ask, 'Can you control your own blood pressure?' It's a little like choosing a swimming coach; start with someone who swims well." Fahrion also pointed out that since learning to relax is a key element in biofeedback, it's important to choose someone with whom you feel comfortable. "That's more important than any degree."

Learning to Relax

If you've read some of the countless articles and books about stress, then you're familiar with the statement that it's not the stress of modern living that is killing us, but our *reaction* to stress. As Dr. Hans Seyle of Montreal, pioneer in stress research, discovered in the mid-1950s, we humans react to stress with an inborn response—the fight or flight response. This causes the heart to beat faster, raises blood pressure, tenses the muscles, and ultimately releases adrenaline and other hormones. It was a lifesaver for the caveman confronted with a saber-toothed tiger; but today, when danger takes the form of a near dented fender, a deadline, or a conversation with an irate spouse, we respond to these emotional stresses the same way the caveman reacted to physical stress. What is so injurious to our health is that we react in this inappropriate manner—our entire system on alert—numerous times a day. As Dr. L. John Mason, author of *Guide to Stress Reduction* (a helpful book on the subject) points out, "If a stress response is chronic, the constant presence of stress hormones begins to wear down the body's immunological systems. . . ."[37]

Back in the 1960s, Herbert Benson, M.D., then a Harvard University fellow in cardiology, was interested in studying the relationship between stress and hypertension.[38] Although people instinctively recognize that getting upset raises your blood pressure, no one had measured the effect of stress on blood pressure. He started with animal studies and showed that monkeys could be trained to control their blood pressure. At this time, he was approached by a group of people who practiced Transcendental Meditation (TM) and who claimed that meditation lowered their blood pressure. After first rejecting their proposal to test this reputed change, Benson finally agreed. After establishing their normal blood pressure, he measured them while they meditated and found that dramatic physiological changes occurred: heart rate and blood pressure decreased; rate of breathing and overall metabolism slowed down; there were changes in brain wave patterns. These findings led to Benson's developing his "relaxation response."

The relaxation response is a four-step procedure that involves (1) finding a quiet place, (2) relaxing the body's muscles, (3) focusing for ten to twenty minutes on a single word or prayer, and (4) ignoring disturbing thoughts. It is described in detail in Benson's *The Relaxation Response* and *Beyond the Relaxation Response*.

Today, the relaxation response is the cornerstone of the Behavioral Medicine Program for Hypertension offered at New England Deaconess Hospital in Boston. (The Behavioral Medicine section, under Benson's direction, also offers other programs for people with a variety of stress-related medical problems.) Participants who attend the hypertension program's group sessions learn how to practice the relaxation response and how to take their own blood pressure. They also receive instruction in nutrition and exercise and stress management techniques.

Over the past five years, more than 700 patients have taken part in this hypertension program. "A study of 100 patients who completed the program showed that 80 percent either reduced their blood pressure or their blood pressure medication."[39] Patients reported that their mental outlook was better—less anxiety and depression: "A major focus of the clinical program was to empower patients to participate in their own care," Benson says.[40]

A group of researchers led by Dr. Vincent DeQuattro at the University of Southern California School of Medicine has been studying the effects of Benson's relaxation response on hypertensive patients and has replicated many of Benson's results.[41]

Fortunately, the components of Benson's program for hypertension—relaxation, diet, and exercise—can all be safely practiced on your own. For up-to-date information about Benson's behavioral techniques, see his latest book, *Your Maximum Mind* (New York: Times Books, 1987).

You may want to investigate other relaxation techniques that have been shown to lower blood pressure. These include autogenic training, progressive relaxation, and self-hypnosis. To locate a licensed professional in your area who is trained in clinical hypnosis, contact the American Society of Clinical Hypnosis, 2250 East Devon Avenue, Des Plaines, IL 60018, (708) 297–3317. If you live in a good-sized city, there may be a hypnosis society in town. Look in the Yellow Pages under "[name of city] hypnosis society."

Dialogue—The Hidden Danger

A friend who's a Freudian-oriented social worker often complains that behavioral techniques "don't go deep enough." If you, too, feel that the high blood pressure therapies we've discussed overlook psychological factors, then you may welcome a treatment for hypertension that's the brainchild of Dr. James J. Lynch, M.D., professor of psychiatry at the University of Maryland School of Medicine and author of *Language of the Heart*.[42] As one might suspect, Lynch is concerned with human relationships and how these relationships affect our health.

Working with patients whose blood pressure was being continuously monitored, Lynch discovered that speech—communicating with others, not talking to oneself or a pet—elevates blood pressure. This rise in blood pressure occurs in everyone, but to a much greater degree in the hypertensive individual. One reason their blood pressure shoots up, often to an alarming degree, is the quality of their speech. People with high blood pressure speak rapidly, with a Type A intensity; they stop breathing when they talk and literally "run out of breath," Lynch says.

But there's a deeper reason for this dramatic increase in blood pressure, according to Lynch. Hypertensive people fear intimacy: despite a social manner, they perceive others as threatening and untrustworthy and therefore keep their distance from others. When forced to discuss emotionally provocative issues, their pressure rises. Lynch describes high blood pressure as a "revolt" on the part of the body—a form of "internal blushing." But unlike blushing, which one can't disguise, the rise in blood pressure is something the hypertensive is completely unaware of. Disassociated from their bodies, they view hypertension as a thing apart from themselves rather than something they are doing to themselves.

Shunning intimacy, avoiding close relationships, which intensifies their sense of loneliness, presents its own dangers. In an earlier book, *The Broken Heart* (New York: Basic Books, 1977) Lynch describes human loneliness as one of the major causes of premature death.

To eliminate the hypertensive's destructive way of speaking, Lynch and associates train their patients to speak slower and lower and to breathe deeply and frequently during conversation. Lynch recommends spending some time each day in quiet reflection or meditation. But Lynch's treatment for hypertension goes much deeper than behavioral training. In his eloquent and deeply moving book, he describes numerous patients who benefited from psychotherapy. By resolving the tensions in their lives that were causing the problem, they learned to control their blood pressure. Lynch's approach, which requires a skilled therapist, is certainly worth considering if you have heart disease or experience chronic pain that interferes with your life.

LOOKING AHEAD

Happily, standard hypertension treatment is moving in the direction that alternative physicians have charted over the past two decades. Mary Marrs, an R.N. in Indianapolis with thirty-five years in public health, recalled what hypertension treatment was like when she was a young nurse: "Drugs were a godsend. Before they were introduced, we didn't know how to help people with high blood pressure." Patients who had no symptoms, she said, naturally balked at taking drugs that made them feel sick, but "quality of life seemed a small price to pay for preventing stroke and heart attack."

Now we initiate treatment with nondrug measures, she said. "We identify a patient's risk factors—ask the patient, 'Which of these do you want to work on?' Often a patient will say, 'I've always wanted to stop smoking—or lose weight.'" Modifying risk factors takes one-on-one counseling—"It's expensive, but if you can prevent a stroke, or other complications, it's worth it.

"We've also changed our ideas about elderly people and high blood pressure. If people control their weight and lipids, exercise and don't smoke, blood pressure doesn't always go up with age."

3

How to Prevent Heart Disease

Heart disease (its proper name is ischemic heart disease) is the number one killer in America. Heart disease kills more people than all forms of cancer combined. This year more than 500,000 people will die of heart attack (myocardial infarction). A heart attack occurs when a blood clot forms in a coronary artery and blocks that artery. This blockage, or occlusion, prevents blood filled with oxygen from reaching the heart muscle and nourishing it. Heart attack is not limited to the elderly; 45 percent of all heart attacks occur in people under age 65. The cost of treating Americans with cardiovascular disease in 1989 will approach $88.2 billion.[1]

Prevention—the Way to Go.   The discouraging thing about heart disease is that by the time the diagnosis is made, it may be too late. As someone recently said to me, "My father's first heart attack was his last." Despite technological achievements and heart drugs, the first heart attack is often fatal.[2] Of the 1.5 million people who suffer heart attacks in the United States each year, only about 350,000 survive.[3] For this reason, "major progress in our battle against this number one killer must rest on finding preventive measures," say representatives of the National Institutes of Health.[4]

Though scientists don't know what causes heart disease, they have identified factors that put you at risk of developing it. One of the three major risk factors for heart disease is high blood pressure (see chapter 2); another is elevated levels of cholesterol in the blood; a third is cigarette smoking. Other less crucial risk factors are diabetes, overweight, lack of exercise, and family history of heart disease.

Modifying risk factors has shown results, says Thomas H. Ainsworth, M.D., author of *Live or Die*. But Ainsworth credits ordinary people, not doctors, for these results. "Beginning in the mid-1960s, on their own, many turned to healthier life-styles. Jogging became a national pastime, health food stores mushroomed, we switched from high-cholesterol animal fats to cholesterol-free vegetable fats. Soon, there was a striking decrease in deaths from coronary heart disease—a 22 percent decline from 1968 to 1977."[5]

Smoking and Your Heart.   Smoking is such an acknowledged threat to health that it may seem preachy to discuss the subject, but its role in heart disease is not as well known as in lung cancer. If you're trying to induce a family member or friend to quit smoking, or have been unable to quit yourself, these new findings about smoking and the heart may be helpful.

If you smoke cigarettes, you are at least twice as likely to develop coronary heart disease as a nonsmoker. One explanation for this is suggested by a recent study at the University of Southern California School of Medicine. Three researchers have shown that long-term smoking alters the production of two critical hormones that regulate blood clotting and the expansion of blood vessels. This change in hormone production may cause development of atherosclerosis (hardening of the arteries) and other cardiovascular diseases in chronic smokers, U.S. studies suggest.[6]

If you're an older person who has smoked most of your life, will quitting really benefit your heart? A Yale University School of Medicine study showed that while cigarette smokers had more than twice nonsmokers' risk of coronary heart disease, this risk declined for those who had quit smoking for as short a period as one year.[7]

If you already have coronary heart disease, stopping smoking can significantly extend your life span. In a University of Washington study, heart disease patients who quit smoking survived almost twice as long as patients who continued to smoke.[8]

MAINSTREAM APPROACHES TO PREVENTING HEART DISEASE

Cholesterol Mania

You can't escape the media blitz—every other product on supermarket shelves proclaims No Cholesterol! TV commercials abound in which one spouse assures the other that the cereal (spread, cooking oil) he/she is serving contains no cholesterol. Book and magazine writers advise on how to lower your cholesterol. Some egg companies, their sales cut in half over the past two decades, are claiming that their eggs are "lower in cholesterol."

Having the lowest cholesterol level has become a new form of one-upmanship at social gatherings.

How has the cholesterol question affected you? Have you given up eggs (or at least the yolks) to maintain or lower your cholesterol? Are you using margarine instead of butter for the same reason? If your husband (like mine) is fond of chicken livers or calves liver, have you renounced high-cholesterol organ meats for the sake of his heart? If your husband's cholesterol is high and diet hasn't lowered it, has your family doctor suggested that he consider taking a cholesterol-lowering drug? If your answers are mostly yes, you'll find plenty to consider in this chapter.

In the spring of 1989 when I began researching the cholesterol question, I had some vague concerns about cholesterol mania. I could remember those halcyon days when no one worried about cholesterol, nutritionists described the egg as the perfect protein, and margarine was merely the "lower priced spread." I was not prepared for what I discovered—hundreds and hundreds of medical articles protesting standard advice about cholesterol. Furthermore, this cholesterol controversy, which at that time had scarcely been mentioned in the popular press, had been simmering since the late 1960s.

Let me be up front about the cholesterol question: Based on my own research (which includes reading articles and books by a great many physicians and researchers trained in nutrition, and interviews with them) I am convinced that we have been given misleading and, in some cases, harmful information about diet and drug treatment to protect the heart. Undoubtedly, the government scientists who established cholesterol policy, specifically the National Cholesterol Education Program launched in December 1984, sincerely believe in the rightness of their cause. (One of the scientists who objects to this program calls them "misguided zealots.") But there is no question that the cholesterol program, which advises your doctor what to tell you about the subject, benefits three powerful groups in our society to the tune of literally billions of dollars. These three are the medical profession, the pharmaceutical industry, and the food companies.

Expressing such views about the cholesterol question sounded like heresy only a few months ago. But since then, the cholesterol controversy, confined for decades to medical journals, has erupted into full view. The catalyst was an article in *The Atlantic,* "The Cholesterol Myth" by Thomas J. Moore (September 1989), excerpted from Moore's book *Heart Failure* (New York: Random House, 1989). At about the same time, a Boston physician, Dr. Allan S. Brett, wrote a hard-hitting article that appeared in *The New England Journal of Medicine* (September 7, 1989), which was highly critical of the government's stance on cholesterol. By the time you read this, these lone voices questioning the cholesterol program may have swelled to a chorus—or been drowned out by the subsequent backlash.

My goal in exploring cholesterol is to help you "liberate yourself from the panic over cholesterol," as Dr. Edward R. Pinckney, coauthor of *The Choles-terol Controversy* (Los Angeles: Sherbourne Press, 1973) put it, and move on to more sensible, time-tested ways to avoid heart disease. These ways, namely a well-balanced diet and appropriate nutrients, are described fully in the section on alternative treatment.

But first, the basics: what exactly is cholesterol?

Cholesterol is a waxy, fatlike substance that is essential to life; it is used to form all cell membranes, certain hormones, and other vital substances. Most of the cholesterol in your blood is manufactured in your body, primarily by the liver. About 93 percent of this cholesterol is contained in the cells of the body and only 7 percent circulates in the blood. Heart specialists are con-cerned about this circulating blood cholesterol, not the 93 percent in the cells.

Experts estimate that those eating the high-fat American diet consume 400 to 500 milligrams of cholesterol each day. This cholesterol is found in foods of animal origin such as meat, eggs, whole milk, cream, butter, and cheese. Organ meats and egg yolks are particularly high in cholesterol. Shellfish, once a no-no, are now considered no worse than chicken. Foods derived from plants do not contain cholesterol.

There are two kinds of cholesterol: the kind we eat in food, called dietary cholesterol, and that made by the body, called serum or plasma cholesterol. Both types, dietary cholesterol and serum cholesterol, are chemically alike and end up in the blood.

Serum cholesterol is one of a number of fats in the blood called lipids. Once in the body, cholesterol is attached to certain proteins and lipids in order to be transported through the bloodstream. These packages made of fats, proteins, and cholesterol are called lipoproteins. They come in two major types: low-density lipoprotein (LDL) and high-density lipoprotein (HDL). Most printouts of blood tests that describe your cholesterol will contain readings for LDL and HDL. LDL is not measured in the lab but is calculated according to a formula based on total cholesterol and HDL.

Low-density lipoprotein (LDL) is considered "bad" because it deposits cholesterol on artery walls, promoting hardening of the arteries. High-density lipoprotein (HDL) is "good" because it carries LDL cholesterol away from artery walls to the liver for disposal, thus preventing its buildup in the arteries.

There's a third type of lipoprotein called very-low-density lipoprotein (VLDL). VLDL transports fats or oils called triglycerides. (Blood chemistry printouts often include triglyceride results.) Too much of these fats increases the risk of heart attack or stroke.

How to interpret the results of cholesterol testing is still being debated. The 1988 report from the National Cholesterol Education Program uses LDL levels as criteria to determine whether treatment is required and, if so, what treatment. But a growing number of studies point to the ratio of total cholesterol to HDL as a better indicator of coronary heart disease risk than LDL levels. Dr. William P. Castelli, medical director of the Framingham heart study, says that "the ideal ratio is probably less than 3.5, but 4.5 is recommended for starters."[9]

Why the Concern about Cholesterol?

Experts say that too much cholesterol circulating in the blood produces thickening and hardening of the arteries, a condition called atherosclerosis. Exactly how atherosclerosis begins or what causes it is still being debated. Until recently, the accepted theory was that fat deposits called plaques line the walls of arteries (blood vessels) and eventually clog the artery, impeding the blood flow through the artery. Blockage of an artery supplying the heart muscle (coronary artery) results in a heart attack. Blockage of an artery leading to the brain causes a stroke. Blockage in an artery leading to the legs leads to difficulty walking (intermittent claudification). Trouble can occur in any part of the body where a blood vessel is blocked.

A newer theory of what causes atherosclerosis is that the process begins with an injury to the wall of the artery. The body then attempts to repair the damage by depositing cholesterol in the artery, like filling in cracks with putty.

Atherosclerosis is a slow, progressive disease that may start in childhood. Autopsies of healthy American soldiers killed in action in Korea showed that three-quarters of them had signs of hardening of the arteries that ranged from thickening of the coronary artery to large deposits of plaque that blocked off blood flow of one or more of the major vessels.[10] Children as young as three years of age have been found to have fatty streaks in the heart's main artery, the aorta.

Studies on Humans.   In the 1950s, scientists began investigating why heart disease was such a threat in our westernized industrial society while relatively uncommon in other cultures. One of these researchers, Dr. Ancel Keyes, along with coworkers from the University of Minnesota, studied a large group of middle-aged men in seven developed countries. They found that Finnish people, who had the highest death rate from coronary heart disease, ate the greatest amount of saturated animal fats and had the highest blood cholesterol levels. (The United States was not far behind.) But in Japan, where people then consumed an exceedingly small amount of saturated fat and cholesterol, their cholesterol levels were very low and deaths from heart disease were uncommon. The difference between Japanese and Americans was not genetic. Japanese who emigrated to the United States developed cholesterol levels similar to native-born Americans and also had a high rate of heart disease.

Other studies of people in underdeveloped countries where cholesterol intake was low appeared to lead to the same conclusion: people who eat a diet high in saturated fats and cholesterol have elevated blood cholesterol levels and a high rate of coronary heart disease.

Not all primitive cultures conform to the lipid theory, which says that consuming large amounts of animal fats and cholesterol raises blood cholesterol, leading to heart disease. The Eskimo, whose traditional diet consists largely of fish and seal and whale blubber, appears to be protected from heart disease. Another exception is the Masai people of East Africa, who are sheep herders and eat mostly milk, blood, and meat. Although the diet is two-thirds saturated animal fat, the Masai have little heart disease.

Studies on Animals.   Animal studies, according to NIH scientists, "offer strong and persuasive evidence" that high blood cholesterol is linked to atherosclerosis. A Russian researcher, N. Anitschkov, first produced atherosclerosis in rabbits in 1913 by feeding them cholesterol. At autopsy he showed that the rabbits had developed yellow, waxlike plaques in their arteries. Since then, researchers have produced hardening of the arteries in monkeys and other species by raising the animals' blood cholesterol.[11] Efforts to raise serum cholesterol levels of human beings by feeding them cholesterol were not successful, however.[12]

Concerning these studies, it should be noted that the type of cholesterol used was a synthetic form easily oxidized when exposed to air; oxidized products are highly toxic and can cause atherosclerosis. In the normal human diet, oxidation of cholesterol is less likely to occur because foods high in cholesterol also contain vitamins and other antioxidants designed to protect the body from harmful oxidation.[13]

How Cholesterol Became a Household Word

Starting in the 1960s, the American Heart Association (AHA) began urging Americans to lower blood cholesterol levels by following a low-fat diet called the Prudent Diet. The public responded with no enthusiasm. Part of the problem, government officials decided, was the attitude of the doctors. As late as 1985, physicians remained unconvinced that cholesterol ranked with hypertension and smoking as a risk factor for coronary heart disease.[14]

What was needed to convince doctors of the danger of cholesterol in the diet was incontrovertible evidence that lowering blood cholesterol levels would reduce the incidence of heart disease. Thus far, this connection had eluded investigators. Nineteen trials conducted over a period of thirty-one years had failed to show that low-fat, low-cholesterol diets would prevent coronary heart attack.[15] But in 1984 the results of a federally sponsored ten-year study appeared to provide such evidence. This $150 million study, called the Lipid Research Clinics Coronary Primary Prevention Trial (I'll call it the LRC study), involved 3,806 middle-aged men, all of whom had abnormally high cholesterol levels. Half of the men followed a low-cholesterol diet and were given a cholesterol-lowering drug (cholestyramine). The control group followed the same low-cholesterol diet but were given a placebo. Those who stuck with the diet and drug program over an eight-year period lowered their cholesterol levels 19 percent. Subjects treated with diet alone experienced only a modest decrease in cholesterol levels.[16]

Critics have charged that investigators made results look more favorable than they were by exaggerating "statistically insignificant" data.[17] For example, if they had looked at absolute or actual risk, results of the LRC trial would have shown that "more than seven years of treatment had reduced the chances of experiencing a heart attack from eight percent to seven percent."[18]

The most disturbing result of the multimillion-dollar study was that the drug-treated group had "a greater number of violent and accidental deaths" than the control group.[19] These deaths, which resulted from gastrointestinal cancers and other gastrointestinal diseases, were described by the investigators as "a chance occurrence," and ignored by the media.

Cholestyramine isn't the only cholesterol-lowering drug that has been shown to cause cancer or other life-threatening diseases. In the Honolulu Heart Program, a low-fat diet was associated with a higher number of deaths from other causes, particularly cancer and stroke.[20] A World Health Organization study, which was done in three European countries at the same time as the American LRC study, showed the same finding: at the end of five years, the investigator reported increased deaths among those who were treated with the cholesterol-lowering drug clofibrate. (Among the ailments that clofibrate caused were gallstones and cancer that affected the liver and digestive system.)[21]

Media reports of the LRC study gave no hint that cholesterol levels in the treated group were lowered an insignificant amount (6.77 percent) and that "a cholesterol-lowering drug seems to have killed more than it saved." Headlines across the country trumpeted "Lowering cholesterol levels in the blood helps to prevent heart attacks."[22] Despite the questionable data, federal health officials interpreted findings of the LRC study as a mandate to take action. In December 1984, at a Consensus Development Conference on Lowering Blood Cholesterol to Prevent Heart Disease held by the National Heart, Lung, and Blood Institute (NHLBI) and a division of the National Institutes of Health, an expert panel concluded that high blood cholesterol is a major cause of coronary artery disease, that lowering elevated blood cholesterol levels (specifically LDL cholesterol) will reduce the risk of heart attacks, and that dietary changes will reduce blood cholesterol levels. This became known as the Lipid Theory.[23]

Although participants in the major clinical trials were middle-aged men with high cholesterol levels, the cholesterol-lowering program was aimed at the general population. The experts recommended that all Americans (except children younger than 2 years of age) reduce total dietary fat intake to 30 percent of total calories, reduce saturated fat intake to less than 10 percent of total calories, increase polyunsaturated fat intake but to no more than 10 percent of total calories, and reduce daily cholesterol intake to 250 to 300 milligrams or less.

The Other Side of the Cholesterol Controversy

In the course of my research on cholesterol, I discovered that a great many experts vehemently opposed the government's National Cholesterol Education Program. Many contended that the dietary recommendations issued by the government's expert panel were not based on scientific evidence and therefore should not be aimed at the general population. Here are some statements by critics of the government's cholesterol-lowering program:

"For the majority of Americans, cholesterol reduction does not appear to make a major contribution to improving life expectancy."—William C. Taylor, M.D., Beth Israel Hospital, Boston, and colleagues. But for those at greater risk of heart attack, cholesterol levels assume an important role in prolonging life.[24]

"In the U.S. about one-half of heart attacks apparently occur in individuals with serum cholesterol levels below 240 mg/dl" (240 mg/dl and above is "high")—D. Mark Hegsted, professor emeritus of nutrition, Harvard Schools of Medicine and Public Health. Hegsted makes the point that screening for serum cholesterol is unlikely to be satisfactory since an individual's cholesterol level varies from time to time.[25]

"For two thirds of people, lowering dietary cholesterol will not affect cholesterol levels."—Donald J. McNamara, Ph.D., professor of nutrition and food science, University of Arizona. The reason that eating an egg has little effect on your cholesterol levels, he says, is because most people have a built-in feedback system that maintains plasma cholesterol levels, irrespective of dietary changes.[26]

"One study showed that the most severe lesions at autopsy occurred in people who had had quite low serum cholesterol values."—H. Kaunitz, Columbia University. Kaunitz suggests that elevated serum cholesterol is "symptomatic of some disease process, not a causative agent."[27]

"The largest part of the general population (perhaps . . . two-thirds) have the least to gain by lowering cholesterol levels."—E. H. Ahrens, Jr.,

Rockefeller University. Ahrens maintains that there's no scientific evidence to show that the "prudent diet" recommended by the American Heart Association will reduce the risk of coronary heart disease.[28]

"Diet does not have a profound influence on plasma cholesterol concentrations in Western populations."—Maria C. Linder, Ph.D., California State University, Fullerton. Restricting cholesterol and saturated fat intake reduces serum cholesterol only 10 to 20 percent. This reduction has been shown to have little effect on risk of heart disease or dying from the disease, Linder says.[29]

What alarms me most about the government's cholesterol program (testing the cholesterol of every adult 20 years of age and over and then giving treatment based on laboratory results) is how easily a healthy person can be diagnosed as having a dangerous condition that needs therapy under a doctor's supervision. Therapy, in an estimated one out of five cases, is a cholesterol-lowering drug; the latest of these drugs is lovastatin, which was introduced in 1987. It's too early to assess the drug's long-term benefits and risks.

Although the editor of a prestigious medical journal, along with other experts, warned that "an intensive trial of dietary intervention is indicated before treatment with lovastatin or other drugs,"[30] doctors appear to be paying more attention to pharmaceutical advertising that "stretches the truth to its limits."[31] Sales of cholesterol-lowering drugs of $202 million in 1987 climbed to $304 million in 1988, an annual growth of about 50 percent. Predicted sales in 1992 are $1.54 billion.[32]

Aspirin and Heart Disease

Since the average doctor is uneasy dealing with a "soft" subject like diet, I imagine there was widespread rejoicing in the medical community at the news, in January 1988, that aspirin could help prevent heart disease. As reported by a research group at Harvard Medical School and Brigham and Women's Hospital in Boston, using aspirin reduced the risk of heart attacks by 47 percent among healthy men. This conclusion was based on results from the Physicians' Health Study, which involved more than 22,000 U.S. physicians 40 to 84 years of age. (One half the group took one aspirin tablet every other day.) In Britain, however, research produced a different conclusion. A study involving 5,000 British doctors "found no strong evidence that regular use of aspirin reduces the risk of heart attack. . . ."[33]

If you, too, question the wisdom of taking a drug ostensibly to prevent developing a serious disease, you'll be interested in a recent study from the University of Southern California. There researchers studying a large group of elderly people who had never had a heart attack concluded that taking aspirin daily increases the risk of kidney cancer and heart disease.[34]

STANDARD TREATMENT FOR HEART DISEASE

Coronary Artery Bypass Surgery

If you learn nothing more from these heart chapters except that a safe and effective alternative to coronary artery bypass surgery exists, you'll be getting your money's worth. (The alternative described in chapter 4 is called chelation therapy.) But in order to appreciate the remarkable benefits of chelation, you need to know a little about the bypass.

The coronary bypass involves bypassing blocked coronary arteries with a graft—either a vein removed from the patient's leg or an internal mammary artery taken from the chest wall.

The coronary bypass is beneficial for patients who have extensive heart disease, known as triple-vessel disease, in which more than two thirds of each artery is blocked.[35] Patients with this life-threatening condition constitute a small proportion of heart disease patients (less than 10 percent). Unless you fall into that 10 percent, *you will do just as well being treated with a cardiac drug as undergoing the trauma of bypass surgery.* That's the finding that emerged from three major long-term studies. One of these, published in 1984, was a multihospital study that followed patients for as long as seven years.[36]

Wouldn't you think that such negative findings would put the bypass out of business? Quite the contrary: the number of bypass operations performed each year escalated from 170,000 in 1982 to 230,000 in 1985 to 332,000 in 1987.[37]

Like any surgical procedure, the bypass presents risks. Depending on the hospital, the death rate ranges from 3 percent or less to as high as 23 percent. The death rate for Medicare patients undergoing bypass in 1984 was 5.47 percent. You may have observed, as I have, that friends who undergo the bypass don't seem as quick as before, have trouble remembering things, and are frequently depressed. These observations have now been corroborated by European researchers who have found that bypass surgery "produces subtle, long-lasting impairment of mental performance in nearly one in five people who undergo the operation." These scientists also find that "up to 20 percent of bypass patients are depressed one year after their operations and that their mood change stemmed from damage sustained in surgery."[38]

Despite the risks of coronary bypass surgery and its limited benefits, a great many doctors perform the operation on patients who don't need it. Doctors and scientists from the University of California and the Rand Corporation found that 14 percent of bypass surgery was clearly not needed, and 30 percent was questionable.[39]

What induces cardiac surgeons and physicians who refer patients to surgeons to ignore the results of published scientific studies? The profit motive undoubtedly figures in these decisions. A surgeon earns $25,000 to $40,000 per bypass operation with hospitals getting a large slice of the pie. Cardiovascular surgeons generated the highest annual revenues per physician for hospitals in 1986—nearly $1 million per year.[40] Insurance companies are questioning the cost of a bypass, with good reason; today the nation spends more than $5 billion a year on bypass operations for more than 200,000 people.[41]

Mindful that other operations have come and gone, the late Robert Mendelsohn took a philosophic view of the coronary bypass. In December, 1979, he wrote, "The First Stage . . . wild and uncritical enthusiasm—now has been tempered by the Second Stage—doubt, skepticism and criticism. . . ." As yet we haven't reached what Mendelsohn prophesied would be "the Third and Final Stage—outright rejection." To explain the delay, Mendelsohn quoted a remark that Dr. Richard Ross, dean of Johns Hopkins University Medical School, made to a Senate Health subcommittee: "We are dealing with a multimillion-dollar enterprise that is very hard to turn off."[42]

Balloon Angioplasty

Spearing a shrimp at a party, Ray, who's in his late 50s, told me that he had had a "balloon treatment" earlier that week. The treatment Ray refers to is balloon angioplasty—a procedure in which a tiny balloon is threaded through an artery and then expanded to clear clogged arteries. Ray apparently has limited coronary disease, which makes him an ideal candidate for the procedure. "They did it under local; I was out in two days," he said happily.

In Ray's case, the angioplasty was performed as preventive treatment— to widen arteries and thus improve blood flow to the heart. But angioplasty, introduced in the late 1970s, has also been used as emergency treatment immediately following a heart attack. Until recently, standard treatment for a heart attack victim was to give a clot-dissolving drug, then use angioplasty to clear away any remaining blockages. Cardiologists "assumed" that angioplasty was necessary—an assumption that was blasted by a 1989 Health study, which found that it was not only unnecessary but did not benefit the patient.[43]

Introduced in the late 1970s as an alternative to the bypass, this procedure with the playful-sounding name has become almost as popular as the coronary bypass. In 1986, 133,000 angioplasties were performed, compared to 32,000 in 1983. The predicted number for 1988 was 200,000.[44]

But the rush to use the procedure on the part of cardiologists (who formerly had to refer patients to surgeons for bypass surgery) raised concerns that it was being overused, that its benefits were unproven, that hospitals were ill equipped to handle it, and that doctors were inadequately trained to perform it. (It's a tricky procedure, experts say.) These concerns were reflected in guidelines issued in August 1988 by the American Heart Association and American College of Cardiology advising doctors not to be too quick to perform the procedure.

The angioplasty has risks: "A coronary artery may be torn during the procedure, or a clot can form in the dilated area. . . ."[45] When performed by the most experienced cardiologists, "about 1 percent of angioplasty patients die, 4.3 percent suffer a heart attack and 3.4 percent require emergency surgery." In one third of patients who undergo angioplasty, the blocked coronary vessels that are reopened will close within a few months and need to be cleared again.[46]

A new tool that is used in conjunction with balloon angioplasty is the laser: the procedure called laser recanalization (LR) wipes out blockages in leg arteries. LR involves threading a tiny fiber-optic catheter through the artery of the leg; the catheter carries a laser beam that burns a tiny hole through fatty deposits in the artery. In most cases, a surgeon uses the tiny hole created by the laser to enlarge the opening with balloon angioplasty, but the opening may be large enough to allow adequate blood flow without further treatment.

Since most patients with peripheral vascular disease (blocked arteries in the legs) are elderly and not good candidates for surgery, the laser has the advantage of being a nonsurgical procedure. But according to the authors of a 1989 study, only 10 to 15 percent of patients with blocked arteries in the legs are suitable for the laser procedure.[47]

As described in chapter 4, chelation therapy is also an alternative to balloon angioplasty.

Cardiac Drugs

In the 1970s, coronary bypass surgery was the "in" operation according to an ABC-TV report. In the 1980s, balloon angioplasty emerged as an option. Today, as these two surgical procedures come under increasing attack, the number of heart drugs is increasing. Front-runners are two new classes of drugs: cholesterol-lowering drugs as preventive treatment and clot-dissolving agents for emergency use when a heart attack occurs.

Cholesterol-Lowering Drugs. The NIH program launched in December 1984 and culminating in the National Cholesterol Education Program served to identify those individuals with high cholesterol and specified how to treat them. ("Drug treatment should be considered for an adult patient who, despite dietary therapy, has an LDL cholesterol level of 190 mg/dl or higher."[48]) The pharmaceutical industry had not had such a windfall since the national effort to control high blood pressure. Like high blood pressure medication, "drug therapy [to lower cholesterol] is likely to continue for many years, or for a lifetime. . . ."[49]

One type of cholesterol-lowering drug is the bile acid-binding resins, including Bristol Laboratories' cholestyramine and Upjohn's colestipol. Cholestyramine was the drug used in the LRC study that triggered the NIH cholesterol program. Colestipol figured in a 1987 study which showed that diet and two cholesterol-lowering agents (colestipol and niacin) could cause regression of atherosclerotic plaque.[50]

Bile acid-binding resins are unpleasant to take; the drug, in the form of a gritty powder that is mixed with a liquid, must be taken three times a day. To increase "patient compliance," Warner-Lambert has introduced Cholybar—a flavored chewable bar containing cholestyramine. The drug in any form causes constipation, among other adverse effects.

A newer type of cholesterol-lowering drug is the HMG-CoA reductase inhibitor. Thus far, the only drug of this type on the market is Merck's lovastatin (mevinolin), which is easier to take than the older drugs because it's a tablet, not a powder. Although adverse effects—headache, diarrhea, gas, and constipation—affect no more than 10 percent of patients, according to Maria C. Linder, editor and principal author of *Nutritional Biochemistry and Metabolism,* "A patient on a cholesterol-lowering drug should be checked for liver damage every two or three months."

This isn't the first time that doctors have turned to cholesterol-lowering drugs as a means of preventing or treating atherosclerosis. In the early 1960s, as Dr. Edward C. Lambert, author of *Modern Medical Mistakes,* tells the story, doctors recognized that patients who died prematurely of heart attacks usually had increased amounts of cholesterol in their blood. These doctors were aware that a diet low in animal fats would reduce blood cholesterol levels, but knowing how difficult it is to get people to change their eating habits, searched for an effective drug to do the job. The drug they hit on was triparanol, produced by the William S. Merrell Company (no longer in existence). After animal studies and one controlled clinical trial had been done, the drug was approved by the FDA for prescription use. "Hundreds of thousands of patients received it, many of them with no apparent disease other than elevation of the blood cholesterol."[51] In the ensuing years, one thousand people developed cataracts as a result of taking the drug. After further investigation revealed that the drug had little value in preventing or reducing atherosclerosis, triparanol was taken off the market.

Clot-Dissolving Drugs. A new class of clot-dissolving drugs can stop a heart attack and lessen damage to the heart in the majority of patients. These drugs accomplish this lifesaving feat by dissolving blood clots that form within blocked arteries to cause heart attacks.

One of these drugs is tissue plasminogen activator, or TPA, which costs

$2,250 per treatment. An older clot-dissolving drug is streptokinase, which costs $76 per dose. In the United States, the more expensive drug has edged out the cheaper alternative, but this may change; a large-scale Italian study, reported on March 8, 1990, found that TPA is no more effective than streptokinase.[52]

Making the Situation Worse. Another type of cardiac drug—the antiarrhythmic—appears to be on its way out. Antiarrhythmic drugs are used to control irregular heartbeat. Since the early 1970s, "scattered reports concerning the incidence of adverse reactions with most antiarrhythmic drugs . . . have appeared in the medical literature."[53] "Scattered reports" sounds innocuous until you look at these reports, described in chilling detail in a 1981 article. One of the common adverse effects of antiarrhythmic drugs is "worsening ventricular arrhythmias" (irregular heartbeats)—the reason the drug was prescribed in the first place. Other adverse effects are dizziness, diarrhea, visual disturbances, convulsions, and coma.[54] A 1986 study conducted at the University of Virginia School of Medicine confirms that adverse reactions to antiarrhythmic drugs occur frequently. The authors of the study conclude that *only patients with life-threatening symptoms of irregular heartbeat should be treated with an antiarrhythmic drug.*[55]

More recently a National Heart, Lung, and Blood Institute clinical trial reported that two of the drugs used to treat heart rhythm irregularities in more than 200,000 Americans have been shown to increase the risk of heart attack and death. These two drugs are Riker Laboratories' Tambocor and Bristol Laboratories' Enkaid. Bristol Laboratories has since issued a "Dear Doctor" letter dated April 25, 1989, advising them to stop prescribing Enkaid for mild or moderate heart rhythm irregularities.

As reported on the ABC television show "20/20," the FDA over the years had sent letters to Riker Laboratories protesting misleading Tambocor advertisements. (The company failed to specify that the drug was only intended for life-threatening situations.) Although the FDA was apparently aware of the drug's lethal effects, the agency took no action.

ALTERNATIVE TREATMENT FOR HEART DISEASE

Your doctor has told you that you have hardening of the arteries, or arteriosclerosis. Arteriosclerosis occurs when fatty deposits in your blood vessels harden, making the arteries increasingly narrow. Both effects—the fatty deposits and their hardening—restrict the flow of blood through the arteries. Your symptoms depend on what part of your body is being deprived of blood.

If you have angina (chest pain) that occurs after physical exertion or emotional stress, your coronary arteries are not supplying your heart with enough oxygen. This condition is called coronary artery disease. Your doctor has most likely made the diagnosis after seeing the results of an electrocardiogram (EKG).

If you have cramping or pain in your legs while walking or during some other form of exercise, the blood vessels in your legs are most likely restricting blood flow to your feet. If nothing is done to improve circulation, you can eventually develop gangrene in one or more extremity.

If you've had a mild stroke that caused slurred speech and dizziness for a day or two, then the carotid artery in the front of your neck may be blocked.

If you've experienced a sudden weakness accompanied by numbness down one side of your body, or distorted vision for a short period of time, this "transient ischemic attack" indicates blockage of blood vessels to the brain. Recurring ischemic attacks often precede a stroke.

That's the bad news. The good news is that chelation (key-LAY-shun) therapy can reverse arteriosclerosis in most patients. Chelation therapy is a series of infusions of a synthetic amino acid called EDTA, which restores circulation to arteries blocked by plaque. In the past forty years, an estimated 400,000 Americans have been treated with chelation therapy with excellent results. No deaths have been attributed to chelation therapy. If you've never heard of chelation, that's not surprising. Reading chapter 4, you'll discover why chelation therapy is the best-kept secret in medicine.

Diet and Your Heart

To understand the alternative approach to protecting the heart through diet, it's helpful to see how it differs from the standard "optimal preventive diet for coronary heart disease" issued by the American Heart Association (AHA).

The AHA's 1988 *Dietary Guidelines for American Healthy Adults* emphasizes reducing total fats (to less than 30 percent of calories) and, in particular, saturated fats (to less than 10 percent of calories). Use of polyunsaturated and monounsaturated fats (both derived from vegetables) is encouraged, although polyunsaturated fat intake is limited to 10 percent of calories. Cholesterol and salt are restricted.

The 1988 AHA diet is similar in many ways to the "prudent diet" that the AMA began recommending in the 1960s. The goal then, as now, was to limit the amount of cholesterol and other fatty substances in the blood. Today saturated fats are considered more harmful than cholesterol in the diet, but cholesterol is still limited to 300 milligrams per day. In view of the fact that an egg yolk contains about 213 milligrams of cholesterol, the AHA diet continues to restrict eggs (no more than four egg yolks a week, including those used in cooking). Minor differences between the AHA's 1988 diet and the AMA's 1967 diet are revealing. Polyunsaturated fats, once considered almost like a medicine to reduce blood cholesterol, are now limited. Soft margarine, derived from vegetable oils, is still preferable to hard margarine, derived from animal fats, but one AHA booklet contains the cryptic statement that "hydrogenation offsets some of the benefits of using unsaturated vegetable oils."[56] (More about the significance of these "minor" changes in recommendations a little later.)

While standard dietary recommendations concentrate on saturated fats and, to a lesser extent, dietary cholesterol, as factors in heart disease, the alternative diet to protect the heart can be distilled into three words: consume *whole foods*. Whole foods refers to the honest, nature-created foods that people ate, as Beatrice Trum Hunter expresses it, before bread resembled "presliced absorbent cotton" and food industry wizards created "new 'wonder' foods . . . made to keep 'forever.'"[57] "Judging by photographs on government pamphlets of green leafy vegetables and healthy milk cows, we harbor the illusion that Americans still eat foods from the four basic groups," says Ross Hume Hall, author of *Food for Naught* (New York: Random House, 1976). "In reality the bulk of American food comes highly processed in brightly colored packages whose contents have little to do with the basic food groups."

These "engineered food products" are what Dr. Roger J. Williams, mentor of a generation of physicians who practice nutritional medicine, called "dismembered" foods. (Williams, a world-famous scientist, was a pioneer in vitamin research and member of the National Academy of Sciences.) According to Dr. Donald R. Davis, editor-in-chief of the *Journal of Applied Nutrition* and director of the Roger J. Williams Nutrition Institute in Austin, Texas, "Americans derive two-thirds of their calories from these dismembered foods."[58]

As Davis explains, all foods are whole when grown, and each contains twenty-five to thirty nutrients. But all or most of these nutrients are lost when a whole food is dismembered. This occurs, for example, when table sugar is extracted from sugar beets and purified, when a grain has its bran and germ removed to make white flour, when oil is separated from nuts and seeds causing a loss of vitamin E, when alcohol is distilled from grains. Don't confuse dismembering with processing, such as freezing, canning, grinding, or cooking, Davis says. Processing causes only a partial loss of a few nutrients.

There are varying degrees of dismembering, says Davis. Sweeteners and products that contain sweeteners, such as soft drinks, are 100 percent dismembered, while orange juice rates as a 75 percent dismembered food. (Drinking a fruit juice instead of eating the whole fruit, you not only lose the fiber, but because it takes a heap of oranges to produce one glass of juice, consume an overabundance of sugar.)

For more information, see Dr. Roger J. Williams, *The Wonderful World within You* (New York: Bantam Books, 1977). A revised edition can be obtained from Bio-Communications Press, 3100 N. Hillside, Wichita, KS 67219, (316) 682–3100.

For a cookbook with recipes high in whole foods, see Nikki and David Goldbeck's *American Wholefoods Cuisine* (New York: New American Library, 1983) and *The New American Diet* by Sonja L. Conner and William E. Conner (New York: Fireside Books, Simon & Schuster, 1986).

For NutriCircles softwear, which enables you to calculate "wholeness," and much more, in over a hundred basic foods, contact Strickland Computer Consulting, P.O. Box 1255, Valley Center, CA 92082.

Cholesterol and Animal Fats Are Not the Problem

What about fats, particularly animal fats and cholesterol, which the AMA recommends keeping to a minimum? Cholesterol appears to be a villain because fatty deposits lining the arteries contain large amounts of cholesterol. But according to Dr. Roger J. Williams, consuming less cholesterol is unwise for two reasons: "If we discard cholesterol-containing foods, we discard the very best foods there are." As an example he gives the egg, the perfect protein, which is an excellent source of amino acids and other nutrients and contains high amounts of lecithin, which helps protect against the deposit of cholesterol in arteries. In addition, reducing the consumption of cholesterol accelerates the production of cholesterol within the body. The way to prevent cholesterol deposits from forming in the arteries is to eat a highly nutritious diet, Williams says.[59]

Another misleading concept, according to Williams, is that one should avoid eating saturated (animal) fats to protect oneself against heart disease: "The evidence shows that high fat consumption, when accompanied by plenty of the essential nutrients that all cells need, does *not* cause atherosclerosis or heart disease."[60] One piece of this evidence is an experiment involving 600 rats observed up to two years that took place at Yale University Nutrition Laboratory in the mid-1950s. Different groups of rats were fed a diet high in animal fats (81 percent of calories) but one that also contained high-quality protein, minerals, and vitamins. The rats experienced no adverse effects on the heart or aorta but gained a lot of weight.[61]

To put Roger Williams's philosophy to work in your kitchen, read *Caring for the Healing Heart: An Eating Plan for Recovery from Heart Attack* by Eleanor Cousins (New York: W. W. Norton, 1988). In this friendly slim book,

Cousins, described by her husband, Norman, as the chief factor in his recovery, points out that egg yolk, as long as it comes from quality eggs, contains "a very fine kind of cholesterol" that the body needs.

Thriving on a Traditional Diet

One of the first scientists to show the devastating effects of modern food "dismembering" was a dentist, Dr. Weston Price. In the 1930s, Price visited peoples all over the world who had remained untouched by modern civilization and followed a traditional diet of whole foods. For example, Swiss peasants in an isolated mountain valley ate mainly whole rye bread, cheese, and fresh goats' or cows' milk. Canadian Indians subsisting in subzero weather ate mostly wild animals but knew how to avoid scurvy by consuming a particular herb. As Price showed in photographs (and with his trained eye), these so-called primitive people had perfect teeth and strong bodies. As Price observed, they also lived in a harmonious manner. Price then visited members of the same groups (including Eskimos, Scots, Polynesians, and Africans) living in more accessible areas who had adopted a modern diet—white flour products, sweet foods, and pastries. In every instance, Price says, tooth decay was rampant and people had badly formed dental arches with crowding of the teeth (a condition that has made orthodontia a rite of puberty in our society). Delinquency and other forms of antisocial behavior had also become a problem.[62]

Fifty years later, Donald O. Rudin, author of *The Omega-3 Phenomenon*, reiterated the same theme: "modern maladies"—heart disease, diabetes, cancer, stroke, to name the killer diseases—struck at the beginning of this century. Surprising as it sounds, the first heart attack was reported in 1896.[63] Dr. Paul Dudley White, the renowned heart specialist, said in 1965, "When I graduated from medical school in 1911, I had never heard of coronary thrombosis . . . (heart attack)."[64] Rudin attributes the sharp rise in these disorders to "significant changes in our diet that took place at the same time these diseases manifested themselves, starting when American diets changed from a rural-local-supply focus to a national food-supply chain of highly processed and imported foods. . . ."[65]

Sweet and Dangerous

Sugar, a hidden ingredient in most processed foods, is, as you know, bad for the teeth and a source of "empty calories." But that's not the whole story. Sugar is one of the causes of coronary heart disease, according to John Yudkin, professor emeritus of nutrition at Queen Elizabeth College, University of London. Studying death rates from heart disease in six countries, Yudkin contends that a better correlation exists between sugar in the diet and heart disease than fats. In Israel, for example, newly arrived immigrants from Yemen had very little heart disease, whereas Yemenites who had lived in Israel twenty-five years or more had a high incidence of heart disease. The traditional diet in Yemen is high in butter and other animal fats but low in sugar. Switching to the high-sugar diet of their adopted country may have caused the rise in coronary disease, according to Yudkin.

Yudkin also based his thesis that the villain in heart disease is refined sugar on experiments with laboratory animals. These experiments showed that a diet high in sugar caused a rise in cholesterol and triglycerides (blood fats that are associated with heart attacks) and made blood platelets clump together more easily. But human subjects did not respond so uniformly to a sugar-rich diet. All young males who participated in studies showed a significant rise in triglycerides from eating excessive amounts of sugar, but only a portion of the men (one quarter to one third) showed other changes. These men gained weight, their insulin went up, and their platelets became stickier. Yudkin concludes that only sugar-sensitive people are in danger of developing coronary disease from eating too much sugar.[66] For more about sugar and heart disease, see Yudkin's *Sweet and Dangerous* (New York: Peer H. Suder, 1972).

Come Back, Little Egg

What about eggs, which are included in a "whole foods" diet but restricted by the American Heart Association? (Incidentally, the AHA's current recommendation of four egg yolks a week is one more than was allowed in the mid-1970s.)

In the early 1970s, Ross Hume Hall, professor of biochemistry at McMaster University, discovered that there were no scientific studies proving that eating eggs increased the risk of heart attack.[67] But plenty of studies exist showing that eating eggs has no effect on heart disease. Williams cites a report in which investigators fed large amounts of egg yolks daily (around fifteen) to 13 subjects. Only 2 subjects showed marked blood cholesterol elevation; the majority showed no change in blood plasma levels.

Eggs can be part of your diet if you prepare them properly, says Dr. Alan Gaby, an authority on vitamin B6. "Cholesterol in your diet is only dangerous when it's exposed to air, or oxidizes. In cooking an egg, oxidation takes place at a much more rapid rate if you break the yolk or expose it to air." Gaby advises, have your eggs poached, boiled, or sunny side up, but forgo scrambled eggs, omelets, and custard.

On the egg question, alternative physicians and cholesterol critics in the scientific community are bedfellows. Said Donald J. McNamara, Ph.D., professor of nutrition and food science at the University of Arizona, "Excluding eggs from the diet is regrettable. Eggs provide good quality protein and are relatively inexpensive. I'm particularly concerned that so many older people are depriving themselves of eggs." In a study that McNamara and coworkers conducted involving 50 middle-aged men who had no symptoms of heart disease, he found that "for two-thirds of people, lowering dietary cholesterol will not affect their plasma cholesterol levels." That's because "most people have built-in feedback mechanisms to maintain their baseline plasma cholesterol levels, irrespective of dietary modification."[68]

Eggphobia has led heart experts, such as Glen C. Griffin and William P. Castelli, authors of *How to Lower Your Cholesterol and Beat the Odds of a Heart Attack* (Fisher Books, 1989) to recommend egg substitutes. But the nutritional shortcomings of egg substitutes were graphically illustrated by two University of Illinois researchers in 1974. The researchers took two groups of rats of the same age and fed one group whole eggs, the other, Egg Beaters. Judging by the list of ingredients on the Egg Beaters label, the only major difference between the product and the real thing is cholesterol; zero cholesterol in one serving of Egg Beaters as contrasted to 240 milligrams of cholesterol in one egg. But a photograph of two rats, one from each lot, taken after three weeks on the diet, tells a different story. The rat fed Egg Beaters is scrawny and frail. (He died the day after the photo was taken.) The rat fed whole eggs is nicely filled out, with luxuriant fur. The researchers conclude, "Obviously there is something in whole eggs that provides nutrients for health which are missing in Egg Beaters."[69] Egg Beaters are one of at least three egg substitutes on the market.

Time-Tested Oils

In 1984 health writer Jane Brody, author of *Jane Brody's Nutrition Book* (New York: Bantam Books, 1984), advised us to use olive oil sparingly. But the following year olive oil came into favor when research led by Dr. Scott Grundy at the University of Texas Medical Center in Dallas showed that olive oil was as effective as vegetable oils, and possibly more so, in lowering cholesterol levels.[70] The AHA now recommends limited amounts of monounsaturated fats, which in addition to olive oil include peanut and avocado oils. Olive oil seems a dependable choice considering, as the AHA notes, that Mediterranean peoples consume a generous amount of this oil and have a low incidence of heart disease. (More about monounsaturated fats on page 99.)

Not-So-Good Oils

Polyunsaturated oils (vegetable oils) are a newcomer on the scene. In the early decades of this century, most Americans used animal fats—butter and lard—for cooking. But this pattern began to change in the 1930s when commercial shortenings made with polyunsaturates were introduced. Polyunsaturates got a further boost in the early 1950s when investigators discovered that a diet high in vegetable fat will lower the amount of cholesterol and fatty substances circulating in the blood. Since then Americans have been consuming increasingly large amounts of vegetable oils. At present, polyunsaturates constitute 42 percent of our fat intake.[71]

Nevertheless, a diet high in polyunsaturates is harmful, according to R. Pinckney, M.D., and Cathey Pinckney, authors of *The Cholesterol Controversy* (Los Angeles: Sherbourne Press, 1973). Polyunsaturated fatty acids (PUFAs) are easily damaged by oxidation and heat; once the process starts, PUFAs form toxic substances, called peroxides, which can promote a deficiency of vitamin E, increase risk of atherosclerosis, cancer, and other diseases, shorten life span, cause premature aging of the skin, and increase the number of skin lesions, the Pinckneys say. PUFAs are even more dangerous when heated, the authors say, because they are then converted to polymers, similar to varnish, shellac, and plastics. If *The Cholesterol Controversy*, published in 1973, had had wider circulation, we might have been spared cholesterol mania. The book is out of print but may be available at your public library.

A Second Look at Those "Good" Vegetable Oils

Dietary recommendations by government agencies for fats and oils have flip-flopped over the past two decades. In 1977 the Heart, Lung, and Blood Institute of the NIH recommended consuming two times as much polyunsaturates as saturates. But in its 1988 *Dietary Guidelines,* the AHA specifies that "polyunsaturated fat intake should not exceed 10 percent of calories." Why the change? The AHA attributes the restriction to "the relatively small amount of data on the long-term use of diets with very high polyunsaturated fat content." A study referenced in the *Dietary Guidelines* describes "increased prevalence of cholelithiasis (gallstones) in men ingesting a serum-cholesterol-lowering diet."[72] Not referenced are animal and human studies showing a link between excessive amounts of polyunsaturates and cancer. Researchers from the University of Hawaii found that tumor incidence in female rats increased 23 percent when they were fed a diet high in corn oil.[73]

Udo Erasmus, author of *Fats and Oils* (Vancouver, Canada: Alive, 1988), criticizes the AHA for failing to distinguish between natural and refined oils. The highly refined oils that we find in transparent bottles on supermarket shelves are unnatural polyunsaturates and should not be used for anything, he says. "They have been degraded by light, have lost much of their nutrient value during the refining processes, which include degumming, bleaching, deodorizing, and the removal of many vital substances, including vitamin E and lecithin, and are usually made from the cheapest, most inferior, most intensely pesticide-sprayed oil plants."[74]

Hydrogenation—What the Government Isn't Telling Us

The use of polyunsaturates is not limited to the oil you pour into your frying pan. When you buy a commercial bakery product—crackers, cookies, pastries, cakes, snack chips, imitation cheese, peanut butter, and candy—the label contains the words *partially hydrogenated oils*. This term refers to the process that a vegetable oil (soybean, corn, canola, cottonseed) undergoes to make it firm enough for commercial use. Another reason for hydrogenating oils is that it gives these synthetic fats a long shelf life, unlike the original liquid vegetable oil, which turns rancid very quickly. Partially hydrogenated oils are used to make all types of margarine.

The process of hydrogenation, as described by Beatrice Trum Hunter, author of *Consumer Beware* (New York: Simon & Schuster, 1971), involves exposing liquid oil or soft fat to a high temperature and placing it under pressure. "Hydrogen is then bubbled through the oil in the presence of nickel, platinum or some other catalyst. . . . The heating of the oil ruins its original character, with destruction of all vitamins and mineral factors as well as an alteration of proteins. The essential fatty acids are destroyed or changed into abnormal toxic fatty acids antagonistic to essential fatty acids."

These toxic fatty acids are a whole new class of substances called trans fatty acids, or trans fats. Research conducted over a ten-year period by University of Maryland biochemist Dr. Mary G. Enig and colleagues demonstrates that when people eat foods containing trans fats, these fats are deposited in varying amounts in some body tissues and affect the way the organs in the body function.[75] Animal studies show that trans fats raise total serum cholesterol levels and lower HDL, the "good" cholesterol; depress the immune system, increasing susceptibility to cancer; stunt growth; decrease the response of red blood cells to insulin, which makes these fats particularly harmful to diabetics; affect the quality of milk of lactating females; and destroy omega-3 fatty acids.[76]

But these harmful effects may be the tip of the iceberg, Enig said, because no one knows the full extent of the damage caused by trans fats. In analyzing fats, the government usually lumps trans fats with *unsaturated* fats, although research clearly shows that trans fats act like *saturated* fats. Furthermore, analysis of the fat content in all foods is faulty; what you read on the label of a box of crackers, for example, bears little or no relationship to its actual fat content. Enig came to this conclusion based on painstaking experiments in which she and her colleagues evaluated the fat content of more than fifty bakery goods. Consequently, all this inaccurate data finds its way into the data banks that nutritionists use for counseling the public.

It would be reassuring to think that trans fat research is proceeding at a fast clip, and the government is poised to warn us about the dangers of partially hydrogenated oils (which constitute 70 percent of the vegetable oils used in foods). Regrettably, this is not the case. As soon as Enig reported the harmful effects of trans fats in food, the food industry exerted pressure on the government to suppress her findings and her funding dried up, she said. "There are multiple layers of people engaged in a conspiracy of not telling the truth."

What to Do About It

To avoid foods containing hydrogenated oils, Beatrice Trum Hunter, who is also food editor of *Consumers' Research,* advises: read labels. Don't be fooled by the term *hardened* oils, for example, which means the same as hydrogenated oils. The best way to avoid these oils and other harmful substances is to limit your use of factory-made foods. Instead of margarine, use a small amount of unsalted butter. To stretch the amount of butter you use, prepare a "butter spread," Hunter said. Here's how: Allow a pound of unsalted butter to soften at room temperature in an electric blender. Gradually add one to one and a half cups of mild vegetable oil (sunflower, safflower, sesame, or a mixture of them) with the motor running. Cream as for a cake until the mixture is smoothly blended. Pour the mixture into a container, cover tightly, and store in the refrigerator.

Hydrogenated oils are not only worthless but deprive us of the essential oils we need, which are called essential fatty acids (EFAs). There are two major types of EFAs: omega-3 oils found in seafood and cold climate plants, and omega-6 oils from plant sources, such as unrefined vegetable oils. A few sources contain both omega-3 and omega-6 oils. (More about essential fatty acids in chapters 5 and 8.)

Fish Oils.   The best-known source of omega-3 oils is fish oils. Fish oils created excitement in the scientific community when three reports about its benefits appeared in a May 9, 1985, issue of the *New England Journal of Medicine.* Two of these reports said that fish oil can prevent heart attacks. The third report suggested that fish oils can benefit patients with inflammatory ailments such as rheumatoid arthritis and migraine headache. This fish oil research was based on studies done more than a decade ago by Danish researchers. These researchers found that Eskimos, who consume large amounts of fat and cholesterol in fatty fish and marine mammals, had a far lower incidence of heart disease than the Danes; when Eskimos moved to

Denmark, their risk of heart disease went up.

Taking a clue from this research, drug manufacturers began to aggressively market fish oil supplements. These commercial goings-on made researchers uneasy, and they began to speculate about harmful effects that might ensue from use of the supplements, such as increased LDL levels or stroke.[77,78]

One researcher who treats patients with fish oil supplements is Dr. Charles Glueck, an authority on blood lipids. Glueck, director of the Cholesterol Center at the Jewish Hospital in Cincinnati, pointed out a common misconception about fish oils: "Taking fish oils will not lower either total cholesterol or LDL [the "bad" cholesterol]. But fish oils have a very significant effect on elevated triglycerides [a type of blood lipid associated with coronary artery disease]. If, despite your efforts to eat a low-fat diet and exercise, these levels remain high, fish oils will enable the body to clear out the major triglycerides from the bloodstream. Fish oils will also often elevate HDL cholesterol [the "good" cholesterol] in people who haven't been able to raise HDL levels with life-style changes."

Another major benefit of fish oils, Glueck said, is their effect on blood platelets (cells involved in clotting). Fish oils make platelets less sticky and thus less likely to clump together and form blockages in blood vessels leading to the heart and brain.

To lower extremely high triglycerides, you need a hefty dose of fish oils, says Glueck, "around 12 to 15 grams per day coupled with a low-fat, low-cholesterol diet. In individuals with low HDL cholesterol, you can often achieve results with a smaller dose, perhaps 4 to 8 grams per day." Glueck recommends two brands of fish oil, Promega (a Parke-Davis product) and MaxEPA, imported from England. "Other fish oil products often have excessive amounts of vitamins A and D, which can be toxic if fish oils are used for long-term treatment."

Glueck cautions against treating yourself with fish oils, even though they are available over the counter. "Fish oils are powerful drugs, and should only be taken under the direction of a physician." An added word of caution: you shouldn't take fish oils if you have an active ulcer, high blood pressure that is poorly controlled, or any history of cerebral vascular bleeding.

One of the alternative physicians who has recommended fish oil capsules to his patients since MaxEPA introduced the product in 1982 is Dr. David Jones of Anderson, Indiana. (Jones's interest in fish and heart disease stems from a year spent in Greenland in 1958.) As a maintenance dose for healthy people, Jones prescribes one capsule three times a day, and larger doses for patients with arteriosclerosis. Jones cautions that fish oil capsules can turn rancid over time and advises that you check expiration date. The only side effect that his patients report, he says, is more frequent copious stools.

Favorite Oil of the Vikings. Udo Erasmus claims that flaxseed oil, a cold-pressed, unrefined variety made from organically grown flaxseed, contains almost twice as much omega-3 oils as fish oils. Erasmus describes the oil as a "rich, deep golden color like liquid sunshine . . . a pleasant nutty bouquet . . . its texture is so light that it is hard to believe that it is oil. . . ."[79] Erasmus endorses Veg-Omega-3 (Spectrum Naturals, 133 Copeland Street, Petaluma, CA 94952). The other quality flax oil is C-leinosan [New Dimensions Distributors, Inc. in Arizona, (800) 624–7114]. Both products are available at health food stores. Unrefrigerated, flax oil has a three-month shelf life; refrigerated, six months. Flax oil is suitable for salad dressing but not cooking; high temperatures destroy the essential fatty acids very rapidly. Recommended daily adult dose is one tablespoon.

Another source of flaxseed is Fortified Flax [distributed by Omega-Life, Inc. in Milwaukee, (414) 786–2070 or P.O. Box 208, Brookfield, WI 53008-0208]. According to Clara Felix, Rudin's coauthor and publisher of *The Felix Letter,* fortified flax is a great source of fiber and omega-3s. Since it has a laxative effect, start with one teaspoon and gradually increase to one tablespoon. (Personal note: Stirred into hot or cold cereal, it has a nice nutty flavor, but anything over a teaspoon makes me feel full and a little burpy.) Refrigerate product after opening. For a sample issue and index to previous issues of *The Felix Letter,* send $1 plus large self-addressed stamped envelope to Clara Felix, P.O. Box 7094, Berkeley, CA 94707.

What an Oil Expert Uses. I asked Ann Louise Gittleman, coauthor of *Beyond Pritikin,* which describes the importance of essential fatty acids, about her favorite oils. "For cooking, one of my favorites is canola oil," she said. Canola oil, made from rape seed, is from the same family (monounsaturates) as olive oil. But don't use a refined canola oil sold in supermarkets, she warned. "The rape seed that the oil is made from has been treated with pesticides and sprays." She recommends an oil labeled "100 percent expeller pressed, unrefined, made from organically grown rape seed." Gittleman's choice is Spectrum's canola oil, from Canada, sold in health food stores. Her other favorite oil is sesame oil. For one thing, sesame oil doesn't go rancid as quickly as polyunsaturated oils like safflower and sunflower; that's because its chemical composition is closer to that of monounsaturated oils. Sesame also has a good taste and can be used for salads, sautéing, and baking. Light cooking with sesame oil is not going to destroy its fatty acids as long as you keep the temperature below 320 degrees—that's the "magic cut-off point." A cooking tip from Gittleman: in following a recipe that calls for shortening or margarine, substitute canola oil but use 20 percent less.

The best source of omega-3 EFAs is fatty fish—salmon, mackerel, and sardines, Gittleman said. For her clients who don't care for fish, she recommends fish oil supplements.

Margarine—Cholesterol-Free but Full of Toxicity

Margarine is advertised as having "no cholesterol" because it's made from "100 percent corn oil" rather than saturated animal fat. But as I've mentioned, margarine is made from hydrogenated oils, which contain harmful trans fatty acids, or trans fats.

Consider an observation made by a physician, Dr. Franklin Bicknell, in World War II and reported by Beatrice Trum Hunter. In Norway, where margarine factories had been destroyed, heart disease decreased. "In England, during the same period, with margarine factories intact, arterial diseases increased."[80] A belief, voiced by Nathan Pritikin and others, is that atherosclerosis decreased in Europe during World War II owing to the scarcity of dairy products and meat. Not so, according to an Oxford University researcher, G. Bourne, who presented documented evidence that countries such as Denmark, Holland, Belgium, and Norway consumed large amounts of partially hydrogenated vegetable fats before the war (they exported their dairy products), but during the war consumed their own butter and meat. It was during this period that atherosclerosis decreased dramatically in those countries. Bourne's argument, long ignored by nutritionists, is that margarine, and other types of hydrogenated oil, are the culprits in heart disease, not animal fats.

The American Heart Association says very little about hydrogenation and trans fats. One of its 1985 brochures states, "Many margarines contain partially hydrogenated oils and may be acceptable if they contain twice as much polyunsaturated as saturated fat." But agencies in other countries are more forthright on the subject. According to Dr. Mary G. Enig, whose research I've mentioned before, in the United Kingdom trans fatty acids are considered the equivalent of saturated fatty acids, and research from Czechoslovakia shows that hydrogenated fats decrease normal sperm in male animals and decrease litter size, among other effects.[81] The sale of margarines containing trans fatty acids is banned in the Netherlands and in Germany, Udo Erasmus said.

Homogenized Milk May Contribute to Heart Attacks

Homogenizing milk to extend its shelf life is another process that damages fats, says Gittleman. According to Dr. Kurt A. Oster, chief of cardiology emeritus at Park City Hospital in Bridgeport, Connecticut, homogenized milk causes the majority of heart attacks in the United States. Here's how Oster describes the problem: Normal milk fat forms large globules, which are easily digested in the intestinal tract. The homogenization process breaks up these globules into tiny droplets, which pass intact through the wall of the intestine and into the bloodstream carrying with them a deadly enzyme called xanthine oxidase (XO). XO attacks artery walls and heart tissue, causing lesions to form and setting the stage for atherosclerosis, or hardening of the arteries. (This process does not take place with skimmed milk, which contains no fat.)

To inhibit XO, take a vitamin called folic acid, Oster says. Folic acid not only blocks the action of XO but helps rebuild cell membranes in arteries damaged by XO. As a self-help measure, Oster recommends 1 to 3 milligrams of folic acid along with a 50- or 100-milligram B complex and brewer's yeast.

For further information about Oster's nutritional program, send $2 for "Homogenized Milk and Atherosclerosis," by Nicholas Sampsidis, M.S., Sunflower Publishing Co., Glen Head, NY 11545.

Foods that Lower Cholesterol

Despite the oat bran craze, no one food has a monopoly on lowering cholesterol, said Dr. Charles E. Elson, professor of nutritional science, University of Wisconsin. "The more cholesterol-lowering compounds we investigate, the more we find. It's not one particular compound that lowers cholesterol but the accumulative effect of, say, fifty of them. You need to eat a variety of foods because no one compound works for everybody."

Fiber. Not so long ago, fiber was dismissed by nutritionists as having no nutritive value. Fiber gained its reputation as a health food when a group of British physicians, each independently studying the total health of rural Africans and other primitive peoples in the 1970s, associated their absence of disease with a high-fiber diet. Since then scientists have shown that soluble fiber lowers cholesterol levels and (important for diabetics) stabilizes blood sugar levels.

There are two kinds of fiber, soluble and insoluble. Standard advice has been that insoluble fiber, such as raw wheat bran, sold in health food stores, speeds up transit time in the bowel but does not lower cholesterol. Now it looks as if one form of insoluble fiber has a dual function. A psyllium preparation, used as a bulk laxative, was shown by James W. Anderson and his team at the University of Kentucky in Lexington to lower blood cholesterol by as much as 15 percent.[82]

Fiber Favorite. Oat bran, the best-known soluble fiber to lower blood cholesterol, burst on the scene in the early 1980s when Anderson and colleagues at the University of Kentucky reported a number of studies in which they gave oat bran to men with high cholesterol levels. A 1984 study showed that a diet high in oat bran decreased serum cholesterol levels by 19 percent and lowered LDL cholesterol approximately 24 percent. (Eating a quantity of cooked beans or bean soup had the same effect.[83]) Food companies, gleeful at finding a new panacea, added oat bran (often minuscule amounts) to cereals and bakery goods.[84]

The oat bran bubble burst when a Boston research team found oat fiber no more effective in lowering people's cholesterol levels than foods made from low-fiber refined wheat flour.[85]

Good Fiber Sources.   In addition to beans, corn, and other complex carbohydrates (starches), fruit ranks high on the list of soluble fibers. According to Dr. Maria C. Linder, editor of *Nutritional Biochemistry and Metabolism,* fruit, owing to an ingredient called pectin, is the most effective cholesterol-lowering food. Large amounts of pectin are found in apples, citrus fruits, cranberries, and sour plums. These can lower cholesterol by 11 percent.[86]

A sure way to lower cholesterol is to become a vegetarian—but not the type who substitutes high-fat cheese and dairy products for meat. According to Dr. Charles E. Elson, professor of nutritional science at the University of Wisconsin, whom I quoted earlier, "For years, we thought that vegetarians had much lower cholesterol levels than others because they didn't eat cholesterol and saturated fat." Instead, Elson's research shows that foods vegetarians eat contain certain compounds that keep cholesterol from accumulating. A low-fat vegetarian diet combined with exercise and stress management techniques has even been shown to reverse atherosclerosis in heart patients.[87] (For more about the vegetarian diet, see chapter 7.)

Guar—A Gum that's Not for Chewing.   For an instant source of soluble fiber, consider guar (pronounced gwar) gum. Until recently, guar gum, made from cluster beans, was chiefly used as a thickening agent in processed foods. But scientific studies conducted over the last decade have shown that guar gum has more important uses. One is lowering serum cholesterol levels. A three-month study done by Finnish researchers showed that guar gum significantly reduced total serum cholesterol and LDL cholesterol.[88]

Guar is available in powder form or capsules, or combined with other sources of soluble fiber. A new fiber drink called Easy Oats (a Futurebiotics product) contains oat bran, psyllium, guar, and pectin. "One heaping tablespoon of Easy Oats . . . gives you the same amount of soluble fiber as four bowls of oatmeal or two good sized oat bran muffins," the company claims.

For further information about Easy Oats, ask your health food store owner or call Futurebiotics, (1/800) 367–5433.

Garlic.   Garlic has been revered as a cure-all since the beginning of recorded history. The *Codex Elbers,* the world's oldest surviving medical text

(1500 B.C.), contains twenty-two garlic-based remedies for ailments ranging from headaches to throat tumor to gynecological problems. Hippocrates prescribed garlic, as did ancient Chinese physicians. The Egyptian slaves who built the pyramids ate garlic daily; the Romans fed garlic to gladiators to give them strength. Through the ages, garlic has been used to protect against plague, traveler's diarrhea, battlefield wounds, and evil spirits.

In more recent years, research conducted by Dr. Benjamin Lau, microbiologist at Loma Linda University, has shown that garlic reduces levels of LDL cholesterol (the "bad" cholesterol) and triglycerides while raising protective HDL cholesterol levels. In a double-blind study published in 1987, Lau and colleagues gave an odorless garlic extract called Kyolic (four capsules a day) to 56 subjects, men and women, over a six-month period. A control group was given a placebo. The majority of subjects (65 percent) had lowered triglycerides and increased HDL. What about the 35 percent who did not respond to garlic treatment? "They were men who ate an extremely high-fat diet—lots of steak, pastry, and ice cream—and drank heavily," Lau said. "You can't expect an herb to achieve miracles." Garlic also did not influence cholesterol levels in subjects whose initial cholesterol levels were low.

If you decide to take a garlic preparation to lower serum cholesterol and triglycerides, don't be alarmed if these levels go up the first month or so. Participants in Lau's experiment experienced this temporary rise, as did subjects in other garlic studies, but levels had dropped considerably by the third month. Lau attributes this initial rise to garlic's ability to dislodge fatty components of cells (lipids) from tissues and move these deposits into the bloodstream.[89]

In addition to garlic's beneficial effect on cholesterol levels, it has been successfully used to treat chronic anemia, arthritis, diabetes, pneumonia, and colitis. Research findings presented at the 71st Annual Meeting of the Federation of American Societies for Experimental Biology indicate it may also help prevent cancer by boosting the immune system.[90] Other studies suggest that garlic's sulfhydryl compounds may bind to and help remove toxic heavy metals such as lead, mercury, and cadmium from the bloodstream.[91] Since raw garlic contains a toxic element called allicin, many doctors who prescribe garlic recommend Kyolic, an allicin-free extract available at health food stores. For further information about Kyolic, call Wakunaga of America Co., Ltd., (1/800) 544–5800 inside California, (1/800) 421–2998 outside California.

Long before I came across these garlic studies, my association with a long-time garlic user, 69-year-old Lena Williams, had convinced me that the legendary powers attributed to the pungent bulb were true. Williams, who has been our cleaning person for close to twenty years, eats ten cloves of garlic a day and has never missed work because of illness. "I make a garlic sandwich—put it in everything I cook," she says.

Onions. Many of the benefits bestowed on the heart by garlic are offered by onions—another member of the allium family—as well.

One of these benefits is the ability (called fibrinolysis) to dissolve blood clots, which can form inside blood vessels and precipitate a heart attack. As Vicki Peterson writes in her charming book, *The Book of Healthy Foods* (New York: St. Martin's Press, 1981), when a horse develops clots in the legs, the owner, if steeped in old-time cures, feeds him garlic and onions. It was this piece of information that led a group of Indian physicians in the late 1960s to investigate onions as a possible source of an anticlotting agent. Their experiment consisted of feeding a group of volunteers a breakfast oozing with butter to which they added onions, either fried or boiled. One would expect all this saturated fat to lower the body's clot-preventing ability. Instead, fibrinolysis actually increased in these subjects.[92] A 1979 study, published in *Lancet,* also showed that onions and garlic keep platelets from sticking together.[93] Another finding from onion researchers is that you can cook onions any way you please, even boil them, without destroying the active principle that protects against heart disease.

VITAMIN SUPPLEMENTS—
WHEN FOODS ARE NOT ENOUGH

Niacin (Vitamin B3)

So you're eating a whole foods diet using good oils and plenty of fiber "extras," but your cholesterol levels are still high. Then take niacin, says Dr. Abram Hoffer. (Hoffer and Dr. Humphrey Osmond, Canadian physicians, pioneered the use of niacin as treatment for schizophrenia in the 1950s.) Much to Hoffer's amusement, "Niacin has become an establishment drug," he said. Official word from the National Heart, Lung, and Blood Institute is that niacin is the preferred cholesterol-lowering agent.[94] (Niacinamide, niacin's twin in many respects, does not have the same ability to lower cholesterol.)

One of the latest niacin studies shows that "you can get significant benefits from giving moderate doses of niacin," according to the study's principal investigator, Dr. Richard C. Pasternak, director of the Coronary Care Unit at Boston's Beth Israel Hospital. In this study, published in *The American Journal of Cardiology,* 101 patients taking 1500 milligrams of niacin each day had a 13 percent reduction in total cholesterol and a 31 percent increase in HDL cholesterol.[95]

But don't take niacin on your own, said Pasternak, who criticized health writers who encourage readers to do so. Pasternak's chief concern is that niacin can cause liver abnormality. "Unless the patient is carefully monitored by a doctor, this side effect can lead to serious problems. I've seen a patient who took large doses of niacin on his own end up in the hospital with hepatic necrosis" (destruction of liver cells).

Hoffer disagrees. "Taking niacin therapeutically, it's best to work with a knowledgeable doctor, but niacin is remarkably safe. Liver problems occur one in two or three thousand people. Unlike other cholesterol-lowering drugs, niacin is a healing vitamin. A national coronary study[96] showed that people who took niacin had a lower death rate." For lowering cholesterol, Hoffer recommends beginning with low doses of niacin and gradually working up to 1 gram three times a day. (A small number of people get the same effect taking half as much while an equally small number require twice the amount, he said.)

Note: Even small doses of niacin can produce a flush. I had read that Nicobid, the time-release form of niacin, produced by Rorer Pharmaceuticals, "completely eliminates the flushing in most people." Not so, said a Rorer spokesperson. "The main advantage of a time-release capsule is that you don't have to take it as often."

Vitamin B6

As Roger J. Williams wrote, "all the nutrients contribute to the prevention of heart trouble,"[97] but vitamins B6, E, and C are particularly important.

If you think bran cereal is for health faddists (he-men eat bacon or sausage), you're likely to be deficient in vitamin B6, says Dr. Alan Gaby, author of *B6: The Natural Healer* (New Canaan, Conn.: Keats Publishing, 1984). Vitamin B6 deficiency is common in our society, he says, and may be closely linked to atherosclerosis. That's the basis of an arresting theory, called the homocystine theory, proposed by a Harvard Medical School professor of pathology, Dr. Kilmer McCully, in the 1970s. Experiments have shown that homocystine, a toxic substance produced by the body, rapidly induces atherosclerosis in rabbits. Normally homocystine is no problem because the body quickly converts it to another compound, cystathionine, which is not toxic. But here's the catch: the conversion of homocystine to cystathionine requires the presence of adequate amounts of vitamin B6; when this vitamin is in short supply, toxic homocystine builds up.[98]

McCully's theory, like so many concepts involving nutrition, hasn't gotten much further than the drawing board. But there's plenty of scientific evidence, Gaby writes, that vitamin B6 not only helps prevent atherosclerosis but keeps blood from clotting and contributes to healthy heart muscle.

Gaby recommends: If you're basically healthy, supplement your diet with 10 to 25 milligrams of vitamin B6 a day. If you have a family history of heart disease or have developed a heart problem, take 50 milligrams of vitamin B6 a day along with the full spectrum of vitamins and minerals. (With any vitamin, the team approach works best, Gaby says.)

Vitamin E

In 1948 the Shute brothers, Drs. Evan and Wilfred, of London, Ontario, Canada, reported in a series of scientific articles that large doses of vitamin E, or alpha tocopherol, could hasten the recovery of heart patients who had not benefited from orthodox treatment. Some of the heart problems that had responded to vitamin E therapy were an inflamed clot in the vein of a leg, early gangrene of the legs, and a clot in the blood vessels of the brain, they said. As might be expected, these encouraging findings were greeted with scientific catcalls, and "this attitude of unhealthy skepticism has persisted for 35 years," Linus Pauling wrote in his book, *How to Live Longer and Feel Better* (New York: W. H. Freeman, 1985).

Lo and behold, the scientific community has discovered vitamin E. Presenters at a 1988 international symposium devoted to vitamin E research (the conference sponsored by the New York Academy of Science) described benefits from vitamin E as diverse as preventing cataracts and protecting against cancer.[99] Pertaining to the heart, Swiss investigators reported population studies that showed low rates of heart disease among men with high levels of vitamin E in their blood. An Austrian study suggests that vitamin E may prevent atherosclerosis.[100] Scientists attribute these benefits to vitamin E's role as an antioxidant, which is precisely what the Shutes maintained. Vitamin E "decreases the oxygen need of the involved tissues," Wilfrid Shute writes.[101]

Said Dr. Gary Price Todd, author of *Nutrition, Health and Disease,* "It's almost impossible to give an optimal dosage for vitamin E since requirements depend on the person's nutritional status. If you have adequate levels of vitamin C and selenium (a rarity) you can get by with as little as 30 or 40 IUs of vitamin E. Another difficulty in giving an accurate optimal amount is that synthetic vitamin E is much less potent than natural E." Given these qualifiers, Todd recommends 400 IUs of vitamin E a day. But mindful that Canadian statistics show taking 800 IUs cuts your risk of heart attack in half, Todd takes the larger amount himself, and ups that amount before strenuous physical exertion.

Vitamin C

Vitamin C (ascorbic acid), the kingpin of antioxidants, is known to benefit conditions from alcoholism to wound healing, so it's not surprising that it also benefits the heart. Four studies show that patients with coronary heart disease have low levels of ascorbic acid; six show that supplementing with vitamin C lowers total cholesterol while raising HDL cholesterol and discouraging platelets from clumping together.[102]

Todd recommends "250 mg per day, increasing that to as much as 10 grams per day in divided doses at the first sign of illness or during stress." As you may be aware, Linus Pauling recommended much higher doses—6 grams as a minimum dose for healthy people. Pauling's mentor, Irwin Stone, recommends 3 to 5 grams a day in several spaced doses.

MINERALS, TRACE ELEMENTS, AND OTHER SUBSTANCES

You may be concerned that you're deficient in certain vitamins, but the most serious deficiencies in our diet are deficiencies of minerals and trace elements, say Richard A. Passwater, Ph.D., and Elmer M. Cranton, M.D., authors of *Trace Elements, Hair Analysis and Nutrition.*[103]

To be precise, there's a difference between minerals and trace elements, the authors explain. Calcium, for example, is classified as a mineral because it becomes part of bone tissue. Other elements, such as selenium, are called trace elements; these don't contribute to the body but affect enzyme reactions and are present in the body in minute "traces." Selenium, which totals less than 1 milligram in an adult, is just a speck or two.

Until recently, scientists didn't pay much attention to mineral and trace element deficiencies—perhaps the minute amounts required put them off— but now it's known that mineral deficiencies make you more susceptible to disease, aggravate existing conditions, and shorten your life.[104] The scary fact is that "these vital minerals are disappearing from modern diet." One of the causes of mineral deficiency is that familiar menace, processed or factory-made foods.

Magnesium

Magnesium deficiency is linked to heart disease, including irregular heartbeat (arrhythmias) and high blood pressure, as well as diabetes and pregnancy problems. That's the conclusion reached by magnesium researchers at a 1988 conference, Trace Substances in Environmental Health.[105] According to Mildred S. Seelig, one of the presenters at the conference, these studies suggest that many people face serious consequences—including death—from preventable magnesium deficiency. Seelig, author of *Magnesium Deficiency in the Pathogenesis of Disease,* believes that 80 to 90 percent of the U.S. population is deficient in magnesium. But because most physicians and nutritionists disregard this condition, magnesium deficiency remains undetected until it is severe, she said.

The main reason for widespread magnesium deficiency is excesses in our diet, she continued: "Sugar and fats increase our need for magnesium. Alcohol, even social drinking, is a magnesium waster. So are soft drinks, which contain large amounts of phosphates. Phosphates bind magnesium in the bowel and prevent its absorption. If you're a diabetic or take diuretics, digitalis, or other heart drugs, you may be at risk of severe magnesium deficiency."

But even if junk food has never passed your lips, you're not home free with magnesium. Fiber causes loss of minerals, including magnesium, Seelig says. Phytase, found in bulk laxatives, interferes with the way we process magnesium. Vitamin D can also interfere with magnesium. As a corollary to her statement about vitamin D, here's a real bombshell: "The amount of vitamin D added to milk . . . is sufficient to cause renal (kidney), cardiovascular, and brain damage in those (children) who are hyperreactive (have a mysterious inability to metabolize vitamin D)."[106] Of particular concern to women, supplementing with calcium depletes magnesium, she says.

Considering all the elements in our diet that rob the body of magnesium, Seelig advises magnesium supplements. Unlike many researchers who balk at offering concrete advice, Seelig recommends "Start with one tablet a day of Slow Mag (G. D. Searle & Co.) and gradually increase to three. (Each tablet is 100 milligrams.) Unless you have kidney damage, even large amounts are safe." Proof of magnesium's safety is the number of people taking laxatives that contain large quantities of magnesium, she said.

For the past decade or more, alternative physicians have used magnesium as a heart drug. Dr. Alan Gaby, who practices nutritional medicine in Pikesville, Maryland, recalled a case in which magnesium was a lifesaver. Mr. H., 83, a retired rabbi, had severe heart failure and gangrene of the legs when Gaby first saw him four years ago:

> He was on his death bed wasted away to nothing. His doctors had told him he needed to have both legs amputated and gave him a month or two to live. His heart muscle was barely pumping; there was no blood flow to the feet. We treated him with an intravenous injection of magnesium combined with the B vitamins and trace minerals once a week for one and a half years. After six weeks, his ejection fraction [a heartbeat measurement] was close to normal, and we reduced his injections to every three weeks.

Today, Mr. H shows no sign of heart failure. "His legs, which were gangrenous, are no longer a problem; areas on the toes that were black and necrotic [dead] have turned into scabs and fallen off. But if he goes more than three weeks without a magnesium injection, he feels tired and his legs start to hurt again."

Magnesium has proved its efficacy in the past. A scientific study published in 1959 clearly shows that giving magnesium injections to critically ill heart patients saves lives.[107] In this study, investigators compared two groups of patients hospitalized with heart disease. The first group of 196 was treated with standard heart drugs. The following year, researchers found that 60 had died. The second group, 117 patients admitted to the hospital the next year with the same diagnosis, was treated with intramuscular injections of magnesium. That year, only one death occurred in that group. Dr. Jonathan Wright, who brought the study to my attention, commented, "These doctors reduced the mortality in heart patients from 30 percent to less than 1 percent!" Although the study was published in an indexed journal, said Wright, "It made no impact on medical treatment, and thirty years later, a magnesium injection for heart patients is far from being standard practice."

Gaby and other alternative physicians use magnesium to treat heart attack victims. As mentioned earlier, clot-dissolving drugs are the current excitement in emergency rooms. Besides being very expensive, these drugs can cause severe bleeding, Gaby said. "Giving magnesium intra venously is safer, more effective, and costs pennies compared to these new drugs."

Dr. Michael Schachter of Nyack, New York, who has practiced nutritional preventive medicine since 1974, uses magnesium to control heart arrhythmias. "We may start with oral magnesium," Schachter—an author of *Food, Mind and Mood* (New York: Warner Books, 1979) and president of the American College of Advancement in Medicine—said. "If that doesn't establish a normal rhythm, then we give injectable magnesium."

Again, scientific studies from the past provide a basis for patient treatment. A magnesium study was reported in 1975 by Dr. Lloyd T. Iseri, then a researcher at the University of California at Davis. Iseri treated two patients, both alcoholics and severely ill with arrhythmias, with magnesium and they recovered.[108]

Today magnesium is on the verge of acceptance in standard medicine. As reported in 1989, cardiologists at the University of Virginia treated 10 patients with varying types of rapid heartbeat with magnesium injections; either their heartbeat slowed or the problem disappeared.[109]

But a friend's recent experience proved to me that magnesium is not standard treatment for arrhythmias. Sandy, a writer struggling to meet a deadline, not only drank excessive amounts of coffee but smoked more than usual. One evening, "I felt faint, blacked out," she said. "When I was lying down, my heart began to race like crazy." She called a neighbor who summoned an ambulance. The emergency room doctor treated her with Calan, a calcium channel blocker. "I'm doing OK now, but my doctor said I may have to take the drug for the rest of my life," she says. Calan can cause chest pain, difficulty breathing, fainting, irregular pounding heartbeat, and confusion, among other side effects.[110] According to Iseri, magnesium is "nature's physiologic calcium blocker."[111]

Copper and Zinc

I've given top billing to magnesium because it's generating so much excitement at the moment, but other trace elements play an important role in heart disease.

Copper and zinc closely interact with one another: too much of one leads to deficiencies in the other. As Dr. Jonathan V. Wright, author of *Dr. Wright's Guide to Healing with Nutrition,* explains, "Too much zinc with too little copper, you get anemia, heart irregularities, cholesterol abnormalities. Too little zinc, you get prostate problems."[112]

Schachter says he is seeing more patients with copper deficiencies, which he attributes to people self-medicating with zinc: "Men take zinc for prostate; women take it for yeast infections."

Schachter's clinical observation that copper deficiency is widespread is corroborated by a U.S. Department of Agriculture researcher, Leslie M. Klevay. The average American diet frequently contains less copper than the daily adult requirement of 2 milligrams, Klevay says. This copper deficiency results in high cholesterol, damage to arteries, and death from heart disease. To prove his theory that a high zinc/low copper ratio is a major factor in heart disease, Klevay compares people with hardening of the arteries and heart disease to animals that are deficient in copper. People with heart disease often die suddenly; so do cattle and rats deficient in copper. Humans with hardening of the arteries develop lesions on the walls of arteries; similar lesions have been produced in animals by depriving them of copper.[113]

I asked Klevay, should we supplement with copper? "It's best to get your copper in the foods you eat," he said. Such foods are liver, oysters, high-fiber cereals, legumes, and, surprise, chocolate and beer. (I've heard lots of excuses for eating a candy bar or drinking a beer, but a need for copper is a new one! Since Klevay's forte is animal research—he relies on other sources for information about human diets—I have no compunction about giving Schachter's recommendation that you supplement with 2 milligrams copper per day. This amount, according to allowances set in 1980 by the Committee on Dietary Allowances of the National Research Council, is "safe and adequate."

Selenium

Keshan's disease is an example of what happens when selenium intake is low. Keshan's disease is a form of congestive heart disease—one that affects children especially—that was prevalent throughout vast areas of rural China. Knowing that the soil in this area was low in selenium, physicians in 1974 set up a controlled study. They gave selenium supplements to one group of children—over 4,000 selected at random—and gave a placebo to another group that served as a control. Results were so dramatic that two years into the study, the control group was discontinued and all children were given selenium supplements.[114]

It's now recognized that if you live in an area with selenium-rich soil (like South Dakota), you're much less likely to develop heart disease or cancer than if you live, say, in Ohio where I do. Here, cattle feed is enriched with selenium, yet, ironically, some authorities still claim that we humans don't need a multivitamin/mineral supplement. Dutch researchers recently found that patients who had suffered a heart attack had low levels of selenium.[115]

Schachter recommends 200 micrograms of selenium a day.

Chromium

Both animal and population studies tell the story about this trace element: a low intake of chromium results in elevated blood cholesterol levels and a buildup of plaque in the arteries. Chromium deficiency is also linked to diabetes; when there's not enough chromium, the body pumps out more insulin.

The bad news is that we Americans are woefully deficient in chromium compared to previous generations and to peoples in other countries. (Asians have five times as much chromium in their bodies as Americans.) The good news is that supplementing with chromium can turn the situation around. An Israeli team of scientists found that giving chromium to laboratory animals with induced atherosclerosis decreased plaque in clogged arteries. Reversing atherosclerosis has not been proven in humans, but the chief investigator of the Israel study said that this was a logical conclusion.[116] The cause of chromium deficiency is, once again, "dismembered" foods, particularly excessive amounts of white sugar. As you probably know, sugar (along with salt) is a major ingredient in almost all processed foods.

Schachter recommends 200 micrograms of chromium daily. Brewer's yeast is an excellent source of chromium, except for those with a yeast sensitivity, he said. One tablespoon of brewer's yeast provides 60 micrograms. When I pointed out to Schachter that you'd have to eat a mess of this bitter-tasting powder to meet his quota, he explained that minerals contained in a natural source are assimilated more easily.

Getting Your Trace Minerals

Obviously a multivitamin/mineral supplement is the most efficient way to take this array of minerals and trace elements. But choosing the right all-in-one supplement depends on the individual, Schachter said. In view of the danger of too much iron, which has been linked with cancer, "I don't give anyone iron until I've tested them. But a menstruating woman probably needs iron." Copper is also an individual matter. "In general people have too little copper, but some have too much copper."

To provide these choices, Dr. Gary Price Todd, a nutritionally oriented ophthalmologist whose work is described in the chapter on cataracts, has devised a multivitamin/mineral supplement with several formulas geared to individual needs. One has copper but no iron. All formulas contain what Todd considers proper amounts. Commercial formulas have too much iron and phosphorus and not enough chromium, selenium, vanadium, and manganese, he said.

For information about nutritional supplements and health care products, call Bio-Zoe, Inc., (1/800) 426–7581.

Coenzyme Q10

In view of a popular 1986 book, *The Miracle Nutrient CoEnzyme Q10,* CoQ10 (its abbreviation) may seem like a new fad, but this is not the case. Thirty years ago, Dr. Karl Folkers, biomedical scientist at the University of Texas in Austin, discovered CoQ10 deficiencies in the hearts of patients suffering from different types of cardiac disease. Folkers, considered the father of CoQ10, had a hunch that giving oral supplements of CoQ10 to heart patients would strengthen the heart muscle and energize the cardiovascular system; his research and that of others has confirmed his prediction. Patients with high blood pressure, hearing disorders, and obesity can be helped with CoQ10 treatment.

Scientific studies conducted mainly here and in Japan have shown that when given CoQ10 treatment, patients with angina pectoris had less pain and greater endurance; patients with cardiomyopathy (weakened heart muscle) improved dramatically, but heart function deteriorated when CoQ10 treatment was temporarily discontinued; and patients with cardiac failure who did not respond to diuretics and digitalis felt better and improved significantly, as confirmed by tests. (All these studies are summarized in Melvyn Werbach's *Nutritional Influences on Illness.*[117])

Today, doctors in Japan routinely prescribe CoQ10 for heart conditions—an estimated 12 million Japanese take the nutrient—but the medical establishment in this country ignores it. ("Claims made on behalf of Coenzyme Q10 have not been substantiated by medical research," says the University of California, Berkeley, *Wellness Letter* [Feb. 1989].) Undeterred by the AMA's usual resistance to nutritional therapy, a growing number of nutritional doctors and cardiologists prescribe CoQ10.

Cardiologist Dr. Steven Korotkin of Birmingham Farms, Michigan, began treating patients with CoQ10 seven years ago. Of the twenty-two patients he has treated, five markedly improved their heart function, he said. One of the five, we'll call him Mr. Smith, had weakness of the heart muscle (cardiomyopathy) and a condition called acute pulmonary edema, which means accumulation of fluid in the lungs. After six years of standard drug treatment, Mr. Smith's condition was still poor. "I started him on the standard dose of CoQ10 (33 milligrams three times a day) and in four months he started showing measurable improvement. In seven months, his heart function was normal."

Patients like Mr. Smith, with weakness of the heart muscle for unknown reasons (idiopathic cardiomyopathy), are most likely to improve with CoQ10, Korotkin said. Patients with diminished blood supply to the heart (ischemic cardiomyopathy) are the least likely to improve. Some patients whose heart valves are diseased respond to CoQ10 treatment, but some do not, he said.

"CoQ10 may take four to six months to start to work," he added. "I give everybody (except patients with diminished blood supply to the heart) a year on CoQ10. If they improve, we continue treatment. I've never had a patient report a side effect from taking CoQ10."

Korotkin learned about CoQ10 from reading an article in a health magazine that described research being done with the nutrient at Scott-White Medical Center in Temple, Texas, and Tufts University in Boston. Contacting researchers at Scott-White, he referred some patients there for CoQ10 treatment. Later, after assuring himself that CoQ10 obtained from a health food store was pure and full strength (he sent a sample to Texas researchers for evaluation), he began treating selected patients with CoQ10. "I was skeptical about CoQ10 before I tried it," he says. "CoQ10 doesn't work for everybody, but it's an option for many patients who have no other road to travel."

CoQ10 is sold over-the-counter as a nutritional supplement.

Thyroid

An underfunctioning thyroid gland may be the cause of many—if not most—heart attacks, says Stephen E. Langer, M.D., coauthor of *Solved: The Riddle of Illness* (New Canaan, Conn.: Keats Publishing Co., 1984). Langer's interest in thyroid function developed when he came across the work of Dr. Broda O. Barnes. After thirty-five years of medical practice, Barnes concluded that at least 40 percent of the American people are deficient in thyroid hormone, a condition called hypothyroidism. Among the many illnesses that result from thyroid deficiency are atherosclerosis and heart attack, according to Barnes.[118]

Langer, who has practiced preventive medicine in Berkeley, California, since 1973, says that most of his patients with low thyroid tend to have high cholesterol and triglyceride levels. Given appropriate amounts of thyroid, their lipid levels go down 10 to 20 percent, he said. Langer uses natural desiccated thyroid, "a more complete substance" than its synthetic counterpart. He starts patients who need thyroid on a quarter- to half-grain supplement; if signs of deficiency persist, he increases the dosage gradually. Along with thyroid, Langer gives vitamin supplements, particularly vitamins B6, C, and E.

As a clue to whether you are hypothyroid, Langer recommends taking the Barnes Basal Temperature Test. To perform this simple test, he says:

Before going to bed tonight, shake down a thermometer. Leave it on the bedside table. As soon as you wake up in the morning after a good night's sleep, tuck the thermometer snugly in your armpit for ten minutes as you lie in bed.

If your thyroid function is normal, your temperature should be in the range from 97.8° to 98.2° F. If it's lower, you are probably hypothyroid, meaning that your thyroid gland is underfunctioning. The test should be done on two consecutive days.

Langer advises a woman to choose a time when she is not menstruating because temperature fluctuates at this time.

A Program to Protect the Heart

In this section we've looked at a whole foods diet to protect the heart along with an assortment of nutrients—and much more. Here's how Schachter puts it all together.

"We look at three areas of a person's life—diet, exercise, and stress management," Schachter said. "Of the three, diet is primary." Schachter explained how he assesses a patient's nutritional status:

> If you were my patient, after doing a physical and the standard lab tests, I'd ask you to keep a food diary for at least a week. I want to find out if you're eating plenty of whole foods—vegetables and fruits and grains—or whether your diet is high in processed foods. Food processing kills a lot of the nutrients, which leads to nutritional deficiencies. Processed food is also high in sugar, which may be as harmful as animal fats. My concern is not about eggs but about fats. The important thing is to avoid the bad fats—margarine is the worst—and make sure you're getting enough of the good oils; that is, the essential fatty acids. I'd recommend that you include plenty of fiber in your diet, especially the soluble fibers, which inhibit absorption of cholesterol.

These recommendations are only broad guidelines, Schachter said. As Roger J. Williams emphasized, we each have our own nutritional needs.

> Although I don't recommend meat-eating to most of my patients, if I were treating an individual, such as an Eskimo, from a very cold climate, I could certainly include a reasonable amount. In the same way, treating an African-American, whose ancestors subsisted on a grain-based diet, I wouldn't hesitate to eliminate meat. In addition to these dietary changes, it's wise to supplement with vitamins, but my greatest concern is mineral deficiencies, which are closely linked to heart disease. Not only food processing but the use of artificial fertilizers removes a good part of these trace minerals. The four minerals I'm most concerned about are magnesium—that's the biggie—selenium, chromium, and copper.

Determining mineral levels is not a simple matter, he said; in some instances, standard tests are inaccurate or not available. At such times, hair analysis or kinesiology can be useful. Kinesiology is a simple arm test to demonstrate which factors in the environment—specific foods, drugs, even music—strengthen or weaken an individual. Here's how Schachter and the coauthors of *Food, Mind and Mood* describe how to do it:

1. To test your muscle strength, stand with your arm outstretched, palm down, while your partner (the test takes two) pushes down quickly and firmly, attempting to force your arm to your side. In most cases you will test strong, meaning that you are able to exert pressure to resist.

2. To test a food for sensitivity, chew a small amount without swallowing, while your partner repeats the arm test. If your arm remains as strong as before, this food "agrees" with your body. But if your arm is weaker, you may be sensitive to this food.

Sometimes clinical signs are the best indications of mineral deficiencies, he said:

> If you have body twitches or muscle cramps, I can be pretty certain you're deficient in one or more of the essential minerals. White spots on the nails is a sign of zinc deficiency. People who have been on diuretics for an extended period of time and complain of weakness and fatigue are low in magnesium and potassium.
>
> Lastly, it's important to evaluate an individual's thyroid function.

How does one's cholesterol level figure in this program? Schachter said, "If you simply attack the cholesterol and try to lower it, you will not be getting to the heart of the problem. But if you correct certain deficiencies and that results in the cholesterol level going down, then it's likely that you will actually reduce the risk of heart attack."

Proof that Nutrition Saves Lives

Can a diet and nutrient program *reverse* heart disease? This was the question that a Johns Hopkins-trained cardiovascular surgeon, Dr. James Pershing Isaacs, set out to answer three decades ago.

In the early 1960s, Isaacs and an associate initiated a study involving 25 heart patients, all of whom had had at least one heart attack and were doing poorly with conventional heart treatment. These patients typified the "high-risk" patient: over half had been heavy smokers and had high blood pressure; one third were overweight; several had cholesterol levels above 330 milligrams. For ten years, the doctors treated them with vitamins E and C, a low-dose multivitamin, and supplements of zinc, copper, and manganese. The regimen also included small doses of estrogen and thyroid hormones. According to accepted predictions (established by Dr. Jeremiah Stamler, professor of cardiology at Northwestern University), at least half of the patients should have been dead after five years, and all after ten years. But this was not the case. At the end of ten years, only two patients had died. One was a construction worker who, after only three months on the program, discontinued the regimen and went back to work; the other patient, a seven-year veteran of the program, underwent extensive surgery and died of complications.

What prompted a heart surgeon to devise a nutritional program for his patients? "In the 1940s, I was convinced that the mechanical approach was the answer to heart disease," Isaacs said. "But after several years in the field, I realized that the key to this major killer—to the entire science of medicine— was nutrition." Isaac's approach was that of a scientist (as evidenced by the book he coauthored, *Complementarity in Biology* (Baltimore: Johns Hopkins Press, 1969), but his concern was with the heart patient.

On February 21, 1974, Isaacs presented what he described as "an encouraging study" to colleagues attending the Texas Heart Institute Symposium on Coronary Artery Medicine and Surgery in Houston (then, as now, the center of cardiac surgery). One can guess how this group of heart specialists reacted to a simple nutritional program that produced such spectacular results. Dr. Robert Vance of Las Vegas, one of Isaacs's many admirers, informed me that Isaacs's presentation was omitted from the printed proceedings of the conference. Later, thanks to support from a group of grateful patients and friends, Isaacs's paper, "Trace Metals, Vitamins, and Hormones in Ten-Year Treatment of Coronary Atherosclerotic Heart Disease," was printed and donated to the Library of Congress.[119]

On the heels of the conference, Isaacs suffered a devastating blow of a different nature. Shortly after the cardiac conference, a front-page story appeared in the *National Enquirer*—"Johns Hopkins surgeon says he can save all heart patients." Crushed by this notoriety, which intensified his estrangement from his colleagues, Isaacs retired to private practice in Fruitland, Maryland. His lifesaving program was gathering dust in the archives until a group of nutritional physicians stumbled on it and incorporated his findings in their practice.

In case you wish to discuss Isaacs's nutritional regimen with your doctor, you can obtain a reprint of his study by sending $2 to Daniel H. Duffy, C.D.C., 1953 S. Broadway, Geneva, Ohio 44041.

LOOKING AHEAD

We know that an uncompromising fresh food diet "works"—prevents heart attacks and even reverses clogged arteries. But will it sell? Can a diet that eschews factory-made food—meaning practically everything in the supermarket except what's in the produce department—compete with attractively packaged "no cholesterol" products? Can such a diet induce doctors not to prescribe a cholesterol-lowering drug? One hopeful note is that today the average American is buying ten pounds more of both fruit and vegetables per year than a decade ago.[120]

4

Chelation Therapy

Over 60 million people have some form of heart disease. This year more than 500,000 people will die of heart attack, while others can't walk more than a few yards without experiencing crushing chest pain called angina. In 1987, 332,000 people underwent surgery because of clogged arteries, but this operation, the coronary bypass, provides temporary relief at best and is not a cure. Another popular procedure used to clear clogged arteries, balloon angioplasty, has to be repeated in one third of patients. But a simple, time-tested procedure exists that can prevent or reverse atherosclerosis (hardening of the arteries), and thus reduce the risk of associated conditions such as heart attack and stroke. The procedure is chelation (key-LAY-shun) therapy. For reasons you'll learn about in this chapter, chelation therapy is one of the world's best-kept secrets but one that could save your life or that of a loved one.

A THUMBNAIL SKETCH OF CHELATION

Chelation comes from the Greek word *chele,* which means "claw." A synthetic amino acid called EDTA (ethylene diamine tetraacetic acid) is slowly dripped into a vein, and once in the bloodstream, claws or grasps heavy toxic metals in the body. This use of chelation—to remove toxic metals such as lead or mercury—was approved by the FDA in the early 1950s. But chelation has another effect, which is to restore circulation to arteries blocked by plaque. And this broader application of chelation is *not* approved by the FDA, for reasons we'll discuss. Chelation therapy is painless, noninvasive, and given in a doctor's office. Patients with hardening of the arteries generally require a

118

minimum of thirty treatments given once or twice a week at a cost of $75 to $120 per treatment. Around one thousand physicians provide chelation therapy. Patients with a severe condition frequently continue having treatments once a month as maintenance. Each IV drip takes three and a half to four hours to allow the infusion of EDTA combined with other nutrients to slowly circulate through the 60,000 miles of blood vessels in the body. During this period patients chat with one another, watch TV, read, or sleep, ensconced in reclining chairs.

I've visited the offices of several chelation specialists and talked to patients there. Without exception, these patients are ardent supporters of chelation therapy and eager to relate their experiences. Here are a few of these patients.

A Heart Attack Victim. Thomas, a 61-year-old general contractor, had a heart attack at age 37, then in 1979 underwent a triple bypass. "I felt fine after the surgery, but five years later, the veins clogged up and I was dragging. The worst part of it was I couldn't think. I'd sit all day over a set of plans and accomplish nothing. I went back to the heart surgeon figuring I needed another operation, but he said it was too risky to operate again." Fortuitously, at this time Tom ran into a friend who had overcome a serious circulatory problem with chelation therapy, and promptly got in touch with his friend's doctor, Dr. H. Richard Casdorph of Long Beach, California, a Mayo Clinic–trained cardiologist. After a few chelation treatments, "My mind began to function," he said. After one year of chelation (thirty treatments plus once-a-month maintenance), "I'm free of chest pains, my blood pressure is normal, and I've been able to reduce my blood pressure medicine."

Gangrene. Ed's problem (he's a 66-year-old truck driver) was severe blockage of the arteries of the legs. "Four years ago, I developed gangrene-type sores on both feet. Walking was very painful. I knew I was in danger of losing my legs—that's what happened to my brother." But Ed didn't suffer his brother's fate. He read about chelation therapy and learned about Dr. Casdorph. "I started chelation in 1983, and after the fifth or sixth treatment I could hardly believe it—the terrible pain was gone. By the sixty-fifth treatment, the sores on my feet had disappeared." Continuing with a monthly maintenance treatment, Ed has had no further problems.

Angina. Four years ago, Darrell, a medical products inventor in Salt Lake City, was rushed to the emergency room with severe angina (chest pain). Darrell was then 46. A cardiologist performed a balloon angioplasty (see pages 85–86) followed by a coronary angiogram (an invasive diagnostic procedure to show the extent of blockage in the arteries). Darrell's doctor then gave him the bad news that his coronary artery disease was incurable, and even if he had a coronary bypass, the odds of his living another ten years were only 50/50. Darrell began reading everything he could find about heart disease, and coming across a book about chelation, tracked down a former Salt Lake City physician, Dr. Robert B. Vance, in Las Vegas. Darrell, skeptical about quick "cures"—as a medical inventor he had seen too many fail—told Vance he wanted to talk to some of Vance's patients. Encouraged by the success stories he heard, Darrell embarked on chelation. After the tenth treatment, "I felt so good I went out and played golf." Darrell now has two treatments every three months and credits chelation with keeping him alive.

Safe and Effective

Chelation has an amazing track record. As Dr. Elmer Cranton, co-author of *Bypassing the Bypass,* describes it, for the past thirty years, "chelation has been used safely over six million times in over 400,000 patients in the U.S. alone. Its success rate in improving blood flow in patients with clogged arteries is close to 82 percent." Cranton, a Harvard Medical School graduate, is proud of his own record. He states that he has been using EDTA to treat patients with hardening of the arteries for twenty years, "with marked and lasting benefit in 75 to 95 percent of patients. . . . No harm has come to any of these patients as a result of EDTA therapy."[1]

As occurs in the beginning phases of any new therapy, there were "serious problems with the early administration [in the late 1950s and early 1960s] of EDTA for atherosclerosis," says Dr. James P. Carter, professor of nutrition at Tulane University School of Public Health and co-investigator in a major chelation study. Giving too high a dosage of EDTA and giving it too fast resulted in several deaths attributed to kidney failure. A small group of physicians who were treating patients with EDTA chelation soon developed a safe protocol. This protocol, Carter estimates, has been used in nearly 500,000 patients.[2]

In 1972 this group of doctors founded an organization now called the American College for Advancement in Medicine (ACAM). ACAM, based in Laguna Hills, California, provides training for physicians in chelation therapy and certifies those who qualify. ACAM holds a twice-a-year annual conference, attended by 200 physicians, which provides the latest findings and procedures in preventive nutritional medicine.

Too Good to be True?   Chelation specialists generally represent chelation as a therapy that reverses atherosclerosis and, by doing so, reduces blood pressure, forestalls heart attacks and strokes, and relieves angina pains. But countless patients have told their doctors that they have improved sexual function, better vision, and reduced symptoms of a whole host of diseases, including arthritis, multiple sclerosis, Parkinson's disease, and psoriasis.

Physicians, according to Cranton, are apt to soft-pedal the benefits of chelation that do not stem directly from atherosclerosis: "It's downright embarrassing to be endorsing a treatment that sounds like a cure-all," Cranton says.[3]

Critics of chelation have derided these multiple benefits as "snake oil," but, as Cranton explained, "these benefits and others naturally occur when blood flow is improved throughout the body."

I've Never Heard of It.   If chelation therapy is such an effective and safe treatment for atherosclerosis, why isn't it better known? Why doesn't your own doctor give chelation treatments or refer patients to a physician who is trained in this procedure? Since the early 1960s, when articles about chelation first appeared in the medical literature, the medical establishment has waged an unrelenting campaign to stamp out the procedure. Spearheading the attack is the American Medical Association, which describes chelation therapy to treat atherosclerosis as "an experimental process without proven efficacy." When investigative reporter Gary Null, in preparation for an article in *Penthouse* (February 1986) requested information about chelation from the AMA, among the materials he received was a reprint of a 1975 article mentioning a death that had occurred before safety procedures for EDTA had been established.

Other divisions of the medical establishment participate in giving a distorted view of chelation. Until very recently, editors of journals rejected articles or letters to the editor favorable to EDTA chelation. The media, taking its clue from the AMA and allied health organizations, ignores chelation or portrays it as quackery. An article in *Science News* compares chelation therapy to patent medicines as "a quick and easy fix to medical problems."[4] The *Harvard Medical School Health Letter* describes chelation as "an elaborate placebo . . . (one that) can afford quite a high income to those who promote it."[5]

What's the motive behind the hostile attitude on the part of the medical establishment? Economics of the marketplace seems a likely answer. Coronary artery bypass surgery is a $3.3-billion-a-year industry "providing a financial windfall to hospitals, drug and equipment manufacturers, and guaranteed employment to a small army of highly specialized, highly paid surgical and postsurgical coronary care teams,"[6] and chelation poses a direct threat to the thriving bypass industry. The author of a *Science News* article highly critical of chelation acknowledges that "chelation therapy is being sought out by many people as an alternative to conventional medical treatments, most notably coronary bypass surgery."[7]

The only disadvantage to choosing chelation therapy is that, without Food and Drug Administration (FDA) approval, health insurance carriers, in most cases, will not cover the cost. A spokesperson at the Fetzer Foundation in Kalamazoo, Michigan, which is supporting research into chelation therapy, described a case that shows the irrationality of the insurance situation. "A woman, who had gangrene in one leg, was advised by several physicians that amputation was the only available option to deal with the condition. Yet, after her leg was saved through chelation therapy, the medical carrier would not cover the $4,000 cost of chelation, but was willing to pay $15,000 if she had had her leg amputated."

This discriminatory situation may soon be ancient history. A long-awaited FDA study (partly funded by the Fetzer Foundation) is under way at Walter Reed Army Medical Center in Washington, D.C., and Letterman Army Medical Center in San Francisco. Two double-blind studies are being conducted at Baylor Medical Center in Houston. One double-blind study, completed in Brazil, is scheduled for publication in *The Journal of the National Medical Association*.

HOW DOES CHELATION WORK?

As we've discussed, chelation therapy removes toxic metals from the body. These toxic metals, primarily iron and copper but also lead, mercury, and cadmium, are troublemakers that interfere with enzyme activity and increase production of free radicals. (Free radicals are unstable oxygen molecules that cause atherosclerosis and other degenerative diseases and accelerate the aging process.) Reducing free radical activity, which causes oxidative damage to the body, is probably the secret of chelation therapy's success, says Dr. J. P. Frackelton of Cleveland, coauthor of a chapter on the subject in *Bypassing Bypass*. Frackelton and Cranton theorized that EDTA binds toxic heavy metal ions, "making them chemically inert and removing them from the body."[8] EDTA then passes out in the urine during the first twenty-four hours following treatment. Other effects of EDTA help alleviate symptoms. Removing calcium from the cell increases circulation in the branch arteries; decreasing the stickiness of the blood cells reduces the tendency of the blood to clot.

The free radical concept that Frackelton and other physicians propose as a scientific basis to explain the diverse benefits of EDTA chelation therapy has been ridiculed by chelation critics. But a growing body of research on the mechanism of disease supports the free radical theory as a rationale for chelation. A landmark article by Dr. Daniel Steinberg and coworkers in *The New England Journal of Medicine* (April 6, 1989) refers to EDTA as a free radical "inhibitor." The authors state that oxidative damage, which requires the presence of large concentrations of copper or iron, can be controlled by reducing amounts of these metals with the use of EDTA "or other metal chelators."[9] Free radical damage contributes to aging as well as disease, which is why so many physicians who administer EDTA chelation therapy to their patients take it themselves as a preventive.

How It All Started

Chelation therapy was first used to treat lead poisoning in the early 1950s and, as I mentioned earlier, it is approved for this use as well as other cases of heavy metal toxicity by the FDA. One of the doctors who first used EDTA to treat factory workers with lead poisoning was Dr. Norman E. Clarke, director of research at Providence Hospital in Detroit. Clarke observed that after a series of chelation treatments, patients' health appeared to improve, including that of a patient with coronary artery disease whose symptoms of angina disappeared. Aware that calcium was involved in plaque formation, Clarke speculated that removing calcium might be beneficial to patients with atherosclerosis and its complications. Clarke and colleagues then treated other heart patients with EDTA and subsequently reported on their results.[10,11]

According to Morton Walker, author of *Chelation Therapy: How to Prevent or Reverse Hardening of the Arteries,* Clarke's reports stirred up interest among other university-based physicians. Lawrence E. Melzer, M.D., and J. Roderick Kitchell, M.D., then head of the Department of Cardiology at the Presbyterian Hospital in Philadelphia, gave 2,000 infusions of EDTA to 81 subjects during a two-year period. In a 1961 scientific article, the authors concluded that "the drug can be used without danger." Two years later, in an interview in *Medical World News,* Kitchell described the remarkable benefits of EDTA in patients with gangrene of the legs who otherwise would have required amputation. But one month after this interview, a negative "reappraisal" of EDTA by the two authors appeared in a medical journal. According to Walker, this 1963 "reappraisal" article "changed all orthodox medical thinking about the therapy."[12]

In 1964 another prominent physician, Dr. Alfred Soffer, then associate in medicine at Northwestern University Medical School, wrote a book, *Chelation Therapy,* in which he stated that atherosclerotic patients suffering from blockage in the blood vessels of the legs appeared to benefit from repeated administration of EDTA, especially those patients with diabetes.[13] But Soffer has since become a leading critic of chelation therapy. Replying to my inquiry about chelation studies, Soffer, now executive director of the American College of Chest Physicians, wrote to say how "disturbed" he was about chelation clinics.[14] Why the turnabout on the part of these influential physicians? Were they "pressured into a change of heart" as Dr. Walker states? Whatever the answer, since the early 1960s, the use of EDTA in the United States as a treatment for circulatory problems has been the province of alternative physicians.

Thus far, most of what you've read here about the benefits of chelation therapy constitutes what standard medicine calls "anecdotal evidence," on a par with gossip. They say these claims of chelation's effectiveness are meaningless without a double-blind study. But clearly this is a Catch-22 situation. Pharmaceutical companies, the big spenders in funding controlled trials to test a marketable drug, have no interest in a substance like EDTA, because its patents have expired. Starting in the mid-1970s, ACAM leaders repeatedly petitioned the FDA to conduct a scientific trial of EDTA, but requests were turned down until 1987 when the FDA approved such a study. For the next two years, the study was delayed by an assortment of bureaucratic roadblocks, however. With no prospects of a trial taking place, chelation specialists with expertise in research methods conducted and paid for their own EDTA studies.

When Casdorph first began chelating patients (he was then chief of internal medicine at the Long Beach Community Hospital and assistant clinical professor of medicine at the University of California Medical School in Irvine), he was amazed by the results he observed. "Those with angina said their chest pains had disappeared, and none of these patients experienced any side effects." Questioning whether chelation therapy might have a placebo effect, Casdorph designed a study, which was conducted by internists at the hospital to avoid investigator bias. "We tested two groups of patients — heart patients and those with brain disorders — before and after twenty chelation treatments. (A basic series has since been upped to thirty treatments.) The tests showed that heart patients, stroke patients, and those with brain disorders (Alzheimer's) improved significantly after chelation therapy."

Casdorph, author of over fifty scientific articles published in prestigious journals, submitted this study to *The New England Journal of Medicine* "with full confidence" that it would be accepted. Then came the rude awakening to the reality of medical politics. "The editor rejected my article, as did every other leading journal." Casdorph's study was finally published in *The Journal of Holistic Medicine.*[15]

A Heart Surgeon Discovers Chelation.   Another chelation study was presented at an ACAM meeting in May 1987 by an unlikely investigator, Dr. Ralph Lev, a Mayo Clinic–trained cardiovascular surgeon. Lev, who was then clinical associate professor of surgery at the University of New Jersey Medical School, thought chelation therapy was "worthless" until his father-in-law suffered a stroke:

> The old gentleman, who had been very active, was completely incapacitated — he couldn't get out of a chair by himself or take care of his bodily functions. After a few months of caring for him at home, his doctor told us there was no hope of recovery, and recommended that we put Sam in a nursing home and let him die. It was then that I remembered the claims that chelation could help stroke victims and others with

circulatory problems. As a last ditch effort, I contacted a doctor who used chelation, and asked him to look at Sam. Much to my surprise, this doctor thought he could help Sam. For the next eight weeks, my father-in-law received thirty-two chelation treatments. Almost at once he showed signs of improvement, but the most dramatic change occurred the fourth week, when he began to walk and talk. By the end of the series he was his old self, even better.

To refute the charges raised by his colleagues that EDTA causes harmful side effects, Lev, who is now certified in chelation, conducted a study of 99 patients with varying degrees of circulatory problems; each received up to forty chelation treatments. Before chelation started and after each series of ten treatments, patients were evaluated by means of blood, urine, kidney, liver, and noninvasive vascular tests. "Results show that chelation did not produce any deleterious effects," Lev said. "There was no variation in red blood count, calcium levels remained constant; in regard to renal (kidney) function, toxicity of EDTA was minimal."

Chelation Study with a Cast of Thousands. A blockbuster of a study, reported in 1988, spanned two continents and involved close to 3,000 patients. The two investigators, Drs. James P. Carter of the Tulane University School of Public Health and Efrain Olszewer, clinical cardiologist at the Clínica Tuffik Mattar in São Paulo, Brazil, treated 2,870 patients who had various types of chronic degenerative disease. Each was examined before and after chelation. The investigators found that patients with peripheral vascular disease and ischemic heart disease benefited the most from chelation. (Peripheral vascular disease is any abnormal condition that affects the blood vessels outside the heart and the lymphatic vessels. Ischemic heart disease is caused by blockage of blood flow through the coronary arteries, resulting in a lack of oxygenated blood reaching the heart muscle.) Of the patients with peripheral vascular disease and blocked arteries of the legs (intermittent claudication), 90 percent showed marked improvement after chelation treatments, as did 76.9 percent of patients with ischemic heart disease.[16]

Proof Positive That Chelation Works. The first double-blind study testing the effectiveness of EDTA as a treatment for patients with peripheral vascular disease (in this case, blocked arteries of the legs) was reported in 1989 by Olszewer and Carter. In this study, 10 male patients with hardening of the arteries of the legs were randomly assigned to receive either EDTA plus magnesium sulfate and vitamin C (a usual combination) or a placebo of magnesium sulfate, B-complex, and vitamin C. Each patient received twenty intravenous infusions. After ten treatments, some patients showed dramatic improvement—they could walk farther and perform better on the bicycle stress test. Laboratory tests confirmed these changes. Therefore, the code specifying who received EDTA or placebo was broken. Those patients who had improved had all been treated with EDTA; those in the placebo group showed no change. During the rest of the trial, patients who had received a placebo were given ten infusions of EDTA and improved to the same degree as those patients in the first group after ten treatments.[17]

Laboratory Evidence. In 1985, members of the Great Lakes Association of Clinical Medicine, Inc. (GLACM) invested in a laboratory study called the Cypher Study (the first major study of its kind). The Cypher Study involved 20,000 patients who had received chelation therapy, along with dietary counseling. (As a control, the study included several hundred patients with atherosclerosis who had not been given chelation.) The study was conducted by Therma Scan, Inc., a laboratory in St. Clair Shores, Michigan, that specializes in thermograph studies. (Thermology, which identifies variations in heat patterns throughout the body, is an established diagnostic technique for peripheral vascular disease and other conditions.)

Chelation patients were studied before and after receiving treatment. Patients in the control group who received no chelation were studied at arbitrary times. The study was "blind," meaning that the examiners did not know which patients had received chelation and which ones had not. The data was then analyzed by statisticians.

The Cypher Study showed that 79 percent of the 20,000 patients who received chelation treatment experienced significant improvement in circulation in the arms and legs. The degree of improvement was dose related; a patient who received only five treatments showed much less improvement than one who received forty treatments. Patients in the control group showed no improvement in blood flow. (The Cypher Study is unpublished as yet.)

The discouraging fact about these impressive studies is that your doctor probably knows nothing about them. As Casdorph discovered early in his career as a chelation specialist, leading medical journals will not publish an article that says anything favorable about chelation therapy. Consequently, many chelation studies are relegated to alternative journals, which are not listed in *Index Medicus,* the guide to medical literature, and are not available for a computer search on chelation therapy. As a result, most doctors never read anything about chelation other than propaganda disseminated by the medical establishment, which calls chelation experimental, ineffective, and a form of quackery.

Where to Find Help

You've learned enough about the benefits of chelation therapy to recognize that chelation is an economic threat to the entire "heart industry." Consequently, the medical establishment uses various tactics to put its potential competitor out of business. One is to harass the chelation specialist.

In some cases, the state medical board charges the doctor with improper behavior. In other cases, hospital boards remove some of the doctors' privileges, or universities demote them. In most instances, justice eventually prevails, but the process is enormously time-consuming and costly for the physician involved.

This campaign on the part of the medical establishment to discredit chelation and suppress information about it may be about to end. In its October 1989 issue, *FDA Consumer* listed chelation therapy as one of "Top 10 Health Frauds." But after an ACAM official alerted the publication to the ongoing clinical trials, *FDA Consumer* apologized for the error.[18]

To locate a qualified chelation specialist in your area, contact The American College of Advancement in Medicine (ACAM), 23121 Verdugo Drive, Suite 204, Laguna Hills, CA 92653, (1/800) 532–3688 (outside California) or (1/800) 435–6199 (inside California). Or, if you live in one of the states surrounding the Great Lakes, contact the Great Lakes Association of Clinical Medicine, Inc. (GLACM), Executive Director Jack Hank, 70 W. Huron Street, Chicago, IL 60610, (312) 266–6246. GLACM members, physicians and osteopaths, practice preventive/nutritional medicine and offer chelation therapy.

THE MANY BENEFITS OF CHELATION

Although most alternative physicians use EDTA chelation primarily as a treatment to reverse hardening of the arteries, some of Casdorph's patients had ailments other than atherosclerosis. Ann, a 58-year-old homemaker with severe arthritis pain in her hips and knees, began having totally pain-free days after only seven treatments. Another plus: Ann's blood pressure, which was too high, dropped 30 points. Casdorph comments, "A common form of arthritis, which may be due to calcium deposits on the joint, seems to be improved by chelation. I have not seen much improvement in patients with rheumatoid arthritis."

Gene, whose blood pressure fluctuated continually and who complained of feeling listless and tired and sleeping badly, was found to have extremely high levels of cadmium and lead in his body. After seven treatments, Gene's blood pressure stabilized for the first time in years, and he felt more energetic.

Alzheimer's Disease

Chelation can help victims in the early stage of Alzheimer's disease. Each year 337,000 people are diagnosed with Alzheimer's, a disease that results in progressive deterioration of brain function.

According to Casdorph, "Chelation performs a dual function. The treatment not only increases blood flow to the brain but chelates and removes aluminum from brain tissue. There's strong evidence that aluminum is a contributory cause of Alzheimer's." A University of Toronto researcher, Dr. Donald McLachlan, has found that the brains of Alzheimer's victims show a much higher concentration of aluminum than is found in people who die of other causes. In chelating patients with Alzheimer's, McLachlan used a chelating substance called deferoxamine, which is even better at removing aluminum than EDTA.[19]

Diabetes

If you are an insulin-dependent diabetic, chelation therapy may enable you to dispense with insulin shots and other diabetes medication. That's the startling preliminary finding of a recently completed Canadian study.

As Dr. Paul Cutler of Willowdale, Ontario, described his study: "I was treating a group of diabetics—32 in all—who were doing poorly; despite diet and medication, their blood sugar was going up and they needed increasing amounts of drugs, either insulin or pills. Testing their mineral levels I found that a number had significantly high levels of iron." This abnormality had not been detected before because doctors don't ordinarily test for iron in diabetics unless they suspect a rather rare disease called hemochromatosis, he said. Although these patients did not have that disease, their iron levels were elevated. Cutler, who was board-certified in chelation in 1983, chelated these 32 patients to remove the iron, using a chelator called deferoxamine (the same chelating agent used by McLachlan with Alzheimer's patients).

Of the 32 patients who were chelated (they averaged two treatments a week), Cutler reports, "24 were totally free of all medication within eight to thirteen weeks. I was amazed! The next step is to run a control—take diabetics who have normal levels of iron and chelate them. This way you can tell whether deferoxamine has some action other than removing iron." (One reason Cutler originally began using deferoxamine was that EDTA, except when used for lead and other metal poisoning, is banned in the province of Ontario in which he practices. EDTA is also banned in the province of British Columbia.)

After an article describing his study was rejected by several medical journals ("Not enough reader interest," one editor wrote), Cutler submitted his paper to *Diabetes,* and it was accepted. In Cutler's estimation, the consequences of this study are mind-boggling: "Chelating with deferoxamine could cure one third of adult diabetes, supposedly an incurable disease."[20]

Cutler's research is not the first use of EDTA to treat diabetes. In the early 1960s, two Philadelphia heart specialists reported that chelating diabetics with EDTA enabled some of these patients to reduce or discontinue insulin injections.[21] But EDTA treatment for diabetes was largely forgotten until now.

Mercury Poisoning

The toxic metals that chelators commonly refer to are iron, lead, and cadmium. But mercury, the second worst toxic metal (number one is plutonium), belongs on this list, says a Reno, Nevada, physician.

Mercury enters your body each time your dentist fills a tooth with a silver amalgam, a filling material that has been in use for 150 years. Mercury is used to harden the filling.

Dentists who advocate mercury-free dentistry contend that even the smallest amount of mercury is highly toxic. These "dissident" dentists (the American Dental Association's term) link continuous absorption of mercury with a range of diseases including multiple sclerosis, Hodgkin's disease (involving the lymph nodes), mental disorders including manic depression, hypoglycemia, and hyperactivity in children. They recommend that patients with "mercury amalgams" (a term they prefer to "silver") who have symptoms indicating mercury toxicity have their amalgams removed and replaced with a composite filling material.

But merely removing the constant source of mercury isn't enough to rid the patient of symptoms, says Dr. Donald E. Soli of Reno, Nevada. Tests show that mercury inhaled over the years is deposited in the pituitary gland, parts of the brain, the kidneys, and the liver. Unless this overload of mercury is removed by chelation, the patient remains sick.

One of Soli's patients, 20-year-old Jonathan, was away at college when his distraught father consulted Soli. According to Soli, "The boy had been an excellent student but now couldn't concentrate, his father said. He slept all the time, was depressed, possibly suicidal. A few months later, Jonathan, who had quit college, came to see me." Checking for silver amalgams, Soli found twelve. "These fillings were shiny, like highly polished metal." On his dentist's recommendation, Jonathan had been rinsing with hydrogen peroxide, which oxidized the fillings, freeing the mercury. (For people who are sensitive to mercury, using hydrogen peroxide in the presence of silver amalgams can create a host of symptoms.) A hair analysis confirmed Soli's suspicions that Jonathan's problem was mercury toxicity. The first step was to initiate chelation treatment before the dentist removed his amalgams. "Removing amalgams, which involves drilling, exposes the patient to large amounts of mercury, which is inhaled and absorbed into the bloodstream," Soli explained. "But chelating the patient the day before his amalgams are removed protects him at a time of high exposure. If he has a high level of EDTA in his bloodstream (EDTA remains in the blood around twenty-four hours), the chelating agent binds to this fresh influx of mercury ions, like handcuffing a criminal."

In addition to a chelation treatment the day before amalgam removal, Soli recommends having another treatment on the day of removal and one the next day as a starter. "In a mercury-sensitive patient, it generally takes twenty treatments to remove the mercury that may have been collecting for years."

After twenty chelation treatments, Jonathan was his old energetic self; his powers of concentration restored, he returned to college. "My last report was that he was a 3.8 student."

More Problems with Metal Toxicity

Another patient of Soli's, 28-year-old Denise, had been plagued with a multitude of symptoms most of her adult life. "She had severe dermatitis—oozing sores on her forehead, infected teeth, inflamed gums. She always felt tired and was agoraphobic; she couldn't walk into a supermarket or ride in an automobile." Tests showed that she had high levels of toxic mercury and nickel in her system. One source was a stainless steel post that a dentist had inserted in a root canal years ago; another was stainless steel posts on earrings. During the course of thirty-seven chelation treatments, Denise improved gradually; her energy returned and her agoraphobia disappeared.

Parents should be aware that wearing braces can be harmful to youngsters who are sensitive to metal toxicity, Soli said. Before orthodontic treatment, 12-year-old Jennifer had been a popular, lively honors student and cheerleader. But soon after being fitted with braces, she developed pains in her stomach, felt nauseated, and had trouble staying awake in class. Most disturbing was the personality change that took place; she locked herself in her room, became a recluse, attempted suicide. Discovering that Jennifer's problem was metal toxicity, Soli identified the sources: one was dental metals, which consisted of stainless steel clasps in plastic retainers and two silver fillings. The other source was nickel jewelry—"She wore three rings on each hand, which left black stains on her fingers." Removing these sources of toxicity (the orthodontist replaced stainless steel clasps with titanium) plus a series of thirty chelation treatments restored Jennifer to her former happy, healthy self.

LOOKING AHEAD

Hopes for acceptance of chelation therapy as an effective and safe treatment are riding on the FDA study taking place at Walter Reed and Letterman Army Medical Centers. Said a Fetzer Foundation spokesperson, "A controlled clinical trial, if successful, will lead to obtaining FDA approval of chelation therapy for atherosclerosis." Cranton said, "This study, if conducted fairly, will be a major breakthrough. Medicare and all the other insurance companies will be compelled to pay for chelation treatment. The cardiovascular surgeon, instead of rushing a heart patient into a bypass, will offer him the option of chelation therapy. Failure to do so will constitute malpractice."

5

Arthritis— Try Nutrition First

In 1983 I interviewed a young woman named Joan (a former beauty contest winner) who was afflicted with rheumatoid arthritis, the most serious form of that disease. Joan was the leader of a self-help group, sponsored by the Arthritis Foundation, where she taught others how to cope with the disease and its many challenges—getting up from a chair, for instance, wringing out a dishcloth, becoming familiar with the spectrum of arthritis drugs. Joan herself was rarely free of pain but had learned to accept her condition. "When I get a flare-up," she said, "I take a nap or cry it out."

She made no mention of diet, which didn't surprise me; I was familiar with the views of the Arthritis Foundation, which for years had assured the public, "There is no special diet for arthritis. No specific food has anything to do with causing it. And no specific diet will cure it." In the 1970 brochure that contained this statement, the agency warned arthritics against "food fanatics" whose main interest was "personal profit." A leading researcher has recently admitted that rheumatologists' skeptical attitude toward nutritional therapy was based on "little objective information."[1]

By the early 1980s, however, a researcher could explore a link between diet and arthritis without being called a quack. The week I met Joan, I had talked to a professor of medicine at Wayne State University in Detroit who reported promising results from prescribing a low-fat diet to arthritic patients. Eager to share this information with Joan, I asked her about her diet. "Sweets are my weakness," she said unconcernedly. "I'm a chocoholic." Aware that chocolate is one of the sweets that is high in fat, I asked her if she

132

had considered cutting down on these foods. "Oh, no," she said, "the Arthritis Foundation says that diet has nothing to do with arthritis."

At the time of our conversation, the Arthritis Foundation was in the process of changing its stance on diet and arthritis. In 1984, in its revised diet guidelines and research brochure, the Arthritis Foundation stated, "Some researchers suspect that there may be a connection between diet and other forms of rheumatic diseases. Until these connections can be proven scientifically, it would be irresponsible for the Arthritis Foundation . . . to offer a diet as either a cure or as helpful in controlling symptoms of arthritis." Its 1988 brochure on arthritis research states that a number of diet-related research studies are in progress.

As of this writing, the diet and nutrition brochure is being revised once again. "It's too early to recommend any special diet," an Arthritis Foundation spokesperson said, "but we're looking at the effect of a low-fat diet, fish oils, food allergies, the question of how diet affects the immune system."

Health agencies apparently play by different rules than ordinary mortals. The Arthritis Foundation feels no need to apologize to the "food fanatics" whom they accused of wrongdoing. But if apologies are in order, it is to the Joans of this country. These millions of arthritis patients, adhering to the dictates of the Arthritis Foundation, either through exposure to the agency or following the recommendations of their doctors, have ignored diet to what may prove to be their peril.

WHAT IS ARTHRITIS?

Arthritis, or joint inflammation, appears in more than a hundred forms and strikes more than 36 million, or 1 in every 7, Americans. Standard doctors say that its cause is unknown. As the population ages, arthritis is likely to afflict larger numbers; a new case is diagnosed every 33 seconds.[2] Let's take a quick look at the two most common forms of arthritis, osteoarthritis and rheumatoid arthritis.

Osteoarthritis (OA) is the milder form of arthritis and afflicts 16 million Americans. According to the Arthritis Foundation, it is "a disease of the joints that involves a breakdown of cartilage and other tissues which make a moveable joint operate properly. The damage from osteoarthritis is confined to the joints and surrounding tissues, with little or no inflammation." Osteoarthritis is often described by standard doctors as a wear-and-tear disease associated with aging, but it can also develop after damage from injury or infection. Its chief symptom is pain, particularly with movement, and inability to move easily and comfortably. Many OA patients experience stiffness upon arising. The cause of the disease varies from person to person. OA is marked by periods of remission that may last for weeks or even years.

Rheumatoid arthritis (RA) is "the most serious, most painful, the most potentially crippling" form of arthritis, says the Arthritis Foundation. Unlike osteoarthritis, which is largely confined to the joints, rheumatoid arthritis is a systemic disease, meaning that it may affect many parts of the body. It causes inflammation and is a chronic condition. Of the nearly 7 million Americans who have rheumatoid arthritis, most are women. Age at onset is usually between 20 and 40 years. Symptoms are stiffness, aching muscles, fatigue, pain that accompanies motion, and tenderness.

STANDARD TREATMENT

According to the Arthritis Foundation, most treatment programs include some combination of medication, rest, exercise, and methods of protecting the joints, but all patients take one or more of the arthritis drugs. Retail sales of such drugs is estimated at $3 billion per year.

The Drugs in Use

Aspirin, says an Arthritis Foundation brochure, is "the most important drug for arthritis and the safest." To reduce inflammation, high doses of aspirin are required over a prolonged period, which commonly causes nausea or stomach pain, ringing in the ears, and decreased hearing.

There are two categories of drugs that reduce inflammation. One is a group of nonsteroidal anti-inflammatory drugs (NSAIDs), which are claimed to reduce pain and inflammation about as effectively as aspirin and were thought to produce fewer side effects until several recent studies revealed some shocking facts. One study estimated that 20,000 hospitalizations and 2,600 deaths each year could be linked to NSAID use in rheumatoid patients. Several other studies linked the drugs with the development of bleeding ulcers, particularly in elderly patients. Most of the time, patients who started bleeding had no warning symptoms. According to the FDA, "200,000 cases of gastrointestinal bleeding, with 10,000 to 20,000 deaths, occur each year due to the 68 million prescriptions of non-steroidal anti-inflammatory drugs, or NSAIDs, used for arthritis."[3] Some of the most widely used NSAIDs are ibuprofen (brand names Motrin, Advil, Nuprin, and more), piroxicam (brand name Feldene), and indomethacin (brand name Indocin).

After approving the drug misoprostol, to prevent stomach ulcers caused by NSAIDs, the FDA strengthened the wording of the label on NSAIDs to include the warning "Serious gastrointestinal toxicity such as bleeding, ulceration, and perforation can occur at any time, with or without warning symptoms, in patients treated chronically with NSAID therapy."[4]

The other category of drugs that reduce inflammation is the cortico-steroids, powerful cortisonelike drugs that cause major side effects. These include ulcers, mental changes, wasting of muscles in arms and legs, and hair growth over the face. Prolonged use causes loss of calcium.

Other types of drugs used only in severe disease are:

- Gold salts—These benefit over two thirds of patients but cause major side effects including kidney damage and blood cell problems that can produce serious bleeding.
- Penicillamine—This antimalarial drug can damage kidney and bone marrow tissue, which produces blood cells.
- Immunosuppressive or cytotoxic drugs—These drugs, developed to treat cancer (*cytotoxic* means "toxic to cells"), suppress the body's immune system.

Rating Standard Treatment

Standard treatment is estimated to be a $10-billion-a-year industry in the United States. How successful is it? To answer this question, a group of English rheumatologists studied 112 rheumatoid arthritis patients who had received "aggressive" drug treatment at a center for rheumatic diseases in Great Britain from 1964 to 1986. What is unique about this report is that the four investigators followed these RA patients for twenty years. At the end of this period, they found that "over one-third of our patients were dead and more than half were either dead or severely disabled." At the ten-year mark these physicians had been more optimistic about their patients' prognosis since the patients' condition and function had improved in the early years of treatment. But after ten years of treatment, their condition declined consider-ably, joint destruction progressed, and after twenty years, 19 percent of the patients were severely disabled. (Apparently, none of the remaining patients showed any improvement.) The authors conclude that the concept that drugs induce a remission in patients is "fallacious." There may be some benefit in early treatment, they say, but using currently accepted drug treatment, "the prognosis of rheumatoid arthritis is not good."[5]

Another long-term study of rheumatoid arthritis patients, by Dr. Theodore Pincus and colleagues of Vanderbilt University, reported in 1984, presents similar findings. In this study, 75 RA patients were evaluated during the course of nine years of conventional drug therapy. At the end of nine years, 20 of the 75 patients had died. Of the 55 surviving patients, 51 had lost significant functional capacity (for example, 93 percent were no longer able to grip well). These patients had not originally been a sickly group. At the onset of disease, 85 percent of the patients under age 65 had been working full time.[6]

The Arthritis Foundation takes a predictably optimistic view of achievements in arthritis treatment. "Many tests have been developed to aid doctors in diagnosing various types of arthritis. . . . Over the past twenty years, new drugs have been developed to slow down the immune system's response in rheumatoid arthritis and lupus. . . ."[7]

ALTERNATIVE TREATMENT

Nutritional therapy, not drugs, is the cornerstone of alternative treatment. One of the popular arthritis diets is the Dong diet, which is based on an age-old Chinese diet. Another, the "no-nightshades" diet, excludes all members of the nightshade family, which includes tomatoes and white potatoes. Still another diet is the low-fat, largely vegetarian diet. One of these widely practiced regimens is the macrobiotic diet; others are the Pritikin and McDougall diets. Those who advocate these various low-fat diets claim that each can prevent and control, or even cure, degenerative diseases, including arthritis. (For more about the therapeutic diet, see chapter 7.)

Another type of therapy that has proven beneficial to arthritic patients for over four decades is the use of various nutritional supplements. Two recent additions to the list of nutritional helpers are evening primrose oil and fish oils, each a rich source of one of the essential fatty acids.

A treatment for arthritis that relieves symptoms in a large percentage of patients is based on the theory that most arthritic symptoms are allergic reactions. Creators of the Dong diet and no-nightshades diet both attribute the success of their respective diets largely to removing unsuspected food allergens from the diet.

Arthritis and Allergy

The theory that arthritis symptoms are a form of allergic reaction is endorsed by a group of 1,500 physicians in the United States who practice "ecologically oriented" medicine. These "clinical ecologists" are mainly specialists in ear, nose, and throat (otolaryngology), pediatrics, and internal medicine.

Standard allergists, also called clinical immunologists, make up a group of 4,000 physicians in the United States who belong to the American Academy of Allergy and Immunology. Allergists do not recognize clinical ecology as a specialty in allergy, calling the principal techniques used by the clinical ecologists "controversial and unproven."[8] Clinical ecologists, in turn, regard the theory and practices of standard allergy as "restricted and limited."[9]

To explore the possibility that your arthritis symptoms are an allergic reaction and to decide what treatment to investigate, it's important to understand the controversy between the standard allergist and the clinical ecologist.

The *allergist* defines an allergen as a substance capable of producing an antibody reaction within the body. It is this reaction that causes allergy symptoms. The only true allergic substance, therefore, is one that can produce antibodies that can be measured by a blood test. Major allergens are dust, pollen, mold spores, and pets. Food allergies exist, the allergist says, but this type of allergy occurs in a small number of people. A severe food allergy, called an anaphylactic reaction, can be fatal.[10]

The *clinical ecologist* defines an allergen as a substance that creates an abnormal response in one person and not another. This substance can be one of the major allergens, or a frequently eaten food, or the additives or chemicals in that food. It can also be an ordinary chemical in use in the home, office, and workplace. Any of these allergens can produce symptoms in almost every area of the body. These symptoms include behavioral disorders, depression, chronic fatigue, arthritis, hypertension, learning disabilities, schizophrenia, gastrointestinal and respiratory problems, and urinary complaints.[11]

Both the allergist and the clinical ecologist take a detailed history, do a complete physical examination, test with different dilutions of allergy extracts for foods, dust, pollens, molds, and pets, and do a skin test to identify safe doses for beginning allergy treatment. There are differences, however, in the way each conducts a test. For example, an allergist tests twenty to forty items at one time; the clinical ecologist tests one item at a time.

The allergist who has recommended diet diaries and elimination diets and administered allergy tests and is still uncertain about what food the patient is sensitive to may recommend a double-blind placebo-controlled oral food challenge test. This involves the patient's ingesting a suspected food allergen and a placebo, both disguised so that neither the patient nor the doctor knows which is which.

The *clinical ecologist* uses several diagnostic techniques that are not approved by the American Academy of Allergy and Immunology. These include provocative testing, in which a drop of an extract from a suspected allergen is placed under the tongue to see if it provokes symptoms; neutralization, which entails giving the patient a dose of allergen too small to produce a reaction but large enough to allow the patient to tolerate offending substances;[12] a diversified rotation diet, which encourages the patient to eat a highly diversified diet and rotate foods that have the potential to cause adverse reactions by eating them at several-day intervals; and fasting, in which the patient fasts for several days in a chemical-free environment, drinking only spring water, and foods are then introduced one at a time to test the patient's reaction to each substance. (Fasting is reserved for severe cases.)

The *allergist* treats the patient with different drugs to control symptoms and advises the patient to avoid problem foods. The *clinical ecologist* recommends one or more of the following: total avoidance of food allergens, ways to make the home as allergy-proof as possible, dose immunization therapy, and the diversified rotation diet. Drugs are avoided as much as possible.

Arthritis as an Allergic Reaction: the Clinical Ecologists.   The theory that arthritis is in most cases allergy related isn't new; it was recognized as early as 1917.[13] Since then, a succession of allergists have attempted to convince their colleagues of the allergy connection in arthritis with little success. In 1949 Michael Zeller, M.D., showed the cause and effect relationship between consuming certain foods and the onset of arthritic symptoms.[14] Another allergist, Theron G. Randolph, M.D., considered the founder of clinical ecology, reported in the 1950s that environmental chemicals such as perfume, hair spray, tobacco smoke, exhaust fumes, insect sprays, and disinfectants can trigger symptoms of arthritis in susceptible individuals. Testing over a thousand arthritic patients using a method called provocative testing, Randolph demonstrated that their arthritis symptoms were caused by an allergylike sensitivity to many common chemical substances and foods.[15]

Tracking Down the Troublemakers.   Provocative testing, or "single-blind testing," is the way clinical ecologists pinpoint the substances that cause allergic reactions in a patient. The term *single blind* means that the patient is unaware of the type of substance being used. Here's an example of how it works.

Soon after moving into a new house, 35-year-old nurse Helen Jones developed arthritis in her hands, feet, knees, and shoulders. It was so severe she needed crutches. For several years prior to the move, she had experienced extreme fatigue. After being admitted to Theron Randolph's contaminant-free hospital unit in Chicago, she fasted for five days on bottled spring water. At the end of this period she was free of swelling, inflammation, and joint pain and able to walk without crutches for the first time in months.

Then, one by one, she was tested with a series of single food extracts given sublingually (placed under the tongue). "Only ten minutes after eating corn and fifteen minutes after eating cane sugar . . . she came down with severe arthritic pains."[16] When Mrs. Jones eliminated these two foods along with other substances, including household chemicals, she remained free of arthritic symptoms.

Reproducing Arthritis with a Food "Challenge."   A Norwalk, Connecticut, clinical ecologist, Marshall Mandell, M.D., who acknowledges Randolph as his mentor, has tested over 6,000 patients in the past thirty years in this manner. Based on his own experience and that of other clinical ecologists, Mandell says that foods and environmental contaminants—a long list that includes pollen, mold, grasses, and all manner of airborne chemicals—trigger allergic or allergylike symptoms in 80 to 90 percent of all arthritics.

Speaking at a meeting of the Huxley Institute (a society of physicians who specialize in nutrition), Mandell showed videotapes of patients being tested in his office. One was a 68-year-old physician, Dr. William H. Johnson, medical director of the health department in Norwalk. As Dr. Johnson said when we talked by phone, "I had noticed that after eating beef for dinner, I was so stiff the next morning I could hardly get out of bed." One of the many food "challenges" that Mandell tested him with was beef. "Within fifteen minutes I couldn't get out of the chair!" Johnson said. "Since eliminating beef from my diet, I've had no trouble with arthritis."

In another video, a 10-year-old boy, normally well behaved, shouted profanities at his mother after being given an extract of milk. For a layperson, it's astonishing to see these videotapes in which patients react, often in bizarre ways, to minuscule amounts of a food or chemical. Yet standard allergists regard this evidence as unscientific or anecdotal. So to convince skeptical colleagues that allergy is a key factor in arthritis, Mandell conducted a double-blind study in which 30 of his arthritic patients volunteered to take part.[17] (Neither patients nor technicians knew the nature of any of the substances being tested.) "When we tested these patients with a series of common allergens—both food and environmental chemicals—we reproduced arthritic symptoms, as well as nonarthritic ones, in 85 percent of patients," he said.

In one patient, Ms. Smith, a middle-aged woman whose arthritic symptoms had been suppressed by medication while under another physician's care, the return of arthritic symptoms was sudden and dramatic. "When we gave her extract of milk, within a few minutes she developed such severe pain in her hips that she couldn't walk." Prior to the test, Mandell had determined, by means of provocative testing, that the patient was allergic to milk. Subsequently, by eliminating all dairy foods from her diet, Ms. Smith has been free of arthritic symptoms without resorting to drugs.

Mandell's double-blind study, published in 1982, also showed that most arthritics react not to a single allergen but to over a dozen substances (50 percent of the subjects reacted, on the average, to sixteen environmental factors each). The most frequent offender was soybeans; other major ones were coffee, milk, and sugar. In most cases, the allergens are favorite foods that the individual eats on a regular basis.

In the same patient, different foods can cause different symptoms. In one patient, milk caused joint and muscle pains, but potato and pork made her extremely tired. In another patient, chicken and egg caused arthritic symptoms, fatigue, and mental confusion.

A patient who is allergic to one member of a food family, let's say corn (a cereal grain), may not be allergic to other cereal grains such as rye and wheat. Mandell has not found that an arthritic who is sensitive to one of the nightshades will be sensitive to all. In Mandell's study, 10 patients reacted to potato and not to tomato; 9 reacted to tomato and not to potato.

A study of rheumatoid arthritic patients, conducted independently by three clinical ecologists in Chicago, Illinois, Dallas, Texas, and Chadbourn, North Carolina, presents more evidence that foods as well as food additives can induce arthritic symptoms.[18]

Playing Allergy Detective.   If you suspect that allergies might be the cause of your arthritis, can you devise an allergy-free diet on your own?

Sallie B. Bigger of Columbus, Ohio, a 72-year-old retired social worker, accomplished this feat. But as Bigger said, this approach was her last hope.

Bigger's first sign of trouble was pain in her ring finger. It began one morning in June 1954, and over the next twenty years, the disease progressed relentlessly. Knees, feet, elbows, and hands became misshapen; she could no longer walk upright; even her throat muscles were affected, and she could only swallow pureed foods. Meanwhile, she was treated with an increasing number of arthritis drugs, beginning with heavy doses of steroids, which failed to halt the progression of the disease. In constant pain, Bigger retired from her beloved profession and "went home to vegetate."

For Bigger, the most devastating aftermath of RA was gangrenous ulcers of the ankles, which in the mid-1970s required having both legs amputated. The gangrene was caused by steroids prescribed two decades earlier, which destroyed the capillary system in her legs.

At this time, June 1976, when Bigger, a hopeless invalid, was contemplating suicide, she read a newspaper story about Dr. Dong and his belief that RA was an allergic disease. (You'll learn about the Dong diet beginning on page 142.) Promptly obtaining a copy of Dr. Dong's book, she stayed up most of the night reading it and the next morning began the diet.

"Within a month, I noticed dramatic improvement, and over the next six months, the pain was under control," she said. Able once again to eat normally, she began experimenting. One by one, she added other foods to the diet and noted any reactions in her log. Broccoli and other members of the cabbage family caused pain within twelve hours that lasted about thirty-six hours. Some weeks later, she tested broccoli two more times, and when it caused pain on both occasions, banned it from her diet. Other "off-diet" foods, such as an ice cream cone, caused no problem when eaten infrequently, but when she consumed three cones in one week, the third one caused pain.

During this period, Bigger also experimented with arthritis drugs. Of the ten drugs she had been taking, she discontinued three and noted withdrawal symptoms (most often, pain, fatigue, and nervousness) that proved to be short-lived. Soon after eliminating these drugs, skin rashes that had plagued her for years disappeared. I'm not suggesting that you stop taking your arthritis drugs, but I certainly admire Bigger's fighting spirit.

As time progressed, other diverse ailments faded away. Chronic constipation was relieved, nasal congestion disappeared, indigestion gave way to a healthy appetite. At night, no longer awakened by pain, she slept well and felt a surge of her old energy returning.

Today, despite two serious falls, in 1981 and 1983, which caused recurrence of severe pain and necessitated resuming stronger painkillers, Bigger has been able to eliminate those drugs once again and is almost pain-free. She is now under the care of an internist, Owen E. Johnson, M.D., who supports her experimentation and monitors her condition. Dr. Johnson attests that his patient "has shown definite improvement with decreased symptomatology from rheumatoid arthritis. . . ."

Bigger's dream is to interest a research foundation in testing arthritics who follow a custom-tailored, allergy-free diet. Although she has prepared a detailed presentation, which over the past ten years she has submitted to the Arthritis Foundation and other organizations, thus far she has had no takers.

For detailed information on how to isolate and eliminate arthritis-triggering foods and chemicals from your home and work environment, as well as a "lifetime arthritis-relief diet," see *Dr. Mandell's Lifetime Arthritis Relief System* (New York: Coward-McCann, 1983).

To locate a clinical ecologist in your area, write to the American Academy of Environmental Medicine, P.O. Box 16106, Denver, CO 80216 or call (303) 622–9755.

The Allergy Connection Gets a Nod from the Establishment. Rheumatologists, as we've mentioned, have been adamantly opposed to the idea that diet affects arthritis. This attitude is changing, due in large measure to the research of Richard S. Panush, M.D., of the University of Florida College of Medicine.

Pursuing an interest in the relationship between arthritis and food-related allergies, Panush prescribed an experimental diet (the Dong diet) to a group of his RA patients for ten weeks and consequently reported that the diet was no better than a placebo.[19] Later he described his examination of the diet as "naive," pointing out that "some patients showed improvement on the experimental (Dong) diet and had recurrence of symptoms when they deviated from it."[20] Next, Panush conducted a study of 97 arthritics who claimed to have food-induced arthritis. Although Panush concluded then that only a small number of people with rheumatoid arthritis—probably less than 5 percent—have food allergies that can aggravate their condition,[21] one year later, in an editorial in the prestigious *Annals of Internal Medicine,* he sounded positively ebullient about the arthritis-allergy connection: "The notion (that) food or food-related environmental antigens induce or perpetuate symptoms . . . is novel, logical and potentially enlightening."[22]

British rheumatologists, at least those engaged in research, have been swifter to acknowledge the allergy factor in arthritis than their American colleagues. In 1981, two researchers described the dramatic case of a 38-year-old RA patient whose condition, over an eleven-year period, deteriorated markedly despite treatment with various medications.[23] Her problem, as the study showed, was an allergy to dairy foods, particularly cheese. This case history confirms the observation of Mandell and others that the foods we're allergic to are the ones we crave; this woman was in the habit of consuming a pound of cheese a day!

Another British researcher described an RA patient whose losing battle with arthritis had gone on for twenty-five years.[24] This patient was allergic to corn, which ironically was an ingredient in the filler of some of her arthritis medication. Within one week of following a corn-free diet, she improved dramatically (except for one mysterious relapse, which was traced to eating a gravy made with cornstarch thickener). She was then (1981) off all medications, her doctor wrote, "looking and feeling better than in twenty years."

Despite these studies, the arthritis-allergy connection is far from being accepted by arthritis specialists. So don't expect your rheumatologist to welcome your suggestion that you should be tested for allergies. As you've seen in other areas of medicine, there's strong resistance to new ideas, particularly when they threaten economic interests. Explaining why an important study concerning allergy and arthritis was rejected by the journal of the Arthritis Foundation, Mandell pointed to the preponderance of pharmaceutical advertisements in the journal. "If doctors knew that arthritis, in many instances, is an allergic reaction and can be controlled by changing the diet and cleaning up the environment, they'd stop prescribing drugs," he said. Mandell pointed out another reason why rheumatologists resist this approach to arthritis: "The allergy factor in arthritis makes almost everything that these specialists learned in their training obsolete."

ARTHRITIS AND DIET

The Dong Diet

Dr. Collin H. Dong, a San Francisco physician who has practiced family medicine there for fifty years, created the Dong diet as an act of desperation. At age 35, having eaten the standard American diet since beginning medical training, Dong had not only gained forty pounds but was stricken with crippling arthritis. In three years of suffering, "there was nothing that physicians could do for me except prescribe large doses of aspirin," which was causing a severe skin disorder.

Searching for answers, Dong went back to his roots and began eating the "poor man's diet" that he had been brought up on—mainly fish, vegetables, rice, and small amounts of chicken. Within a few months he had shed excess weight, was free of stiffness and joint pain, and could play golf again. Over the years he has recommended the diet to thousands of patients and says that a high percentage have achieved the same favorable results as he. Dong is his own best testimonial; at 85, he continues to practice medicine full time and play golf.

Why It Works.   According to Dong, his diet works for arthritics because arthritis is caused by allergic reactions to certain foods and chemical additives in the food. "It's what you don't eat that counts," he says. The Dong diet excludes (1) meat, (2) fruits, including tomatoes, (3) dairy products of all kinds, (4) vinegar or any other acid, (5) pepper of any variety, (6) hot spices, (7) chocolate, (8) dry roasted nuts, (9) alcoholic beverages, particularly wine, (10) soft drinks, and (11) all additives, preservatives, and chemicals, especially monosodium glutamate.

In light of current information about diet, the Dong diet, devised in the early 1940s, seems almost trendy. First, it wins points as a fish-centered diet. There's good reason why Anne M. Fletcher, M.S., R.D., author of *Eat Fish, Live Better* (New York: Harper & Row, 1989), describes fish as the number one health food. Dutch investigators, who studied 852 middle-aged men over a period of twenty years, made headlines when they reported in 1985 that consuming as little as one ounce of fish a day cut one's risk of dying from heart disease in half.[25] Fish oils also appear to benefit arthritics. (More about fish oil and arthritis on pages 146–147.) Being meatless, the Dong diet is also low in fat. Owing to liberal amounts of vegetables and rice, the diet is high in fiber. The foods that are excluded from the diet—tomatoes, chocolate, and nuts—are all common allergens. Restricting processed foods removes preservatives and chemicals that cause allergic reactions in sensitive people.

One Woman's Experience.   One of the thousands of patients who has benefited from the Dong diet is Tudi Sprague of Atlanta, age 44, an executive's wife and mother of two daughters, 15 and 18. Tudi Sprague's battle with arthritis began one January day ten years ago:

> The first twinge was in my right index finger—it felt as if it were asleep. A few days later, the index finger on my left hand began to tingle. I went to our family doctor. After blood tests and such, he told me I had osteoarthritis. "That's the mild kind," he said. "The type you don't want is rheumatoid arthritis." At that point, I felt I needed a specialist and consulted a rheumatologist. After running more extensive tests, he gave me the verdict—I had rheumatoid arthritis.

The disease came on so fast. When my fingers first bothered me, tennis was a big part of my life—I played on our club team. Within a week or so, I could hardly grip the racket. Before long it was an effort to get up from a chair; my husband had to help me dress, take a bath. Housekeeping chores became increasingly difficult. My fingers were so stiff I had trouble putting the car key in the ignition; I couldn't open a pickle jar or fix my daughters' ponytails. As the disease progressed, I had constant pulsating pain in my wrists, elbows, shoulders; I never got a good night's sleep. My feet were so swollen I could only shuffle around in bedroom slippers. The doctor gave me different medications to try—nothing helped. One of the drugs caused oozing sores on my chest that soiled my blouse. I felt life slipping away from me; what would I be like one year, two years from now? The following Christmas, I hit rock bottom. I told my husband, I can't take it much longer. We prayed.

The next day, my college roommate, whom I hadn't seen in years, called. I told her my troubles. "I'm going to put you in touch with Jean," she said. Jean, a friend who also had severe arthritis, went on a special diet and is fine now. When I talked to Jean by phone, I learned that she was a patient of a Dr. Dong in San Francisco, who had written a book about his diet for arthritis—she sent me a copy. The day the book arrived, I had prepared lasagna and cheesecake for dinner. As I soon learned, these were some of the foods that aggravated my arthritis symptoms.

The next day, as Jean advised, I fixed Dr. Dong's "magic mixture" soup, made of cooked rice, vegetables, and tuna whipped up in the blender, and ate nothing but that soup for five days. I noticed that my feet were less swollen and I moved more easily. Next month, I went to San Francisco to see Dr. Dong. I had been to four doctors that year and asked each one, "Will I ever play tennis again?" In each case the answer was the same: "You learn to live with your condition." Dr. Dong smiled at me: "You'll be out on the tennis court before you know it." Then he added, "Have you ever considered golf? There's much less wear and tear on the body." That first appointment, Dr. Dong gave me an acupuncture treatment, which he repeated at my periodic checkups.

One year on the diet, I soon felt well enough to exercise—mainly walking and swimming. A few years ago, I followed Dr. Dong's advice and took up golf—my husband's favorite sport. This year, exactly ten years after I met Dr. Dong, I won the Ladies Nine-Hole Championship at our club, and since then I've graduated to the eighteen-hole group.

Following the Dong diet isn't difficult. I fix lots of brown rice, kasha, and other grains, steam vegetables or stir fry them with slivers of chicken breast. We have fish twice a week plus tuna sandwiches and salmon dishes. Any time I go off the diet— now and then at a friend's house—I suffer for it. Cheese is the worst; the next day my left foot is very painful. (I once broke a bone in that foot.)

For further information about the Dong Diet, see *The Arthritic Cookbook* (New York: Thomas Y. Crowell, 1973) and *New Hope for the Arthritic* (New York: Thomas Y. Crowell, 1976).

The No-Nightshades Diet

Another diet that has an impressive track record is the no-nightshades diet; more than 70 percent of arthritics who faithfully follow the diet have experienced some degree of relief. Nightshades include tomatoes, the white potato, eggplant, peppers of all kinds (except black and white), and tobacco.

How It Began.　As in the case of the Dong diet, the no-nightshades diet was devised by a victim of arthritis as a self-help measure. The suffering patient, Norman F. Childers, Ph.D., then a professor of horticulture at Rutgers University, had developed a series of disabling conditions, which started with diverticulitis and culminated in severe joint pains and stiffness.

Examining his diet, he noted that a few hours after consuming tomatoes in any form, he developed sore muscles and joints. Being aware that the nightshade family of plants could be toxic—he had observed livestock kneeling, their knee joints too painful to support them, after consuming solanine-containing weeds—he then tested the nightshade foods one by one. Finding that each one aggravated his arthritic symptoms, he eliminated all of them from his diet, and within a few months his aches and pains were gone.

Frustrated by lack of interest in his diet on the part of Arthritis Foundation officials and arthritis specialists, he placed a notice in a few small-circulation magazines asking for cooperators to test the no-nightshades diet. Over the years, Childers, now professor of horticulture at the University of Florida, Gainesville, has collected case histories of 763 cooperators. Based on these data, Childers concludes that totally eliminating nightshades will prevent, reduce, or cure the muscle stiffness and aches and pains of arthritis in people who are sensitive to nightshades—about 10 percent of the population. (Childers prefers the term *sensitive* to *allergic;* the meaning is the same.) The rate and extent of improvement is dependent on the age of the individual and the duration of the illness.

Other foods that should be avoided or limited are dairy products, including cows' milk and eggs, as well as vitamins A and D and foods fortified with these vitamins, such as margarine.

Although data are incomplete, Childers says that a great many cooperators report improvement in heart problems, high blood pressure, hearing, sight, and other conditions.[26]

Story of a Cooperator.　What is it like to follow the no-nightshades diet in our pizza-happy society? To find out, I talked to one of Childers' staunch cooperators, Emily Osterman, 68, who has been on the diet since 1976.

"Before starting the diet, I could hardly walk," Osterman said. "I had pain in both hips, neck, elbows—you name it. An orthopedic surgeon told me I would need a hip replacement." She worked assisting her husband, owner of a landscape nursery, but "My hands were so bad I couldn't type a bill before noon. When my ankle swelled up, the doctor put me on Indocin—it didn't help."

Living near Rutgers University, where Childers was teaching, she learned about the no-nightshades diet and began following it faithfully. "After three to four months, I noticed a change in my fingers—I could hook my bra, put on panty hose without using the heels of my palms. That first year, I saw the greatest improvement." Osterman's mother, who was unable to stand owing to arthritic knees, also went on the diet. "Her knees were too bent to support her, but the pain in her legs went away."

Is the diet difficult to follow? "Not when you hurt enough," she said. "But you must read labels. Cream of mushroom soup contains potato flour as thickener; so do some breads."

ANTIARTHRITIS FOODS

Fish Oils—
Good for More than the Heart

Fish oils are rich in omega-3 fatty acids, one of the two major types of essential fatty acids. (The other type is omega-6 fatty acids, found in unrefined vegetable oils and evening primrose oil.)

The big excitement over fish oils is the discovery that the omega-3 oils found in cold-water fish, such as cod, mackerel, sardines, bluefish and salmon, protect against heart disease. Two of three articles about fish oils reported in the May 9, 1985, issue of *The New England Journal of Medicine* show that fish oils have a beneficial effect on triglycerides but, more significantly, thin blood, making blood platelet cells less likely to clump together and form a clot that can cause heart attack or stroke. Fish oils have also been shown to benefit patients with rheumatoid arthritis and other immune system–related disorders. The third article concludes that a diet enriched with fish oils may have an anti-inflammatory effect.[27]

That same year, an Albany Medical College researcher, Dr. Joel M. Kremer, reported that consuming daily doses of fish oil supplements produced a "modest but significant" improvement of arthritic symptoms in a small group of patients.[28] A follow-up study that appeared two years later confirmed the beneficial effects of fish oil supplements for RA patients.[29] In this double-blind study, 20 arthritic patients received fifteen capsules a day of MaxEPA (a dose equal to a salmon dinner or a can of sardines), while a group of patients with similar symptoms received a placebo. Patients taking supplements experienced less pain, fatigue, and swelling than usual; patients receiving placebos showed no improvement. After fourteen weeks, the groups were switched—those who had been receiving fish oil received placebos, and vice versa. Again, only members of the group taking the supplements improved.

Omega-3 fatty acids appear to relieve arthritic symptoms by suppressing production of leukotrienes (a group of compounds derived from unsaturated fatty acids), which cause pain and inflammation, but the precise mechanism is not known.

The Down Side of Popping a Pill

As soon as stories about the marvels of fish supplements began appearing in the press, researchers quickly pointed out that the supplements could cause adverse effects. An Oregon Health Sciences University physician warns that "blood clotting changes have been reported in people on high doses of fish oil supplements that could lead to bleeding problems in some individuals.[30] Greenland Eskimos, who consume quantities of fish, are prone to bleeding in the brain. A Harvard Medical School researcher cautions that a small group of healthy people who were given large quantities of fish oil supplements experienced changes in their white blood cells, which are involved in inflammatory reactions in the body.[31] Furthermore, in view of the "modest" benefits of fish oils in arthritis, these pills are expensive, say the authors of the Tufts University *Diet and Nutrition Letter*. They estimate that one month's supply of MaxEPA costs around $50.

By way of comparison, a month's supply of Feldene, one of the most popular anti-inflammatory drugs, costs about the same. Feldene "has caused serious side effects and numerous deaths, especially in older adults."[32]

Kremer, whose research we described, does not recommend fish oil supplements to his patients. "A lot more research has to be done. We don't know how it works, whether the benefits we've reported are sustained. Fish oil treatment is not a dramatic cure or a breakthrough that will enable patients to discontinue standard medications. I think it will turn out to be an adjunct to other medications."

Eating fish is undoubtedly the best way to get your fish oils. As Anne M. Fletcher, author of *Eat Fish, Live Better* (New York: Harper & Row, 1989), points out, fish is high in protein and low in fat and calories, which helps keep your weight down. In addition, "marine fish are the richest natural food source of iodine, a mineral needed for proper thyroid function [and] are also a reliable source of selenium, which may play a role in preventing heart disease and possibly cancer."

If eating a sufficient amount of fish—Fletcher advises three to seven times a week—isn't feasible for you, and you're considering taking fish oil supplements, here's a clue on dosage. Stuart M. Berger, M.D., author of *How to Be Your Own Nutritionist* (New York: William Morrow, 1987), recommends three capsules of MaxEPA for arthritics, along with several vitamins and minerals.

As part of a nutritional program for arthritis, James Braly, M.D., coauthor of *Dr. Braly's Optimum Health Program* (New York: Times Books, 1985), recommends increasing MaxEPA to nine capsules daily.

Supplementing the diet with fish oils isn't a new wrinkle. If you're of a "certain age," you may remember your mother standing over you with a spoonful of cod liver oil every morning. (My mother "disguised" the oily solution in chilled orange juice, which may account for my continued aversion to that beverage.) Cod liver oil has one worrisome aspect, which I'll mention shortly, but judging from countless testimonials and a scientific study, it has helped a great many arthritis sufferers.

Dale Alexander, author of *Arthritis and Common Sense #2,* is a tireless proponent of cod liver oil as the "key weapon" in controlling arthritis. Alexander, a self-taught health educator, discovered the benefit of cod liver oil for arthritis in the early 1950s when searching for something to help his mother, who was crippled with rheumatism. Based on some early research, he treated her with cod liver oil, and in five months she was able to move freely without pain.

Arthritis is a disease of dryness, says Alexander. To combat this oil deficiency, you need to lubricate the joints in the same way that your automobile requires a "lube" job. Alexander recommends taking one tablespoon of emulsified cod liver oil mixed with freshly squeezed orange juice (not the frozen variety, which is acidic) or cool milk. The oil must be taken on an empty stomach, either at bedtime (three to four hours after your evening meal) or upon arising (one to two hours before breakfast). After following this regime for three months, continue on a maintenance dose—one tablespoon of cod liver oil at least twice a month.

In addition to daily doses of cod liver oil, Alexander advises avoiding foods that have a drying effect, such as citrus juices, carbonated drinks, and sugary foods, and consuming foods that contain the right oils—the ideal beverage being homogenized vitamin D whole milk. (This advice, admittedly, runs counter to recommendations from the American Heart Association and every other health agency to substitute low-fat milk for whole milk.) It's also essential, says Alexander, to refrain from drinking oil-free liquids, such as water, coffee, and alcoholic beverages, at meals. Why? These "free" liquids reroute the good oils into the liver, depriving the joints of lubrication. Of these free liquids, the worst offender is ice water, which congeals the oils, Alexander says.[33]

Cod liver oil's popularity as a health maintenance measure for children in the previtamin era was undoubtedly due to its being a rich source of vitamins A and D. But today, when milk and many cereals are fortified with vitamin D and 40 percent of the population takes a multivitamin containing both A and D, the need for these vitamins is less acute. In addition, as mentioned in chapter 3, magnesium authority Dr. Mildred S. Seelig warns that milk fortified with vitamin D can be toxic to some children.

Let's look at vitamin D, the most toxic of the vitamins. One tablespoon of cod liver oil (the dose that Alexander recommends initially) contains 1,275 international units (IUs) of vitamin D. Patricia Hausman, M.S., author of *The Right Dose* (Emmaus, Penn.: Rodale Press, 1989), describes an intake of up to 1,000 IUs of vitamin D as a safe range, except for pregnant and nursing women and the elderly, who require only 600 to 800 IUs. Is there a danger of overdosing on vitamin D if you also take vitamin D supplements? "In a healthy adult 1,300 IUs of vitamin D is not enough to cause a problem, particularly when you're only taking that amount for three months," says Hausman. "But some question remains about this size dose because a few studies have shown that doses in the 1,200-unit range may have contributed to kidney stones and elevated serum cholesterol. Personally, I wouldn't take a dose that high unless I were under medical supervision."

The amount of vitamin A in cod liver oil—one tablespoon contains 12,750 IUs—is well within what Hausman considers a safe limit, which is 25,000 IUs. But Hausman cautions that if you were to combine cod liver oil with a high-potency multivitamin, or vitamin A alone, there might be a problem with vitamin A toxicity.

E. R. Squibb, which makes a mint-flavored cod liver oil, plays it safe. "The only condition that calls for cod liver oil is a vitamin A or D deficiency," said a Squibb pharmacist. (He was vague as to how one determines such a deficiency.)

Alexander is not concerned about vitamin toxicity, because vitamins contained in a natural source, like cod liver oil, have a different effect than synthetic vitamins, he said. "Best proof is that cod liver oil has been taken for four hundred years with no evidence of toxicity."

One of Alexander's many grateful followers is Sister M. Rosalia of the Sacred Heart Convent in Lisle, Illinois, who suffered for years with arthritis. In a letter, she writes, "I had given up hope of finding any help for arthritis until I heard Mr. Alexander on the radio. I followed his advice faithfully for six months and since then, thank God, I've had no pain."

Here's how Sister Rosalia describes her regimen: "On an empty stomach, I combine two tablespoons of milk with one tablespoon of oil in a small jar, shake for two minutes, then sip with a straw." She uses Norwegian cod liver oil, flavored orange or cherry.

In the 1950s, cod liver oil as a treatment for arthritis was "widely recommended in many textbooks of medicine and therapeutics," according to two physicians who conducted a study on the value of cod liver oil reported in 1959. Dr. Charles A. Brusch, medical director of the Brusch Medical Center in Cambridge, Massachusetts, and a co-investigator treated a series of 98 arthritic patients for six months on a dietary regimen that included giving cod liver oil on a fasting stomach and restricting water intake. After six months, 92 of the 98 patients showed major improvement. "The majority of our patients evidenced increased warmth in their extremities, less swelling, and more energy after four to five months."[34]

Evening Primrose Oil

This poetic-sounding substance is better known as a treatment for eczema, premenstrual stress, schizophrenia, and alcoholism, but there's some scientific evidence that it may help in RA.

Seeds of evening primrose produce an oil that contains an essential fatty acid called gamma-linolenic acid, or GLA. GLA is a building block for the formation of prostaglandins, hormonelike substances made in virtually every cell of the body, which help regulate the immune system, the nervous system, and the cardiovascular system.[35] Owing to our life-style and diet, most of us are deficient in GLA, said Dr. David Horrobin, director of the Efamol Research Institute in Nova Scotia, and a pioneer researcher in prostaglandins.

A trial in which 60 patients with RA were treated with Efamol, trade name for evening primrose oil, was carried out by researchers at Glasgow University Medical School. In phase one of the trial, the double-blind portion, patients whose symptoms were controlled with anti-inflammatory drugs (NSAIDs) were given either Efamol, Efamol Marine (a mixture of Efamol and fish oil), or placebo capsules along with their NSAID therapy for three months. Then, for the next nine months, the NSAID dose was gradually reduced.

In phase two, those patients taking Efamol or Efamol Marine were switched, without their knowledge, to placebo for the final six months of the trial. Of the 34 patients who completed the full 18-month trial, 18 improved sufficiently in phase one to stop or substantially reduce NSAID therapy. Of these 18 patients, 16 relapsed in phase two (when on placebo) and had to be restored to full doses of NSAIDs.[36]

Says Horrobin, author of 660 published scientific articles, "Results of this trial demonstrate that Efamol enables arthritics to either reduce NSAID dosage or discontinue the drug." The advantage of Efamol, as compared to NSAIDs, is that it causes no discernible side effects and may stimulate the healing process rather than suppress symptoms, Horrobin said. For these reasons, Horrobin urges other researchers to corroborate his findings, a request that has gone unheeded in the United States. (Considerable research on evening primrose oil has taken place in the Scandinavian countries and Germany.)

If you decide to take Efamol, here's advice from Horrobin: Because NSAIDs as well as stronger arthritis drugs inhibit prostaglandin formation, it's necessary to take GLA, a slow-acting substance, for several months to realize its full benefits. In his experience, some of the patients who in the long term respond best have a transient worsening in the first one to two weeks of nutritional therapy.

What dosage of Efamol should you take? "Most people need to take six to eight capsules a day for two to three months, but once you see some improvement, then you can cut down to one or two capsules a day. Dosage is an individual matter that you have to work out for yourself."

To obtain scientific literature about Efamol, contact Efamol Research Institute, POB 818, Kentville, Nova Scotia, B4N 4H8, Canada, (902) 678–5534.

To obtain Efamol's evening primrose oil, contact Nature's Way, P.O. Box 4000, Springville, UT 84663 (1/800) 453–1468.

Another source of gamma-linolenic acid (GLA) and linoleic acid is borage oil, derived from the seeds of the borage plant. The company that imports the oil from France claims that borage oil contains 24 percent GLA as compared to 7 to 10 percent GLA in evening primrose oil.

For further information about borage oil, contact American Health, 15 Dexter Plaza, Pearl River, NY 10965, (914) 735–0640 or (1/800) 445–7137.

Alfalfa

I first learned about the benefits of alfalfa when a Covington, Kentucky, physician, Dr. W. Thomas McElhinney, told me that his nightly leg cramps disappeared when he started eating a handful of alfalfa sprouts twice a day. Prescribing fresh sprouts to many of his patients, several reported that sprouts relieved their arthritic pains.

This came as no surprise to McElhinney; an Iowa farm boy, he was familiar with the food value of alfalfa and other grasses. Alfalfa's roots reach deep into the soil, fifty feet or more, which makes the crop a rich source of trace minerals. Alfalfa is particularly high in calcium and magnesium, in vitamins A and K and other vitamins, and contains eight essential enzymes. In comparing amino acids (the building blocks of protein) in common crops, a University of Wisconsin biochemist gave highest marks to alfalfa.[37]

If considering alfalfa, should you grow sprouts or take a tablet? According to Brian Robert Clement, director of the Hippocrates Health Institute in West Palm Beach, Florida, "When sprouts are alive and growing, all of the nutrients—enzymes, vitamins, minerals—are intact. Furthermore, the chlorophyll content of the sprouts carries oxygen molecules into the body; diseases cannot exist in an oxygen-rich environment."

The mainstay of the Hippocrates health program, devised by Ann Wigmore in 1957, is live, enzyme-rich wheatgrass and leafy green sprouts. For further information about the health program, write Hippocrates Health Institute, 1443 Palmdale Court, West Palm Beach, FL 33411, (407) 471–8876.

Les G. Wong, biochemist with the Shaklee Corporation in Hayward,

California, described the advantages of taking alfalfa in tablet form: "Alfalfa sprouts are 80 to 90 percent water—like lettuce. A concentrated form of alfalfa that contains the mature leaf cutting contains more nutrients than those found in sprouts." Dosage is individual; find out what works for you. As for toxicity, Shaklee's product, Alfalfa Tabs, has been sold for over fifteen years, he said. "No ill effects have ever been reported."

Royal Jelly

Royal jelly, a substance produced by bees and fed to the queen bee, can prevent and relieve arthritic symptoms, says Woodrow Whidden, a veteran beekeeper in Titusville, Florida. Whidden bases his claims on the research of a British physician, Dr. E. C. Barton-Wright. In the early 1960s, Barton-Wright discovered that his arthritic patients were deficient in pantothenic acid, one of the B-complex vitamins, and concluded that arthritis was a vitamin deficiency disease. In an article in *The Lancet,* Barton-Wright reported excellent results from treating arthritics with a daily injection of pantothenic acid and royal jelly, a rich source of pantothenic acid.[38] The treatment also included following a vegetarian diet. As an alternative to injections, Barton-Wright recommended oral doses of royal jelly.

Whidden heard Barton-Wright lecture in Atlanta thirty years ago, and ever since, the beekeeper has extracted royal jelly from his hives and shipped the product worldwide. The substance tastes bitter and peppery, Whidden said, so it's sweetened with honey. Whidden, an energetic 78, and his wife each take a teaspoon of royal jelly every day. To order royal jelly, contact Whidden's Royal Jelly & Honey Co., 1005 Tudor Lane, Titusville, FL 32780, (407) 267–0560, or inquire about a commercial product at your health food store.

Vitamins that Can Help You

Vitamin therapy has received so little attention from rheumatologists that you would think the treatment was a Johnny-come-lately, but that is not the case; vitamin therapy for arthritis is fifty years old.

Although the following information on prescribing vitamin megadoses for arthritis is emphatically *not* for self-care, to help you evaluate these amounts I've quoted safety results provided by Patricia Hausman, M.S., author of *The Right Dose, How to Take Vitamins and Minerals Safely.* Hausman, who has written four other excellent books on nutrition, served on the Surgeon General's office work group on nutrition and testified before Congress on the inadequacies of the Recommended Daily Allowances. Hausman is executive vice president of the American Nutritionists Association, 6710 Bradley Blvd., Bethesda, MD 20817.

Niacinamide. In 1943 a Stratford, Connecticut, physician, Dr. William Kaufman, reported that by giving massive doses of niacinamide to a large number of his arthritic patients, most improved greatly. Niacinamide is one of two forms of niacin, or vitamin B3. The other form of niacin is nicotinic acid. Niacinamide is used more often in multiple vitamin products since it does not produce the "niacin flush" that results from substantial doses of nicotinic acid. Chalk one up for niacinamide for sparing the patient this mildly unpleasant side effect. But nicotinic acid has the major advantage of lowering levels of "bad" cholesterol (LDL and triglycerides) and raising "good" cholesterol (HDL) levels. Niacinamide does not perform this function.

In assessing a patient's degree of impairment and monitoring the patient's progress, Kaufman did not rely on the patient's subjective reports or his own impressions; he carefully measured the flexibility of twenty joints, then established a joint range index (JRI) as a criterion. Based on each patient's JRI, sense of balance (Kaufman related impaired balance to niacinamide deficiency), and sedimentation of the red corpuscles of the blood, Kaufman determined the appropriate dosage. In addition to niacinamide (1,500 to 4,000 milligrams per day in divided doses), Kaufman often prescribed other B vitamins.

In most patients, vitamin B therapy was able to stop or reverse or control degenerative changes in joints, Kaufman said, provided that injury had not progressed too far. Kaufman also stipulated that to achieve good results, patients must eat a nourishing diet and not overuse the affected joints.

Hausman's safety results for niacinamide: Little research has been published on this subject. Hausman relates the case of Stephen, a 35-year-old graduate student, who, after taking 3,000 milligrams of niacinamide daily, landed in the hospital on five different occasions complaining of nausea and vomiting. On his fifth admission, Stephen was jaundiced and tests revealed abnormal liver function. Happily, his liver function was restored to normal after he was off the vitamin for three weeks. "Only a small minority of healthy adults have developed side effects at doses below 1,000 milligrams," Hausman says.[39]

Dr. Abram Hoffer, who has close to forty years of experience using megadoses of niacin, says that the dose range for nicotinic acid is 2 to 6 grams per day. (A gram is 1,000 milligrams.) Exceeding the "optimum dose" (what the patient needs) will produce nausea, he says. Note: Discuss this discrepancy in dosage with your nutritional physician.

As self-treatment with niacinamide, Stuart Berger, M.D., recommends 100 milligrams per day for arthritics, the amount found in high-potency multivitamins.[40] James Braly, M.D., recommends 250 milligrams per day.[41]

Vitamin B6. In the 1960s, another small-town family doctor, Dr. John M. Ellis from Mt. Pleasant, Texas, discovered the value of another B vitamin,

vitamin B6 (pyridoxine) for arthritis.[42] In treating a large number of patients
who suffered from the various muscle and joint aches that used to be called
rheumatism, he discovered that patients with specific symptoms responded
to B6 treatment. These symptoms included numbing, tingling, and a "dead"
sensation in the hands that impaired hand movements and caused patients to
drop things. Some reported pain in finger joints and puffy swelling in that
area. Many middle-aged women developed reddened bony knobs on the sides
of finger joints, called Heberden's nodes. Skin on the hands was glistening
and shiny, without wrinkles. As patients worsened, they often developed pain
and stiffness in the shoulders and sometimes the elbows. Some patients
reported being roused from sleep night after night with excruciating leg and
foot cramps.

For patients who fit the rheumatism picture, Ellis's treatment was simple: a daily oral dose of 50 milligrams of pyridoxine. Patients were also told to
continue eating their regular diet. Within a few days, many experienced some
improvement, and within a few weeks, most patients were much better: they
had less pain, reduced swelling and stiffness, their joint function and grip
strength increased, and nocturnal leg cramps either disappeared or were
much less severe.

Alan Gaby, M.D., author of *The Doctor's Guide to Vitamin B6* (Emmaus,
Penn.: Rodale Press, 1984), says he has found B6 helpful for patients
with what he calls "vitamin-B6 responsive arthritis." According to Gaby,
50 milligrams of pyridoxine (Ellis's prescription) is safe to take on your own,
but you should not take more than that a day unless you are under a doctor's
care.

Hausman's safety results for Vitamin B6: Huge doses of vitamin B6
(2,000 to 6,000 milligrams daily) can cause nerve damage. Doses in the 50- to
200-milligram range will be well tolerated by many.

Vitamin B1 (Thiamine).   Another B vitamin, thiamine (B1), also benefits
arthritics, according to a Cleveland physician, Dr. Derrick Lonsdale, author
of *A Nutritionist's Guide to Clinical Use of Vitamin B-1* (Tacoma, Wash.: Life
Sciences Press, 1987). "A 10-year-old girl came to me with classic symptoms
of rheumatoid arthritis; she had swollen fingers, bent knees—she walked like
an old lady. After treating her for one year with a form of vitamin B1 called
TTFD—it's absorbed more easily than the original vitamin—she stands
straight and moves easily."

One of Lonsdale's early successes using this new form of thiamine was
his wife, Adele:

> For years, Adele had complained of severe shoulder pain which I dismissed as
> bursitis—"You'll have to live with it." When pain spread to her hips, I sent her to an
> orthopedist who treated her with cortisone, which did not help. She then consulted a
> rheumatologist who ridiculed her symptoms as neurotic.

I became aware of the extent of her suffering the night of our club dance. Adele loves dancing but she hurt too much to dance and, at the end of the evening, had to be carried to the car.

By this time, I had learned about TTFD, a form of vitamin B that is absorbed more easily than the original vitamin and is nontoxic. [TTFD, which stands for tetrahydrofurfuryl disulfide, is manufactured by Takeda Chemical Industries Ltd., Osaka, Japan.] I started Adele on a maintenance dose of 200 milligrams of TTFD a day, and since then she has been virtually free of pain. Now and then, a change in weather or becoming fatigued may cause her to stiffen up. When that happens, she takes a little extra TTFD.

Owing to FDA regulations, TTFD can only be imported by a researcher with an "investigational new drug" license. A physician who wishes to give a dose of regular thiamine that's comparable to Lonsdale's treatment must use ten times that amount, or 2 grams of thiamine, Lonsdale said.

According to Hausman, 5 milligrams daily of regular thiamine is the lowest oral dose known to have caused ill effects.

Lonsdale, incidentally, is adamant about the dangers of a patient's self-prescribing supplements—"I hate vitamin peddlers!" If you have arthritis, seek the care of a physician trained in nutrition, he says.

Vitamin C.   Ascorbic acid (vitamin C), which is so essential for the workings of the immune system, also plays an important role in arthritis. A relation between deficient amounts of ascorbic acid and rheumatoid disease was noted back in the 1930s, but this research made little impact on treatment. (According to the late Dr. Irwin Stone, author of *Vitamin C Against Disease* (New York: Grosset & Dunlap, 1972), investigators used doses too small to show significant improvement.) Today, "It's well known that arthritis can be greatly relieved by giving adequate amounts of vitamin C," says Richard A. Kunin, M.D., specialist in orthomolecular medicine.[43] A dramatic example of vitamin C's healing power in arthritis was Norman Cousins's recovery from an arthritic condition called ankylosing spondylitis. Cousins persuaded his physician to give him intravenous infusions of ascorbate (35 grams per day), which along with generous doses of laughter, cheerful surroundings, and a good diet, apparently led to his recovery.

Dr. Robert F. Cathcart of Los Angeles, a physician with extensive clinical experience with vitamin C, said that vitamin C is "critical" in treating arthritis, lupus, and other autoimmune diseases, "but should be used in conjunction with other treatment."

Minerals

Vitamins are only part of the nutritional picture. According to Roger J. Williams, vitamin pioneer, in some individuals "an inappropriate mineral balance may cause arthritis." One of these minerals is copper. For the past two decades, a University of Arkansas researcher, John R. J. Sorenson, Ph.D., has been investigating the results of copper deficiency in arthritis. When arthritics exhaust their stores of copper, "most likely they enter the chronic stage of the disease," he said. Sorenson advocates copper chelates (compounds) as an antiarthritic drug and to treat epileptics.[44] "Copper complexes are more effective and less toxic than drugs being used to treat arthritis," he says. Sorenson has been preaching this message since 1974, but drug companies don't seem to be listening.

The Copper Bracelet: Superstition or Scientific Treatment?   You may be one of the legion of arthritis patients who swears by the copper bracelet, which the Arthritis Foundation calls an unproven remedy.

Is there any scientific validity to the belief that wearing a copper bracelet relieves arthritis pain?

An Australian chemist, Dr. W. Ray Walker of the University of Newcastle, decided to find some answers for himself. He was aware that a copper-aspirin compound was known to have an anti-inflammatory effect, and that copper chelates were used as arthritis drugs from the 1940s to the 1950s in France and Germany. He knew that the world's oldest medical text, the Egyptian Ebers papyrus, recommends pulverized copper to treat various types of inflammation.[45] Walker also knew that when copper is in contact with the skin, it forms chelates with components of human sweat and is thus absorbed through the skin.

So, to find out if copper bracelet users knew something that scientists ought to know, Walker embarked on a study with 300 arthritis sufferers, half of whom had previously worn copper bracelets. Copper bracelet users were asked not to wear their bracelets for one month. Other subjects who had never worn a copper bracelet were given two bracelets—one made of copper, the other a placebo (aluminum)—and asked to wear each bracelet for one month. Subjects did not know which bracelet was copper and which the placebo. As a check on whether subjects wore their bracelets, each copper bracelet was weighed before and after a month's use. (A bracelet decreases in weight as it is worn owing to absorption of copper.)

During the course of the study, previous copper bracelet users reported that they were significantly worse when not wearing their copper bracelets. The majority of the other subjects said that they felt their best during the month when they wore the copper bracelet.[46] Said Walker, a copper bracelet may not release as much copper as a copper-aspirin chelate, but think of it as a "time-release" source of copper that desensitizes the individual to irritants associated with chronic inflammation.[47]

The following advice on buying a copper bracelet comes from 36-year-old Sergio Lub, artist/craftsman in Walnut Creek, California. Lub's copper bracelets, executed by a staff of forty artists, can be seen at many craft galleries and quality gift shops.

- Buy only pure copper, which is a red-gold shiny color. If uncertain whether the bracelet is a fake (iron-plated) or the real thing, test with a magnet. Iron will be attracted to a magnet, copper will not.
- Buy a cuff bracelet, not a bangle; you want the maximum surface of the bracelet to be in contact with your skin.
- Buy a handmade bracelet, not one that is machinemade. To tell the difference, look for the artist's signature, smooth-finished edges, and the ability to conform to your wrist. Only handmade bracelets are "annealed" (heat treated) to make them malleable.

Another mineral deficiency that contributes to arthritis is calcium, says Dr. Richard A. Kunin. When calcium is in short supply, the body withdraws calcium from the bones, where it belongs, and it may settle in the areas around the joints causing irritation and joint pain, he says.

In learning about these various vitamins and minerals, all of which play a role in arthritis, it's tempting to seize on one or the other as a panacea for this painful and frustrating condition. But Dr. Roger J. Williams, ever the sensible oracle in nutritional matters, reminds us, "No nutrient by itself can be effective. . . . It is like a nut or a bolt in a complicated machine; by itself it cannot operate."[48]

Physicians who use nutritional therapy in treating patients with arthritis emphasize how these "nuts and bolts" interact with one another: Copper in the serum rises because of a lack of zinc and manganese in the diet and blood.[49] Copper is required to convert vitamin C into usable form.[50] Vitamin A and zinc are essential in repairing inflamed and damaged tissues. And so on.

What an Alternative Doctor Can Do

Appreciating how complicated (and endlessly fascinating) the body's biochemistry is points up the need for an analysis of one's nutritional status and needs. This can best be accomplished by consulting a nutritionally trained physician, who will conduct such an evaluation by means of clinical observations and laboratory tests.

If you've read other chapters in this book, you know that I've sounded this theme elsewhere. Another constant refrain in this book (this one voiced by the medical establishment) is "the cause of this disease [be it arthritis, or cancer, or heart disease] is unknown." Physicians who specialize in nutrition don't agree. "If you look hard enough you'll find the cause of the patient's problem," says Dr. Hugh D. Riordan, president of the Olive W. Garvey Center for the Improvement of Human Functioning, Inc., in Wichita, Kansas. For many of its patients, the Center is a "last resort"; only patients who have been seen by one or more physicians elsewhere and have not done well with standard therapy are accepted.

The three-day evaluation that's standard procedure at the Center includes extensive laboratory testing to precisely measure nutrient levels, says Riordan. "We want to know your vitamin levels, trace mineral levels, your enzyme saturation, amino acid patterns; these factors all contribute to your biochemical profile. It's important to determine if your body is overloaded with toxic metals. It's helpful to know your biological age, which is an indicator of your life expectancy. If it's higher than your actual age, there are strategies to improve it."

One of the arthritis patients treated at the Center who benefited from this biochemical approach is Robert Alford, retired Wichita businessman. "My arthritis came on [in the] fall of 1987," Alford said. "At first I couldn't raise my arm. By Christmas I was an invalid! Once I timed myself; it took me five minutes to put on a sock."

First Alford consulted an arthritis specialist: "He put me on fourteen drugs." Reading a book describing the side effects of these drugs, Alford learned that one of the drugs could cause blindness. ("I already had progressive blindness in one eye.")

In February of 1988 Alford became a patient at the Center. After test results were in, he was given a diet and a nutrient prescription based on his nutritional needs: "I take zinc lozenges, L-histidine, nystatin, calcium, and acidophilus capsules." By April his arthritis problems were over, he said. "Some time if I move my arm I have a little pain—just enough to tell me to keep on taking my nutritional medicine."

Another Center patient, Marge L. Page, 67, of Wichita, a golf and music enthusiast, had suffered from arthritis for almost thirty years. "At age 40 I had trouble getting out of a chair—I was in so much pain. I went to bed exhausted and woke up tired." She consulted doctors at the Mayo Clinic; "They gave me aspirin and told me I had to live with my arthritis." Ten years ago, Page discovered the Center. Tests revealed, among other findings, that Page was allergic to several foods (corn, lettuce, potatoes, mushrooms, and peanuts) and had high levels of lead in her system.

"As long as I abide by my diet I have no problem with arthritis. But if I go off my diet—eating in a restaurant you never know what you're getting—within twenty-four to thirty-six hours, my arthritis is back." Page also has a chelation treatment every three weeks to keep her system free of lead. (Chelation, as described in chapter 4, is an intravenous infusion that removes toxic metals.) Today, Page is back playing golf and performing with an instrumental ensemble. "I'm sure I'd be in a wheelchair if I hadn't learned about my food allergies."

To apply for the Center's Achievable Benefit Not Achieved (ABNA)

Clinical Services, write to ABNA, 3100 North Hillside Avenue, Wichita, KS 67219.

To locate a physician who practices nutritional medicine, contact the Academy of Orthomolecular Medicine or other organizations listed in the Resources section.

LOOKING AHEAD

If you take an anti-inflammatory drug (NSAID) regularly, you are at serious risk of developing a bleeding ulcer. That shocking fact about NSAIDs, the most common drugs for arthritis, is now widely known thanks to a hard-hitting segment on ABC's "20/20," aired November 29, 1989. But given the facts about NSAIDs, where to go from here? One doctor interviewed on the show said that he would continue to prescribe NSAIDs—in most cases "we've tried everything else," he said. The only solution that the show offered was a new drug called Cytotec that appears to reduce the risk of bleeding from NSAIDs in certain patients. (A year from now, will they need a drug to counteract the risks of Cytotec?)

If you've read this chapter, you know there are doctors who are concerned about finding the cause of arthritic symptoms (most often something in the diet) and treating the patient accordingly. You may have discovered the link between diet and arthritis on your own. Dava Sobel and Arthur Klein, coauthors of *Arthritis: What Works,* surveyed over a thousand arthritis patients and found that almost half had changed the way they ate because of their arthritis. Of these, 20 percent said the dietary changes had helped their condition, in some cases dramatically.[51]

6

Constipation—
How to Banish It
from Your Life

As those who suffer from it can testify, constipation, which affects almost all Americans at some time, can make you feel miserable. Defined as difficult or infrequent bowel movements, constipation can cause headaches, diminish your appetite, distend your abdomen adding inches to your waistline, and make you feel logy, out of sorts, or mildly depressed. Faced with these unpleasant symptoms, those with chronic constipation can become obsessed with the ailment, counting a "good" day one when their bowels move. Constipation can also make you reluctant to travel: will you be able to function in a strange bathroom or have enough time?

Don't Be a Laxative Junkie. Judging by the preponderance of laxative commercials shown in prime time television, it should come as no surprise that 40 million people take laxatives, 8 million of whom are "heavy" users. The tab for this addictive practice is $500 million a year.

Recently, Nancy, a 34-year-old computer analyst, asked my advice about her constipation problem. "I've taken a laxative every night since I was in my early 20s. The trouble is I have to take bigger doses all the time, and sometimes that doesn't work. If I'm in this condition at my age—what's going to happen when I'm older?"

I assured Nancy that there are plenty of things she can do to kick the laxative habit, and even a colon tortured by years of abuse can be restored to normal function. To help do the job, alternative practitioners have developed many successful "internal cleansing programs." A half dozen such programs are available that make it easy to detoxify and rejuvenate the colon. In addition, colon authorities can advise you on what you should eat to aid the process and maintain healthy bowel function.

What Goes On in the Colon.   Before venturing into the subject of colon therapy, it's helpful to understand what bowel function entails. The prime function of the small intestine is to digest food and absorb nutrients. The remaining waste matter, a watery fluid containing only nondigestible material such as fiber, passes into the five-foot-long large intestine, gut, or colon. There, rhythmic contractions known as peristalsis propel the bowel contents up, across, and down (graphically called the ascending, transverse, and descending colon), then into the rectum (the last six inches of the colon), and ultimately through the anal canal. In the process, the wall of the intestine soaks up excess water so that the longer the waste remains in the large intestine, the harder and drier the feces.

STANDARD VIEW OF CONSTIPATION

Standard doctors regard the American preoccupation with constipation as much ado about nothing—advertising hype perpetrated by the laxative makers. They say, "A bowel movement once every two to three days is as normal a schedule for some people as twice a day for others." According to *The Physicians' Manual for Patients* (New York: Times Books, 1984), "Daily bowel movements are not essential to health," and the only time to be concerned is if you notice a dramatic change in bowel habits.

ALTERNATIVE VIEW OF CONSTIPATION

Alternative practitioners strongly disagree with the establishment point of view that it's "normal" to have a bowel movement every few days. On the contrary, they say a daily bowel movement is essential to prevent the buildup of caked waste matter in the colon. They go so far as to say that *ideally* we should function as babies do, or animals or members of "primitive" cultures— eliminate wastes after each meal.

Retaining stool in the colon is harmful for a number of reasons. The longer that dregs of digestion remain in the colon, the more moisture is absorbed from the fecal mass, which results in dry hard stools. The straining needed to expel these hard stools can cause hemorrhoids as well as hiatus hernia and varicose veins. A life-threatening disease that is linked with sluggish bowel function is colon cancer, the commonest cause of death from cancer apart from lung cancer.

The Modern Plague

For at least sixty years, a few indomitable nutritionists have been preaching the message that disease begins in the colon. Bernard Jensen, an 80-year-old former chiropractor and author of over twenty-five books on health, describes constipation as a "modern plague" that "cripples and kills more people in our country than any other single morbid condition."[1] Constipation causes a multitude of diseases including cancer, diverticulosis, even breast cancer in women, he says, owing to "autointoxication"—the body poisoning itself on its own toxins. "When the bowel is underactive, toxic wastes are more likely to be absorbed through the bowel wall and into the bloodstream from which they become deposited in the tissues. . . . As toxins accumulate in the tissues, increasing degrees of cell destruction take place [and] digestion becomes poor. . . . Proper function is slowed in all body tissues in which toxins have settled."[2]

Where Constipation Does Not Exist

Jensen's idea that disease begins in the colon was given new credence by the research of world-famous scientist Dr. Denis Burkitt, published in the mid-1970s. Originally known for his discovery of Burkitt's lymphoma, a form of cancer, Burkitt was largely responsible for changing the image of roughage, or dietary fiber—the portion of plants not digested in the small intestines—from that of an animal feed to that of an essential health food for humans.

Note: In the late 1970s, when Burkitt's book appeared, all edible fiber was lumped together as "dietary fiber." Dietary fiber is now divided into two types, soluble and insoluble. Water-soluble fiber, from fruits, vegetables, peas, beans, and oats, stabilizes blood sugar levels and inhibits cholesterol absorption. Insoluble fiber, from wheat bran, whole grains, and beans, assists in elimination and fits Burkitt's definition of fiber as the food that "passes through the large intestines virtually unchanged."

As one of a small group of British epidemiologists (those who study the geographical distribution of noninfectious diseases) working in rural Africa in the early 1970s, Burkitt observed that the bowel habits of African villagers were very different from those of the British. Africans passed soft odorless stools four times the weight of the British bowel movement, which consisted of small dry stools that had a rotten smell. Furthermore, the scientists noted that intestinal transit time—interval from eating food to expelling it—among the Africans was as short as one day, compared to a full three days or more for the British. Comparing the Africans' diet of starchy carbohydrates, such as cereals, beans, peas, and root vegetables like potatoes or yams, with the British diet, predominantly white flour products high in sugar, researchers calculated that the Africans consumed as much as 120 grams of fiber a day as compared to the British intake of 25 grams or less a day. Obviously, the Africans' high-fiber diet accounted for their copious and frequent bowel movements. The significance of the difference in bowel habits between the Africans and British became apparent when the scientists discovered that an African village was a "medical Garden of Eden."[3] The villagers were not only free of colon cancer but all the noninfectious diseases that are so common in the Western world. In addition, no one was fat.

Constipation Causes Disease

Based on the African study and others he has conducted in different parts of the world, Burkitt relates five common diseases to constipation: diverticular disease, appendicitis, hemorrhoids, hiatus hernia, and varicose veins. Each is caused by straining at stool to expel hard fecal matter, he says.[4]

In addition, a host of more serious diseases "characteristic of modern Western civilization" have been shown to be related to intestinal transit time and to the bulk and consistency of stools.[5] Colon cancer, one of the most dangerous of these diseases, is related to "bowel behavior and content," Burkitt says. Here's why: A low-fiber diet, which causes constipation, increases the number of harmful bacteria in the stool. These bacteria (predominantly Bacteroides and Bifidobacteria) convert harmless bile acids into powerful cancer-producing compounds. Thus, in a constipated person, the dregs of digestion and its store of cancer chemicals wash over the colon for seventy-two hours or longer. In a healthy colon, however, waste matter moves along at a fast clip, reducing prolonged contact with the lining of the intestine in which the cancer forms.

In view of Burkitt's research and that of others, reported at least fifteen years ago, it seems inconceivable that standard doctors should continue to take a laissez-faire attitude toward constipation. Dr. Burkitt himself says that the prevailing view among doctors "that it does not matter whether you have two motions a day, or three a week," is wrong.[6]

What They Knew Back Then

Linking disease to poor bowel function is not a new idea. Hippocrates, the father of medicine, urged the citizens of Athens to "Cleanse the bowels!"[7] Maimonides, twelfth-century physician, said, "If the body does not eliminate properly, first the mind becomes tense and nervous, and then the body becomes diseased."[8] In India, the ancient system of medicine called ayurveda relates elimination to mental health. Dr. Michael Gerber of Reno, Nevada, learned this lesson as an intern on a mental ward. As Gerber tells the story, he asked an Indian friend, " 'How do you treat schizophrenics in India?' The friend replied, 'When someone is crazy, we give them seven liters of saline.' 'But why?' I asked. My friend looked at me as if I were a backward child. 'They have bowel movements continuously and then they feel better.'" Gerber subsequently discovered that many of his schizophrenic patients were severely constipated, and when bowel function was restored, their behavior improved, he said.

In the early 1900s, a Russian scientist and Nobel Prize winner, Dr. Élie Metchnikoff, propounded the theory that much disease is due to "microbial putrefaction in the intestines which literally poisoned the body by releasing toxins that destroyed artery walls and caused senility and early death."[9] (Incidentally, Metchnikoff's solution to this life-threatening condition was "sour milk," later renamed "yogurt.") This theory, that constipation leads to intestinal toxemia, was held by physicians here and abroad. In 1914, at the invitation of the Royal Society of Medicine of Great Britain, fifty-seven of the world's leading physicians met to discuss the subject of alimentary toxemia. "Every organ of the body is affected by these poisons . . . constantly bathing the delicate body cells," one said.[10] In the United States, Dr. John Harvey Kellogg, dynamic surgeon and long-time director of the prestigious Battle Creek Sanitarium in Battle Creek, Michigan (later the home of Kellogg's Corn Flakes), preached the dangers of constipation. In his 403-page book, *Colon Hygiene,* published in 1916, Kellogg attributes a long list of diseases— gallstones, hemorrhoids, and skin diseases such as acne, eczema, and psoriasis—to the digestive system's becoming saturated with poisons from bacteria in the colon. If intestinal toxemia continues, he said, worse conditions such as rheumatism, gout, and cancer of the colon develop. Constipation was becoming more prevalent, Kellogg said, mainly because of modern milling methods, which separated the bran from the bread. He advocated "reform of the bowel" with diet, including bran.

The Pendulum Swings in One Direction . . .

By the 1930s and 1940s, "wonder drugs" and surgery were in full sway, and doctors had little use for such time-consuming practices as "reforming" the colon. During this period, when laboratory equipment failed to identify any toxic substances in the blood of constipated people, the concept of intestinal toxemia fell out of favor with mainstream physicians.

But ordinary people instinctively feel there's something unhealthy about those dregs sitting in the gut. When you were a child and had a headache or a stomachache, if your mother was like mine, the first thing she did was quiz you about your bowels.

And Back Again

Today, researchers are recognizing the importance of the intestines as a "key target organ."[11] In a 1984 medical text that explores the effect of environmental chemicals on the alimentary tract, Carol Schiller, Ph.D., senior scientist at the National Institutes of Health, comments on our "relatively limited understanding of many basic intestinal processes" and the need for future studies.

One such study was undertaken by two University of California physicians. Drs. Nicholas L. Petrakis and Eileen B. King of the University of California, as reported in *Lancet,* have found that women who have two or fewer bowel movements per week have four times the risk of breast disease (benign or malignant) as women who have one or more bowel movements per day.[12]

With scientists and a small number of physicians taking more of an interest in problems of the digestive tract, researchers have devised tests that measure bacterial flora in the colon. One such test, the comprehensive digestive stool analysis (developed by the Great Smokies Medical Laboratory in Leicester, North Carolina), shows that slow transit time causes a change in flora balance, said Steve Barrie, naturopathic physician and president of the laboratory. "In most cases, sluggish elimination increases the number of unfriendly bacteria in the intestinal tract, and secondly, increases the time that harmful chemical byproducts are in contact with the intestinal wall," he says.

Now that the phenomenon of bowel toxicity can be observed under the microscope, it's probably only a matter of time before the medical profession becomes more concerned about constipation.

STANDARD TREATMENT FOR CONSTIPATION

The standard treatment for constipation is to add foods high in fiber to the diet, such as whole grain breads and cereals and fresh fruits and vegetables. If necessary, eat a small amount of bran cereal. In addition, drink six to eight glasses of fluids each day, exercise, and promptly obey the urge to move the bowels. Authors of *The Physicians' Manual for Patients* (New York Times Books, 1984) advise, "For people whose constipation is not adequately controlled by diet and exercise, careful use of a laxative can resolve the immediate problem."

Both standard doctors and alternative practitioners agree that laxatives that chemically stimulate the colon are harmful. These harsh chemical laxatives, such as Dulcolax, Ex-Lax and Senokot, and herbal preparations that contain senna and cascara sagrada, cause the colon muscle to contract, thereby propelling stool toward the rectum.[13] By completely emptying the bowel, these chemical agents eliminate water and nutrients as well as stool, which weakens colonic muscles and induces dehydration. Dehydration in itself causes constipation, creating a vicious cycle. There are two types of laxatives that are considered safe: one is a stool softener, such as Colace and Surfax, which does its job by allowing moisture to penetrate the stool; the other is a bulk-forming laxative (best known of which is Metamucil), which draws water into the colon.

ALTERNATIVE TREATMENT FOR CONSTIPATION

To restore and maintain normal bowel function, the essential element, as always, is diet, along with exercise. Unlike standard physicians, alternative physicians say that these measures are not enough. Owing to the condition of the colon, which in most Americans is like a "clogged sewer," to quote Norman W. Walker, grandfather of colon therapy, the first step in colon therapy is "internal cleansing" to detoxify the colon. This can be done with commercial products made of herbs and fiber, and by colonic irrigation and enema, ancient forms of hydrotherapy.

Diet

The role of diet in disease is seldom clear-cut. For example, many researchers suspect that breast cancer is linked to dietary fats, but it's hard to prove the association. But when it comes to constipation, there is no question about the culprit. "Lack of fiber, and of cereal fibre in particular, is . . . the most important single cause of constipation," says Dr. Denis Burkitt.[14]

A significant benefit of fiber that was not appreciated in the past is that fiber promotes the growth of friendly bacteria in the colon, Burkitt says. "The smooth muscular movements of the large bowel and the passage at least once a day of soft, fairly large feces depends almost entirely on whether these bacteria get enough to eat in the form of fiber."

Compared to the Africans that Burkitt studied, who were free of constipation and other degenerative diseases, our diet is woefully deficient in fiber. We consume about 20 grams of fiber a day, compared to 60 to 90 grams contained in third world diets. What we should aim for, Burkitt says, is to increase our intake of fiber to 40 grams or more per day.

To increase your fiber intake, eat as your ancestors did two hundred years ago, Burkitt says. Increase grains, potatoes, cereal fiber found in whole grain bread, coarse hot cereals, brown rice, and bran. At the same time, reduce fats, particularly animal fats, and refined white flour products. These changes reinforce one another. Filling up on starchy carbohydrates like rice, pasta, and potatoes doesn't leave much room for bacon, Danish, ice cream, and other fatty favorites. It's like a seesaw. As starchy foods in your diet go up, fats, oils, and sugar come down.

Where to start increasing fiber? In his concise and clearly written book *Don't Forget Fiber in Your Diet,* Burkitt advises:

1. Increase whole grain bread, which is 8.5 percent dietary fiber. Look for 100-percent whole wheat, not pseudo "wheat bread" or others that contain mostly white flour.

2. Add miller's bran (44 percent dietary fiber) to breakfast cereals, hot or cold. (Since these flakes have the consistency of sawdust, I like to moisten bran with milk and allow it to become mushy before adding it to cereal.) Start with one heaped teaspoonful a day; increase gradually until at least one soft stool is passed daily, and keep to this daily amount. Two tablespoons a day is average. In a study in Britain of 62 patients with diverticular disease who were chronically constipated, two tablespoons of bran daily as part of a high-fiber diet restored normal bowel function in all.[15]

3. Eat more legumes; that is, peas, beans, and lentils, the next best source of fiber after cereals. (Peas contain 12 percent dietary fiber.)

Next on the fiber scale are root vegetables, such as potatoes and carrots. (A boiled yam is 3.9 percent dietary fiber.) Fresh fruits and vegetables also contain fiber, but since they're composed largely of water, you have to eat an enormous quantity to meet your fiber requirements. (Spinach tops the list of vegetables at 6.3 percent dietary fiber.)

Several chiropractors and nutritionists who specialize in colon therapy emphasize the need to "feed" the friendly bacteria in the intestinal tract. The friendly bacteria, called Lactobacilli, keep harmful bacteria in the colon in check as well as promoting good digestion and synthesizing B vitamins.[16] Best known of the friendly bacteria is *L. acidophilus,* but recent research shows that another type of good bacteria in the colon, called Bifidobacteria, promotes proper elimination.

Intestinal Cleansing. To control "putrefaction" within the intestinal tract ("a process of decay in which foul odors and toxic substances are generated"), Robert Gray, author of *The Colon Health Handbook,* recommends what he calls a "mucoidless" diet. (*Mucoid* refers to unhealthy mucus, which sticks like glue to the walls of the colon and small intestines.) Gray's mucoidless diet is a severely restrictive one, which eliminates meat, fish, eggs, dairy products including yogurt, and soy products, and permits only vegetables, fruit, and moderate amounts of grains. One way to produce good bacteria is by eating cabbage. Since you would have to eat a pound of cabbage a day to notice any appreciable difference, Gray recommends one half to one cup of cabbage juice two or three times a day. Another good nonmucoid food is the Jerusalem artichoke, he says.

For literature about the Robert Gray intestinal cleansing program, write Holistic Horizons, Box 2868, Oakland, CA 94618-0068.

Supplements.   A simpler way to grow friendly bacteria in your colon is by taking supplements containing the microorganisms normally found in the healthy colon. Bernard Jensen recommends acidophilus supplements as well as alfalfa tablets (four or five with each meal) and liquid chlorophyll. To obtain literature about Jensen's colon cleansing program, write Bernard Jensen International, 24360 Old Wagon Road, Escondido, CA 92027.

The president of a nutrition company that specializes in cultured dairy products claims that another type of friendly bacteria, Bifidobacteria, is best suited to the vegetarian. For more information about this new area of Lactobacillus supplements, write Natren, Inc., 10935 Camarillo Street, North Hollywood, CA 91602.

Laxative Foods.   Dick Gregory, comedian and health guru, says that the best natural laxative is a glass of warm water containing the juice of one half lemon taken upon arising. Other favorite laxative foods, in addition to bran and drinking quantities of nonchlorinated water, are:

> Stewed prunes
> Plums
> Apricots
> Pears
> Rhubarb
> Figs
> Sauerkraut juice
> Other raw vegetable juices:
> > Spinach
> > Watercress
> > Carrot
> > Cucumber
> > Tomato
> > Celery
> > Red beets
> Yogurt
> Buttermilk
> Olive oil (one spoonful) mixed with lemon juice
> Glass of salt water (occasional use only)
> Agar-agar (commercially prepared seaweed)

Food Combining.   The diet recommended by many of the "new wave" of colon therapists whom we will meet shortly involves food combining. As indicated by the name, this technique refers to a method of combining types of foods—protein, starch, and fruits—to improve digestion. Proteins should not be eaten with starches; fruits are not to be eaten with other foods. One of the reasons for these rules is that each type of food has a different digestive timetable—the amount of time spent in the stomach. Starches require 2 to 3 hours to complete digestion, proteins take around 4 hours, while fruits whiz from stomach to small intestine in less than an hour. But if you break these rules—eat your morning cereal topped with sliced bananas—the fruit has to sit in the stomach waiting for the starch to digest, which causes fruit sugars to ferment.[17]

Information about the food-combining diet, introduced by a chiropractic physician, Dr. Herbert M. Shelton, in the 1940s, is disseminated by several resources. One, headed by a long-time spokesperson of the natural hygiene movement, Jo Willard, is Natural Hygiene, Inc., P.O. Box 2132, Huntington, CT 06484. A booklet, "Food Combining Simplified," can be obtained by sending $3.50 to Dennis Nelson, P.O. Box 2302, Santa Cruz, CA 95063.

Milk May Not Be Good for You.   Is there such a thing as a constipating food? I first became aware that milk had earned this dubious distinction by talking to Suzanne Kircher, Romanian-born R.N. and owner of Sans Souci, a much acclaimed spa in Bellbrook, Ohio.

"For years, I suffered with constipation, so severe that I consulted a colon specialist," Kircher said. "I did all the right things—included lots of fiber in my diet, drank quantities of water, devised special abdominal exercises—but nothing helped." Kircher even developed cramps, she said, from eating too much fiber. The one time that her bowels functioned like clockwork was when she attended an annual yoga retreat. At first she attributed this happy occurrence to the concentrated exercise, but then realized that it might be the diet she consumed at such times, which was strict vegan fare—no dairy products, including milk. Returning home from one of these retreats, Kircher eliminated milk from her diet. "This was three years ago, and I've had no problems since." Apparently, a milk sensitivity caused a spastic colon, she said.

Jensen is one of the colon authorities who says that milk is a common allergen and can be constipating. Another is world-renowned physician Dr. Albert T. W. Simeons, author of *Man's Presumptuous Brain* (New York: Dutton, 1960). Milk is constipating, he says, because it withdraws excessive water from the lower portion of the colon. Simeons's recommendation: for every glass of milk consumed, drink a glass or more of water.

Colonic Irrigation

According to Norman W. Walker, a pioneer of colon therapy and author of *Colon Health* (Phoenix: O'Sullivan Woodside, 1979), a colonic irrigation is the best means of removing accumulated waste in the colon that results from faulty diet. "These foods (processed, fried and overcooked) leave a coating of slime on the inner walls of the colon like plaster on a wall." (Walker, who died at age 120, obviously knew something about a healthy life-style; at age 110, when I talked to him by phone, he was revising his colon book.)

Colonic irrigation, which requires a machine and a trained operator, "is a safe, effective method for cleansing the colon of waste material by repeated gentle flushing with water," says Dr. Mark A. Baker, a chiropractic physician in Bridgeton, Missouri, who specializes in colon therapy and has written an excellent new booklet on the subject. To obtain the booklet, "Colon Irrigation: A Forgotten Key to Health," send $3 to Mark A. Baker, D.C., 11558 St. Charles Rock Road, Bridgeton, MO 63044.

If you lived some of your adult life before World War II, you may remember when a hospital patient, prior to undergoing barium studies or surgery, was routinely given a colonic irrigation. The colonic was also used as a means of delivering nutrients or medication to the patient who could not eat. During the 1920s and 1930s, physicians published scientific studies describing the benefits of colon therapy in a great many diseases, including hypertension, heart disease, and depression. The most dramatic improvement, according to these physician-authors, occurred in arthritic patients.[18] "That's because arthritis is an accumulation of toxins in the joints," Baker explained. "Colon therapy helps to reduce those toxins."

With the emergence of antibiotics in the 1940s and a drug-centered approach to treatment, colonic irrigation was regarded as time-consuming and unnecessary, and colonic equipment gathered dust.

Today, standard doctors say that the colonic has no medical value, and can be dangerous. As proof, they point to an outbreak of amoebic dysentery that occurred in Colorado in 1981, where seven persons died. All had received colonic irrigation at a chiropractic clinic in which personnel neglected proper sterilization techniques. Today, several types of colon machines are available that eliminate any possibility of contamination; they use a disposable plastic applicator and a drainage system that prevents backup of water.

As a consequence of the backlash against the colonic, in most states only medical doctors, osteopaths, and chiropractors are permitted to offer this treatment. (An exception is Florida, where licensed massage therapists are permitted to give colonics.)

Naturopathic physicians, whose system of natural healing is founded on the belief that disease originates in the colon, have helped keep this "old-fashioned" treatment alive. The John Bastyr College in Seattle, one of two naturopathic schools in the United States, continues to instruct its students in the colonic, and many naturopaths in this country provide the treatment.

Despite restrictive laws governing use of the colonic, which have relegated the treatment to the alternative "underground," a modest revival of the colonic is taking place.

Chiropractic physicians, like Baker, are offering colon therapy, although they are still a minority. (A member of the Ohio Board of Chiropractic Examiners said that, to his knowledge, none of his colleagues were involved in treatment.)

The Multi-Health Group in Mesa, Arizona, whose staff includes physicians who specialize in homeopathy, naturopathy, and acupuncture, provides colon therapy. The colonic is one of several ways we detoxify the system, said Dr. Harvey Bigelsen, the group's director. Other detox measures include homeopathic treatment.

Bigelsen, trained as an ophthalmologist, emphasized that colonic irrigation is not limited to the patient who is constipated: "Anyone who is toxic should have a series of colonic irrigations." Diagnostic measures used at the clinic to reveal toxicity, he said, include electrodiagnosis (for a discussion of ED see chapter 10) and a type of live cell microscopy that originated in Germany. Every patient at the clinic who requires concentrated detoxification (except those who have had a heart attack or are at risk for one) undergoes colon therapy. When I asked Bigelsen why heart patients are exempt from the colonic, he said that a reflux from the anus to the heart can precipitate a heart attack. "Once the patient is detoxified, we employ measures to revitalize the organs and tissues and let the body heal itself."

How can you tell if you're toxic and require colonic treatment?

Colonic treatment is indicated, said Shirley Jones, the group's colon therapist, if you have chronic constipation, diarrhea, or flatulence, your skin is broken out, you're extremely fatigued but have trouble sleeping, are overweight, or suffer from muscle and joint pain or colitis. Jones, a licensed nurse practitioner for twenty-seven years, said she was skeptical at first about the colonic treatment "since it wasn't mentioned in medical books," but that taking a training course provided by a colon equipment company, Health Products, Inc., in Phoenix, changed her mind. "Almost anyone can retrain the bowel if he changes his diet along with a series of colonics," she said. Most clinic patients undergo six to ten colonic treatments.

Here and there, colon therapists have been quietly plying their trade for decades. One of these veteran colon therapists, the best in the business according to a faculty member of the John Bastyr College, is Bob Rogers of Seattle. Rogers' interest in colonic therapy began thirty years ago when he was a surgical assistant preparing a young man with a colon disease for a colostomy. Rogers also had a colon problem at the time and, suddenly realizing what might be in store for him, doggedly tracked down a colonic machine. After treating himself, he trained with a therapist who had practiced during the heyday of colon therapy and opened shop.

Colonic irrigation involves more than using water to flush out toxic wastes from the colon, Rogers said. The treatment can also restore proper acid/alkaline balance to the colon by adding various herbs and substances to the water. "The health of the colon depends on its pH—acid/alkaline balance. Friendly bacteria flourish in a predominantly alkaline colon. If the colon is too acid, bad bacteria outnumber the good."

In a client's first session, Rogers uses "the formula that Mae West gave me—one tablespoon of baking soda, air-dried sea salt, one cup brewed coffee. Soda makes the colon more alkaline so bad bacteria won't grow. Coffee helps to drain the liver and gallbladder." (As described on page 31, a coffee enema is part of the Gerson Therapy for cancer patients.)

After determining the client's acid/alkaline ratio by means of a simple litmus test, Rogers devises an herbal formula that will correct the imbalance. (For a sampling of herbal formulas, see Jethro Koss's *Back to Eden* (Loma Linda, Calif.: Eden Books, 1939).

The colonic helps the body overcome any disease more easily, Rogers said. Candida occurs in persons who have been heavy users of penicillin, because the antibiotic remains in the body: "Candida is yeast, and penicillin thrives on yeast. A colonic removes the penicillin." A colonic is useful in drug withdrawal for the same reason, he continues. "I treated a woman who after twenty years on tranquilizers was like a zombie. After a series of colonics, she came back to life."

Since the skin is an important organ of elimination, skin problems also respond to colonic treatment, he said. Recalling a client with psoriasis, "His skin lesions smelled so bad he was in danger of losing his job. After one year of treatment, he had gorgeous skin. Adolescent acne improves dramatically when you keep the gut and blood clean."

To locate a colon therapist:

- Look in the Yellow Pages under *colonic* or *colon therapy*.
- Ask alternative health practitioners if they can refer you to a colon therapist.
- Confer with the owner of your favorite health food store or bookstore that specializes in health books.
- Contact the National Colon Therapists' Association, 1010 Deep Creek Avenue, Arnold, MD 21012, (301) 974–1181, or a west coast group, the California Colon Hygenists' Society, 209 Morning Sun Avenue, Mill Valley, CA 94941, (415) 383–7224.

Since colon therapists are not certified, it seems wise to spend some time talking with them before making an appointment, unless they are recommended by someone whose judgment you trust. Ann Robinson, founder of the National Colon Therapists' Association, advises:

1. Ask about their training, their experience, how they became involved in colon therapy. Ask whether any health professionals in the area refer patients to them. Look for someone you feel comfortable with, since this is an intimate procedure.

2. Inquire about the equipment they use. Ask whether the machine has a disposable speculum and hoses. If it's an older model without disposable parts, ask what hygienic procedures are followed. (Parts should be sterilized!)

If you cannot locate a colon therapist and are willing to expend considerable effort in pursuit of treatment, several do-it-yourself colonic methods are available. The Colema board, "a safe and easy way to take a high enema or colonic," is part of the Vit-Ra-Tox Seven Day Cleansing Program. Dr. Bernard Jensen incorporates this program in his treatment and describes it in detail in *Tissue Cleansing through Bowel Management*. For further information about the program, write V. E. Irons, Inc., P.O. Box 296, Natick, MA 01760.

Another self-use colonic is the Wood Method Colonic Irrigation System developed by the late Dr. Robert A. Wood, known as "the father of colon therapy." The unit is distributed by Judith A. DuFresne, who worked with Dr. Wood and trains medical professionals in the Wood method. For further information, write Dr. Robert A. Wood Institute, P.O. Box 530, Valparaiso, IN 46384.

Although the Fleet Enema, a ready-to-use enema containing a saline laxative, is the number one seller among the top one hundred over-the-counter drugstore products,[19] colon therapists I've talked to recommend the old-fashioned hot water bottle equipped with a syringe. If you're having any abdominal pain, particularly in the right lower side (that could indicate appendicitis), do not give yourself an enema or have a colonic.

For directions on how to give yourself an enema, see *Introduction to Patient Care; a Comprehensive Approach to Nursing*, by Beverly Witter DuGas (Philadelphia: W. B. Saunders, 1983). For an informal description of what he calls an "internal bath," read chapter 4 of *Dick Gregory's Natural Diet for Folks Who Eat: Cookin' with Mother Nature* (New York: Harper & Row, 1973).

Internal Cleansers

Today, the colonic and old-style enema are unfamiliar to most Americans, but the need for colon cleansing is greater than ever at a time when we're exposed to a tremendous number of environmental contaminants. As a result, colon experts have devised internal cleansing in the form we're accustomed to—taken by mouth.

An internal cleanser contains a mixture of herbs and a bulking agent; together, they loosen stagnant matter in the colon and accelerate its removal. (Products such as Metamucil and Perdiem, which contain psyllium seeds, are bulking agents only.) Of the half dozen internal cleansers on the market, one of the best known is the Yerba Prima Internal Cleansing Program, which was introduced in 1980 and tested at the Linus Pauling Institute under the supervision of Jeffrey Bland, Ph.D., professor of nutritional biochemistry at the University of Puget Sound. In a study of 12 healthy subjects, all under 40, who followed the program for three months, all experienced a reduction in harmful bacteria in the colon and an increase in absorption of water-soluble vitamins and protein.

The skin being a primary organ of elimination, the Yerba Prima program and others recommend daily skin brushing to cleanse the lymphatic system and stimulate circulation. Linda Berry, chiropractor, gives directions as follows.[20] Use a long-handled bath brush with natural bristles, and keep it dry. With long sweeping motions (not back and forth or circular) brush from hands and feet toward the abdomen, then across your upper back and down the front and back of the torso. For the face, use a soft cosmetic brush. Begin in the center of your face and stroke outward, then up the side of your face and neck.

For information about the Yerba Prima Internal Cleansing Program, contact P.O. Box 2569, Oakland CA 94614, (800) 421–9972.

Other internal cleansers include Triphala (formulated by Michael Tierra, author of *The Way of Herbs*), available from Planetary Formulas, P.O. Box 533, Soquel, CA 95073; and Vit-Ra-Tox, Seven Day Cleansing Program, V. E. Irons, Inc., P.O. Box 296, Natick, MA 01760.

LOOKING AHEAD

Although the subject is still an unmentionable, Americans are becoming more conscious of colon health. According to pharmacist Forrest E. Pack (he's chairman of the Ohio Association for Independent Pharmacy), sales of Ex-Lax, Senokot, and other chemical stimulants are declining, and more of his customers are buying stool softeners and bulk-forming laxatives. So, the day may come when the colonic irrigation is once again recognized therapy and you can discuss the treatment as freely as you would a massage.

7

The Therapeutic Diet

It was a promise that still sounds outrageous: if you are afflicted with heart disease, hypertension, diabetes, hardening of the arteries, or obesity, and you follow my program of diet and exercise, you can reverse any of these conditions and increase your chances of living a long healthy life.

This was the message that Nathan Pritikin, engineer and lifelong student of medicine, delivered in the mid-1970s. Since that time, an estimated 40,000 people have attended one of the three Pritikin Longevity Centers (in Santa Monica, California, Downingtown, Pennsylvania, and Miami Beach, Florida) and experienced the results Pritikin predicted.

A decade before Pritikin appeared on the scene, Michio Kushi was expounding the benefits of an Oriental-type life-style and diet called macrobiotics.

In the early 1980s, John A. McDougall, M.D., one of Pritikin's protégés, introduced the McDougall Plan "for super health and life-long weight loss."[1]

All three diets — Pritikin, McDougall, and macrobiotics — I've called "therapeutic" because each is designed not only to prevent disease but to treat it.

In standard medicine, diet is strictly a preventive measure. Three well-known preventive diets are the U.S. Dietary Goals (issued by the U.S. Department of Agriculture in 1980), the American Heart Association diet ("an eating plan for healthy Americans"), and the National Cancer Institute's guidelines (published in a report, *Diet, Nutrition and Cancer*). All three diets advise Americans to reduce total amount of fat, reduce animal fats, increase polyunsaturated fats, eat starchy foods, reduce cholesterol, and increase fiber-rich foods.

For some time, I had the rosy impression that we Americans were on a health kick. Look at the profusion of health books, health foods, running shoes. These signs appear to be misleading. Based on a large-scale nation-wide telephone survey conducted by the *New York Times,* "The dramatic nutrition revolution that was going to change the way Americans eat is not happening," says *Times* food editor Marian Burros. "The results of the survey . . . indicate that most Americans, regardless of age, have not re-sponded in a significant fashion to calls for decreasing fat in the diet, reducing sodium, taking in fewer calories, or otherwise eating more healthfully."[2]

Further evidence about the eating habits of Americans—that more people are eating out (over 42 percent of meals) and eating more fast food, most of which is loaded with fat, that the family dinner is extinct—contributes to the impression that the "fitness revolution" is more of a merchandising ploy than actual life-style change.

So the therapeutic diet fills a real need. But do these therapeutic diets work? If you're considering one of these diets, you'll want to know whether there are significant differences between them and if they are so restrictive that people have difficulty sticking to them.

To answer some of these questions, I "audited" the program at the Pritikin Longevity Center in Santa Monica and took part in the McDougall Program at St. Helena Hospital and Health Center in Deer Park, California, 75 miles north of San Francisco. Investigating macrobiotics, I've talked to a great many macrobiotic counselors, teachers, and people who practice mac-robiotics and over the years, attended lectures on the subject and classes in macrobiotic cooking, and taken part in pot luck suppers.

A word of warning before you sample these three therapeutic diets: Pro-ponents of these eating plans are in a sense explorers charting a path that others have taken but one that has become overgrown and hidden from sight. These present-day health trailblazers have some of the traditional explorer's characteristics, including a dose of arrogance. (Years ago, I attended a lecture of Nathan Pritikin's in which he described the harmful foods. Apparently I missed some of the discussion, because afterwards I went up to him and asked, "What's wrong with eggs?" He gave me a withering look. "Eggs are for raising chickens," he snapped.) So, reading this chapter, you may find yourself irri-tated or impatient and looking for loopholes in their arguments. (I've indulged in a little of that.) But keep in mind that these three therapeutic diets have an excellent track record and may work for you as they have for countless others.

THE PRITIKIN PROGRAM

During a lecture on heart disease at the Pritikin Longevity Center in Santa Monica, the woman next to me rests her hand (long red nails, gold rings, a bracelet) on her husband's ample back and rubs protectively. The information that the youthful bespeckled physician imparts is scary:

- Cardiovascular or heart disease is the number one killer of adult Americans, and the major cause of heart disease is atherosclerosis.

- High blood pressure, or hypertension, which afflicts 50 percent of people over 40, often leads to heart attack, stroke, congestive heart failure, and kidney disease.

- Diabetes is one of the leading causes of death, but most diabetics do not die of diabetes; they die of the complications that result from diabetes, such as heart attack, stroke, kidney diseases, and gangrene.

But the grim statistics are offset by the encouraging message that has brought these people to the Center: diet combined with exercise can control and even reverse these diseases.

Participants with "mild" diseases—hypertension, weight problems, diabetes—pay $4,190 to spend thirteen days at the Center, a six-story 1920s red brick hotel set on the beach a stone's throw from the ocean. The twenty-six-day program ($7,200) is for those with advanced heart conditions or insulin-dependent diabetes. At any one time, there are 100 to 125 people at the Center.

Eating Wrong and Right

Lectures at the Pritikin Center, some with slide presentations as technical as a medical paper, compare two diets: the American diet and the Pritikin diet. The American diet is high in fat (40 percent of calories from fat), high in cholesterol (450 to 500 milligrams per day), contains more than three times the amount of salt we need, and is low in fiber. This diet is the primary cause of the diseases that cripple and kill us. The Pritikin Lifetime Eating Plan diet is low in total fat (10 percent of calories), low in sodium (1,600 milligrams per day), and high in fiber. This diet consists mainly of whole grains (*whole* meaning not refined) and fruits and vegetables (legumes, among others). It also permits "modest" amounts (three and one-half ounces per day) of "high protein," meaning fish, fowl, or meat, and two servings each day of dairy foods. (A dairy serving is eight ounces of skimmed milk, six ounces of yogurt, or two ounces of hoop cheese.)

The Pritikin Lifetime Eating Plan, as its name implies, is forever. Ideally this diet should be started at age 2 and followed for a lifetime "to maintain good cardiovascular health." Pritikin named this diet the maintenance diet. But the Lifetime Eating Plan is not the diet that participants at the Center follow. For those who need to regress or reverse atherosclerosis and also lose weight, Pritikin designed a more spartan diet that is now called a "therapeutic modification" of the Lifetime Eating Plan. This modified diet limits high protein to three and one-half ounces per week. Following this diet, a woman is allowed 1,000 calories per day, a man, 1,200 calories per day.

If, at the end of your stay, your cholesterol level is still too high and you have not yet achieved a normal weight (as determined by the physician conducting your final examination), you will be advised to continue on the modified eating plan. But if your cholesterol levels and weight are within desirable limits, then you graduate to the Pritikin Lifetime Eating Plan.

Proof Is in the Pudding Substitute

My first Pritikin meal was the evening meal. The high-ceilinged dining room, which accommodates 150, overlooks the ocean; I was greeted with a picture postcard view of the sun, a red ball, disappearing into the horizon. I stood in line at the salad bar, which offered an array of crisp raw vegetables and three no-fat Pritikin dressings, then joined two women, mother and daughter, in velour warm-up suits and heavy eye makeup, at a table set with a white tablecloth and fresh flowers. The mood of gracious dining was dispelled by the menu—a one-page computer printout with a column "Exchanges," containing mysterious abbreviations. I learned that one tablespoon of salad dressing equals approximately 10 calories. Being extremely hungry, having missed lunch that day, I had trouble making my choice among the three entrées, which were halibut in dill sauce, vegetable cutlet, or steamed vegetable plate; the choice of starch was baby potato or bulgur and wild rice pilaf. I finally asked the waiter if I could have both the vegetable plate and the vegetable cutlet. My two tablemates, Florence and Debbie, ordered the halibut and then, pencils in hand, made notations on their menus.

My concern that I had been greedy ordering the extra entrée vanished when the waiter brought our orders. The vegetable cutlet was about two inches square, and the vegetable plate consisted of two slices each of zucchini, yellow squash, and turnips. Florence and Debbie joked good-naturedly about their halibut portion; covered with a yogurt sauce, it looked like a bite-size piece of pickled herring. Dessert was four spoonfuls of watermelon served in a sherbet glass. Hot beverages—herbal tea and decaffeinated coffee—were available.

At breakfast, which offered a bountiful choice of fruit, breads (pita, English muffin, toast, or bagel) and both hot and cold cereals, portion sizes seemed less restrictive. (But maybe you'd feel deprived having half a bagel or banana.) Lunch was raw vegetables from the salad bar, a cup of split pea soup, a well-seasoned macaroni and bean dish, a few cubes of squash, and a one-ounce piece of pita bread.

In accordance with the Pritikin philosophy of small frequent meals, morning and afternoon snacks were available in the dining room. The morning snack was an orange or raw vegetables. Afternoons, more raw vegetables or a vegetable-based soup such as mushroom bisque (made with skimmed milk), zucchini, or gazpacho.

Nothing Is Left to Chance

The next morning, attending a lecture given by Kathleen, a dietician, I learned the rules that govern portion size. Vegetables and grains are each served in one-half-cup portions. A fruit serving is three-fourths of a cup. Twice a week, you're permitted a one and one half ounce portion of high protein. Within the confines of your daily allowance (1,200 calories, if you're a man, 1,000 calories for a woman), you can "exchange" a specified amount of a certain food—say, a slice of bread—for a specified amount of another starch, such as cereal. As a newcomer, I found this slide rule approach to eating tedious and confusing, but others, who had been there a few days, seemed to have no difficulty.

The Workout

Exercise is a twice-a-day activity. Based on results of a treadmill test, you're assigned to a class with people of similar fitness levels. First, gentle stretching, after which you progress to forty-five minutes of aerobic exercise. Afternoons, your choices include aerobic dancing, aerobic weight training, or yoga, or you can take an hour's walk on the beach. (I chose the beach walk, but the spectacle of individuals unconcernedly drinking soft drinks and beer and licking ice cream cones might be hard on a dieter.) The exercise class I observed took place in the Center's high-school-size gymnasium. There, class members strode with a purposeful air on motorized treadmills while a crew of exercise physiologists in gray coverups buzzed about reaching for a wrist to check the pulse or wrapping a blood pressure cuff on an upper arm.

Results

The Pritikin Program of Diet and Exercise appears to live up to the Pritikin Promise, at least on a short-term basis. In a study (in conjunction with Loma Linda University) of the first 893 participants attending the twenty-six-day program:

- 85 percent of hypertensives who entered the program on hypertensive medication lowered their blood pressure and left drug-free.
- 50 percent of insulin-taking adult-onset diabetics lowered blood sugar and left the Center insulin-free.
- 62 percent of drug-taking angina patients left the Center drug-free, while many others reduced their medication.
- 70 percent of those who came in on gout medication were drug-free at the end of the program and showed normal uric acid levels.

- Cholesterol and triglycerides were each reduced 25 percent.
- Men lost 10 to 14 pounds, and women lost 8 to 12 pounds.[3]

The Dark Ages

A great many changes have occurred in medicine since Nathan Pritikin opened his first Longevity Center in 1976. At that time, few doctors thought there was a link between cholesterol and heart disease, and research showing the importance of fiber was in its infancy. Today, the American Diabetes Association (ADA) recommends a high-carbohydrate, high-fiber diet; back then, the ADA recommended a diet high in fat and protein and low in carbohydrates. Nutrition experts emphasized the need for protein in the diet and described animal protein, which they called "complete" protein, as superior to plant protein ("incomplete or of poor biologic value").[4] Obesity was commonly regarded as being "all in the head." Researchers contended that people became fat because they used food to satisfy unmet psychological needs.

The American Heart Association (AHA), to its credit, had been telling the American public to reduce its level of fat since 1961, but the fat intake that the AHA recommended in 1976 (45 percent of calories) seems a large amount by today's standards. Today the AHA recommends a fat intake of 30 percent of calories, still very high compared to the Pritikin diet, which restricts fat to 10 percent of daily calories.

Nathan the Revolutionary

In 1976 Nathan Pritikin, then a successful 60-year-old engineer and inventor, seemed an unlikely contender to challenge medical authorities. But Pritikin was no ordinary nutrition guru; his knowledge of medicine rivaled that of most medical specialists.[5] Pritikin also had the unshakable confidence in his ideas about diet and disease that springs from personal experience. At age 42, diagnosed with heart disease, he had been prescribed a drug to increase blood flow to the heart and warned to avoid strenuous exercise. Rejecting the wisdom of the day, he searched the medical literature for studies that related to heart disease, and he found several dating from the 1940s that implicated fat and cholesterol as the culprits in heart disease. Based on this scientific evidence, Pritikin painstakingly devised a low-fat, low-cholesterol diet that would also provide optimum nourishment.

The diet worked. In less than three years, he lowered his cholesterol level, originally 280 milligrams, to 120 milligrams. Although he was elated at this achievement, an EKG showed that he was not fully cured of heart disease, and other measures were needed. Again the medical literature supplied an answer. Finding long-forgotten animal studies showing that exercise could induce the growth of new capillaries, he developed an exercise program for himself to improve the circulation of blood and oxygen. As a starter, he took short frequent walks and gradually extended the distances. When a stress test showed that his heart rate was almost normal, he began running a few laps and eventually progressed to ten miles a day.

Convinced that his program of diet and exercise was the answer to hypertension and diabetes as well as heart disease,[6] he began counseling anyone who sought his help free of charge. During these years others following his program experienced the same benefits as he, and the concept of a Pritikin Center took shape. In 1976, having gained the support of a group of eminent progressive physicians (among them two British scientists, Dr. Denis Burkitt and Dr. Hugh Trowell), he opened the first Pritikin Center, several rooms at a Howard Johnson Motor Inn in Santa Barbara, California.

Not So Common Sense

Two years before the Center was established, a book called *Live Longer Now* (New York: Grosset & Dunlap, 1974), which Pritikin coauthored, had introduced his incendiary ideas about diet and disease. We have a massive health problem in the United States, the authors wrote. Heart disease and other degenerative diseases all stem from atherosclerosis, "a disease that clogs the body's arteries, just like rust clogs water pipes in the house."[7] Atherosclerosis, in turn, is caused by a high-fat, high-cholesterol diet. In subsequent books and interviews, Pritikin delighted in shooting down myths of the day.[8] A sampling:

- Blood cholesterol "norms," 150 to 330 milligrams at the time, are far too high for good health. To determine your normal cholesterol level, add 100 to your age with a maximum of 160.

- Unsaturated fats (such as safflower and corn oils), which the American Heart Association recommends as a substitute for saturated fat, are harmful. Although eating unsaturated fats makes cholesterol levels go down, it increases cholesterol in arterial plaque and other body tissue.

- Our body's need for protein has been grossly exaggerated; excessive protein causes the body to excrete important minerals such as calcium in the urine and also raises insulin blood levels and uric acid levels. Milk, being high in protein, is an inappropriate food for humans after weaning.

- The yolk of an egg, being high in fats and cholesterol, is like cyanide. Consuming minute amounts of cyanide, as found in lima beans, is safe, but it is extremely harmful when taken in larger quantities.

- Animal protein is not superior to vegetable protein. This erroneous idea was based on early studies with rats, whose nutritional needs are different from those of humans. The Tarahumora Indians of Central Mexico, who can run one hundred miles at a stretch and have no heart disease, subsist on a diet of corn, wild plants, beans, squash, and small amounts of fish and meat.

Meanwhile, Back at the Establishment

In the mid-1970s, when Pritikin went public with his ideas, nutritionists had already become critical of the American diet. "Diets high in saturated fat, high in cholesterol, or too high in calories are among the factors leading to coronary disease," wrote Corinne H. Robinson, professor emeritus of nutrition and formerly head of the Department of Nutrition and Food at the Drexel Institute of Technology in Philadelphia. At the same time, Robinson commended the "greater wealth of food choices, more snack items, and more convenience foods" available at the market. She also identified the "food quack" as one who tells you "that the food in grocery stores is robbed of its nutritional values because it has been grown on depleted soil or because processes such as canning or dehydration have removed most of the nutrients."[9] But Pritikin had no compunction about describing food products in a supermarket as garbage! Leading the "good life," characterized by lack of exercise and eating the wrong kind of food, is causing a modern plague of degenerative diseases, he said.

Members of the medical establishment, incensed by an outsider challenging their beliefs (and attracting so much media attention), criticized his program and rejected medical papers submitted by physicians at the Pritikin Center. Medical societies authorized dieticians to assess the Pritikin diet. One described the diet as "unsound . . . experimental." Another said it was "restrictive, austere, and dreary." A leading clinical professor of medicine reported in 1980 that the Pritikin program offered no more relief from peripheral vascular disease (atherosclerosis) than did the moderate diet proposed for many years by the American Heart Association.[10]

But Pritikin's ideas have triumphed. In the ensuing years, the medical establishment has edged closer and closer to Pritikin's views on diet. In 1984, a panel convened by the National Institutes of Health concluded "beyond a reasonable doubt" that lowering elevated blood cholesterol levels will reduce the risk of heart attack. The panel advised all Americans, except children under 2, to adopt a diet lower in total fat, saturated fat, and cholesterol. In October 1987, new guidelines issued by the National Heart, Lung, and Blood Institute (NHLBI), a federal agency, in cooperation with twenty-three major medical and health organizations, defined the risks of high cholesterol and suggested treatment. For persons with high cholesterol levels, the NHLBI recommended a cholesterol-lowering diet as the initial treatment. Pritikin's warning that heart disease starts at an early age in the United States is now well accepted. According to a *Science News* article (October 8, 1988),

"Circumstantial evidence has now accumulated to the point where many physicians believe mass interventions to lower children's cholesterol levels will save lives."

Doubts about Pritikin's Program

One leading authority on heart disease has reservations about the Pritikin program on two counts. First is the effectiveness of the program. "The Pritikin diet is largely unproven," says Dr. John C. LaRosa, dean for clinical affairs at the George Washington University Medical Center. "In many patients, it is an effective short-term way to lose weight and lower cholesterol, but I'm not convinced that it has any beneficial effect on heart disease."

The problem is that to provide irrefutable proof that a particular treatment has improved the condition of a group of heart patients, it is necessary to perform multiple angiograms on these patients. An angiogram consists of inserting a plastic tube through a large artery in the leg, which is fed up to the heart, where dye is injected into the heart chambers and arteries. X rays taken during the procedure show if a coronary artery is narrowed or blocked and where. According to Dr. Robert C. Atkins, "One person in a thousand dies from the procedure and countless more suffer nonfatal but serious complications."[11] In any case, Pritikin participants, who are paying $280 a day to improve their health, would hardly be willing to submit to such tests.

"I'm convinced that the Pritikin program can reverse atherosclerosis," said Dr. Stephen Inkeles, director of clinical nutrition at Santa Monica's Pritikin Center, "but we don't have the evidence that the medical profession insists on."

Ironically, proof that the Pritikin program can reverse atherosclerosis (at least in one individual) was provided at Nathan Pritikin's death. Pritikin took his own life in 1985, at age 69, when the leukemia that he had battled for many years worsened. Autopsy findings showed that his arteries, which had been severely blocked with atherosclerotic plaque in 1958, were almost completely free of atherosclerosis.[12]

Can You Keep Up the Good Work? Dr. LaRosa's other objection to the Pritikin diet is that "people fall off the wagon when they return to the everyday world." The Pritikin organization agrees. A recent survey of Pritikin graduates showed that 20 to 25 percent adhered fully to the program, another 25 percent adhered part of the time, while 50 percent abandoned the program.

To improve compliance, Robert Pritikin, Nathan's son, who directs the Pritikin enterprises, is trying to make the Pritikin diet less restrictive. He has added a new category of "caution" foods, such as sweeteners, decaffeinated coffee, and tea, to the diet ("If consumed occasionally or in small amounts, they pose little danger"). Participants at the Center are deluged with tips on how to dine out, compile a marketing list, and organize their kitchen. Lifetime counselors teach stress reduction techniques. Alumni can keep in touch by toll-free hot line and monthly newsletter. A line of Pritikin Foods—sauces, salad dressings, rice mixes, and soups—is available. An evening program, part exercise, part nutrition, called Pritikin P.M., is being instituted at health clubs around the country.

The "Good" Fats.   Criticism that raises serious concerns about the Pritikin diet comes from a Pritikin insider, Ann Louise Gittleman, M.S. Gittleman is a former director of nutrition at the Pritikin Center in Santa Monica and coauthor of *Beyond Pritikin* (New York: Bantam Books, 1987). The point in question is the extremely low fat content of the Pritikin diet. In restricting all fat, Gittleman says, the Pritikin diet deprives the individual of fats that are necessary for health.

One of the two major types of essential fats is omega-3 oils from fish and other marine animals, she says. These marine oils are high in two fatty acids called eicosapentaenoic acid, or EPA, and docosahexaenoic acid, or DHA. It is these fatty acids that keep Eskimos, whose traditional diet contains over 70 percent of its calories in fat, free of heart disease.

The other essential fat is omega-6 oils from plant and botanical sources such as unrefined vegetable oils, borage, and evening primrose oil. The omega-6 fatty acid called gamma linolenic acid, or GLA, helps cardiovascular problems, weight loss, and immune disorders such as arthritis, among others. "Both omega-3 and omega-6 fatty acids work in the body by forming hormonelike substances called prostaglandins [which] control the human body's daily function."

Gittleman first became aware of the downside of the Pritikin diet when some participants, while at the Center and afterwards, complained about gaining weight despite feeling hungry all the time. Although Gittleman acknowledges dramatic improvements in many who followed the Pritikin diet, she also noticed that participants who were on the program for a year or more developed vertical ridges on the fingernails, "a syndrome that signals a nutritional deficiency."

Gittleman's chief criticism of the Pritikin diet is that it restricts all fats, thereby also excluding the "good" fats, but she differs on some other issues. If you're sensitive to gluten, "excessive eating of carbohydrates" (80 percent in the Pritikin diet) can irritate the intestines, she says. Gittleman also contends that cholesterol is not all bad. "Cholesterol is such a vital substance to the body that if sufficient amounts are not ingested from the diet, the body's own tissue (primarily the liver) will produce more to compensate for dietary lack."

A Cardiologist Defends Pritikin

Dr. Charles Tam, former director of cardiology at St. Helena Hospital in Deer Park, California, who lectures widely on the subject of essential fatty acids, strongly endorses the Pritikin diet.

In assessing the Pritikin diet from the standpoint of the two essential fatty acids omega-6 (GLA) and omega-3 (EPA), Tam emphasizes the role of an enzyme, Delta 6-Desaturase, which is necessary to convert the omega-6 cis linoleic acid into gamma linolenic acid (GLA). "This same Delta 6 enzyme is also required to change alpha linoleic acid to fish oil (EPA)."

The problem is not that we're lacking these two essential fatty acids in our diet, Tam said. Unless you are malnourished to the point of starvation, you have an ample supply of omega-6 and omega-3 oils. "The problem is that our diet is so full of things that inhibit the Delta 6 enzyme from converting these essential fatty acids into prostaglandins." Some of these damaging substances are alcohol, caffeine, saturated fats, refined (vegetable) oils, and cholesterol, he said. Factors in our diet that activate the Delta 6 enzyme are vitamins, minerals, and essential amino acids.

"The Pritikin diet achieves such good results mainly because it restricts refined oils and saturated fats, two of the substances that are most damaging to the Delta 6 enzyme. Ironically, Pritikin knew nothing about essential fatty acids and prostaglandins."

Conclusion

Pritikin's insistence on a spartan regime for heart patients seems to be the way to go. In a recent study of a group of patients with severe coronary artery disease, those who stuck with the demanding regimen of a vegetarian diet, meditation, and exercise for one year reduced the plaque in their arteries.[13] Jane E. Brody, *New York Times* health columnist, wrote on December 7, 1989, that "the most effective way to limit and even reverse fatty deposits in arteries is to consume a diet very low in all fats, on the order of 15 percent of calories from fat."

THE MCDOUGALL PLAN

In January of 1988 I spent three days taking part in the twelve-day McDougall Program (cost, with private room, $3,700). It's given at the St. Helena Hospital and Health Center, which is set on top of a hill overlooking the Napa Valley and looks more like a health spa than a hospital. I arrived in late afternoon, and a friendly young man carried my suitcase to my room on the

McDougall floor, which is well lit and decorated in soft pastels. Opening the sliding doors, I stood on the terrace breathing in cool mountain air, with a view of fir-tree-covered hills.

The next morning, I was one of ten gathered in a classroom awaiting Dr. McDougall's introductory talk. My classmates, men and women ranging from their late 20s to their 60s, appeared to be professional people. (Everyone I talked to produced a business card from the pocket of a warm-up suit.) Judging from the four participants I became acquainted with, the McDougall Plan attracts people who have some serious health problems.

Four McDougall Participants

Carl, 58, a realtor given to deadpan quips, weighs 214 pounds, has a hernia, and wants to improve his "terrible" eating habits, which he attributes to a divorce some years ago and job stress.

Stan, 66, a newly retired professor, appears to be the least likely candidate for a heart problem; he's wiry, has an outgoing personality, eats very little meat, and describes a happy marriage and a close-knit family. But last month, when he was taking a routine exam, "They stopped the treadmill test and told me to get an angiogram right away. When my doctor saw the results, he said I needed a bypass and scheduled me for surgery the following week." Stan consulted Dr. McDougall for a second opinion, and "He told me, 'Your arteries are no worse than most men your age; you can fix that with diet.' So I turned down the surgery and signed up for this program."

Catherine, 48, a computer specialist, weighs 210 pounds and is on medication for high blood pressure. She first became aware that she had a health problem one and a half years ago. "I'd nod off in the middle of a meeting, and I was often very thirsty." At her initial examination, McDougall discovered she was diabetic. She too has poor eating habits and blames this on job stress and a recent marital separation. "I snack a lot, drink too much coffee."

Dorothy, 52, president of a mental health organization, weighs 200 pounds and has been plagued with health problems all her life. "I had a mastoid at 6 years, appendicitis at 21." In addition, she has undergone several major operations, including heart surgery. She now suffers from abdominal pain— "They can't find what it is"—and arthritis. Dorothy's childhood was unhappy—"I've been on my own since I was 16"—and she's married to a man "who is negative like my father."

McDougall's Story

McDougall, boyish-looking at 40, six feet tall, wearing a sport shirt and jacket, greeted us in a friendly, relaxed manner. "I have a right to talk to you about disease," he said. "As a child, I ate eggs, bacon, milk, hot dogs, and had stomach problems and constipation. I went off to college and ate more of the same." At 18, he had a stroke (he still walks with a limp) and at 26 underwent abdominal surgery.

As a family practitioner, McDougall spent three years on the island of Hawaii, where "Eventually, I became involved in diet because I was a frustrated physician—my patients were not getting better. I could help someone who was injured—stop the bleeding, set a bone—but my chronic disease patients got sicker and sicker." One of his patients, a young newlywed, had high blood pressure so McDougall treated him with one of the standard drugs. "The next visit, he told me he couldn't get an erection. Some time later he had a stroke, so the drug didn't help him anyway."

During that period, his patients taught him a valuable lesson. "Many of my patients living on the Big Island were first-generation Chinese, Japanese, Filipino. They ate the traditional Oriental diet of rice and vegetables and were trim, hardworking, and healthy. Their offspring ate the American diet. These second-generation Americans were fat and had the usual American diseases—high blood pressure, diabetes, heart disease. I had been taught that chronic disease is genetic—inherited from one generation to another— but I could see with my own eyes that this wasn't true."

Struck with this discovery, McDougall, then a resident in internal medicine, began spending long hours at the medical library combing the literature for studies dealing with diet and disease. A wealth of studies published prior to the 1950s contained the same message: when sick people change to a diet of simple foods, they get well.

A Royal Feast

"How can eating a simple diet restore people to health?" McDougall asks. "To find the cure for a disease, look for the cause. All the diseases we suffer from,"—here a long list fell trippingly from his tongue— "atherosclerosis, heart attack, strokes, high blood pressure, obesity, adult diabetes, gout, gallstones, kidney stones, osteoporosis, hemorrhoids, constipation, colitis, appendicitis, diverticular diseases, psoriasis, multiple sclerosis, and cancer—all have the same cause: eating a diet of rich foods." Rich foods, he explains, are primarily animal foods and dairy products. These foods are high in fat and cholesterol, which clog our arteries, causing hardening of the arteries, or atherosclerosis.

"The type of life-threatening disease you develop depends on which arteries are involved. When hardening of the arteries takes place in arteries that lead to the heart, heart disease results. When arteries to the brain are clogged, a stroke can occur. When clogged arteries prevent adequate blood reaching the kidneys, kidney failure results. When the legs don't get enough blood, walking becomes painful. Eventually the foot or the entire leg may die from lack of blood, and gangrene develops."

The Culprit—Cholesterol. Taking his cue from his mentor, Nathan Pritikin, McDougall blames all this misery caused by hardening of the arteries on too much cholesterol in the diet. "Your body produces enough cholesterol to do its job; you don't need to consume additional cholesterol. But when you eat the flesh of animals or animal by-products—milk, ice cream, cheese, and eggs—you are ingesting large quantities of cholesterol. The body has a limited ability to excrete cholesterol; much is excreted by the liver, but excess amounts are deposited in the tissues. When cholesterol settles in the lining of the arteries, the stage is set for atherosclerosis."

The Good News. "If you can intervene before these diseased arteries cause irreparable harm to the heart and major blood vessels, then you can actually reverse hardening of the arteries. Plaque does not harden like cement, as we were once told. If you eliminate the dietary fat and cholesterol that caused the buildup of plaque in the first place, and replace this diet of rich foods with a health-supporting diet, you can reduce the plaque in your arteries."

McDougall's Diet

The McDougall diet is a vegan diet (a total vegetarian diet that excludes poultry, fish, seafood, and dairy products). It is a starch-centered diet; starches make up the largest portion of the meal. McDougall defines starches as whole grains, legumes, flour, pasta, root vegetables, and winter squashes. Smaller amounts of vegetables and fruits are added to complement the starch main dish. This is not a fad diet, McDougall says, but the traditional diet that people have thrived on since prehistoric times. The starch varies from one culture to another—rice in Asia, corn in North and Central America, sweet potatoes in New Guinea—but the proportion of starch (80 percent) remains the same.

McDougall seeks to eliminate excess fat, the most harmful element of a "rich" (animal food) diet. "After we eat a meal high in any type of fat, our blood cells can actually stick together in clumps that plug the blood vessels."[14] Animal foods and products contain large amounts of fat and cholesterol, but plant foods are low in fat and contain no cholesterol. The only dietary fat we need, McDougall says, is a polyunsaturated fatty acid called linoleic acid; adequate amounts of this oil are found in a grain-based diet. (For example, linoleic acid comprises 50 percent of the total calories of barley.)

To eradicate every speck of fat in the diet, no oil is used in cooking. (Both *The McDougall Plan* and his second book, *McDougall's Medicine* [Piscataway, N.J.: New Century Publishers, 1983 and 1985], contain a recipe section.) To "sauté" vegetables (as a change from steaming, the usual method), use a small amount of water or vegetable stock, McDougall advises. In cooking class, our teacher suggested spraying the pan with a light coating of Pam no-stick cooking spray and wiping off the excess.

Sampling McDougall Fare

We ten participants sat at the same table in a cheerful, homey dining room and served ourselves from a buffet reserved for our use. My first breakfast consisted of fresh orange and grapefruit sections, hot oatmeal with nut milk, baked hash brown potatoes, and thick slabs of a dense whole grain bread, chewy and satisfying. All the breads are baked without oil. Applesauce and a sugarless jam are breakfast staples. Another morning, we had slices of pineapple and melon, hot apple granola cereal, potato patties (a little heavy on the onion for my taste), and home-baked raisin cinnamon bread. Lunch one day was a tossed salad, whole wheat bread, and a fruit salad. Another lunch consisted of pasta salad garnished with raw vegetables, a tofu burger on a roll with tomato slices (burger a bit dry), a tofu dip with onion, and rice raisin pudding. Salsa and various herb seasonings are available at lunch and dinner.

The three dinners I had were all delicious, including the plainest, which consisted of vegetable split pea soup with whole wheat croutons and potatoes, carrots, and brussels sprouts, cold potato salad with snow peas, and herb bread with applesauce and jam. One of several meals with a Mexican theme was baked tortilla chips with "broccomoli" (a dip with the consistency of guacamole), pinto beans mixed with vegetables, whole wheat bread, and salad. The day I left, lunch included paella with swiss chard and strawberry-banana tapioca. (A seafood lover might feel a little cheated discovering that McDougall-style paella contains everything but lobster, shrimp, or clams.) According to my menu plan, dinner that evening was whole wheat spaghetti with mushrooms and spinach with pesto sauce.

My companions, who were not accustomed to vegetarian fare, enjoyed the food as much as I, although this was not the case the first evening (so I was told), when dinner was stir-fried vegetables and brown rice (the blandest offering in a menu plan that leans heavily on spicy ethnic dishes). "Stan and I were ready to pack our bags," Carl said. But by the third day, when we prepared our own dinner in a cooking class, we were congratulating each other's efforts and swapping recipes.

All You Can Eat Within Reason

Although most of the participants were considerably overweight, there wasn't a calorie chart in sight. All heaped their plates full, and most went back for second helpings. According to McDougall, when you limit your diet to healthy foods (starches and vegetables), you can eat all you want within reason. A starch-based diet is an ideal weight loss diet, McDougall explains, because starches are so filling and low in calories. In a portion of potatoes, only 1 percent of the calories come from fat. McDougall participants, on the average, lose ten pounds a month. If weight loss is too slow, eliminate bread and possibly beans, he says.

The only food restriction in our group applied to persons who were diabetic or hypoglycemic; they were not allowed fruit at every meal.

As in the Pritikin Program, exercise is an important part of the McDougall Plan. The first few mornings, participants (who have passed a treadmill test) walk laps around a track—eighteen laps to a mile—for thirty to forty minutes. Those sufficiently fit progress to a hike as long as five miles. Afternoons, participants engage in thirty minutes of pool exercises— relaxing and easy on the joints, said Ed Haver, exercise physiologist at St. Helena Hospital and Health Center. "Diet and exercise go together. If a person continues exercising at home, he's more apt to stick to the diet."

Dieticians and the Vegetarian Diet

During the 1970s, the American Dietetic Association (ADA) viewed the vegetarian diet as inferior ("The quality of vegetable protein is less than animal protein").[15] But in its July 1980 "Position Paper on the Vegetarian Approach to Eating," the ADA acknowledged that "most of mankind for much of human history has subsisted on a near-vegetarian diet," and recognized that "well-planned vegetarian diets are consistent with good nutritional status."[16] In 1988 the ADA went one step further: "A considerable body of scientific data suggests positive relationships between vegetarian life-styles and risk reduction for several chronic degenerative diseases, such as obesity, coronary artery disease, hypertension, diabetes mellitus, colon cancer, and others."[17] Furthermore, the ADA states in comparing vegetarians to non-vegetarians that the former are less apt to die of heart disease, generally have lower blood pressure, are not as prone to adult-onset diabetes, maintain a desirable weight, and "have lower rates of osteoporosis, kidney stones, gallstones, and diverticular disease."

But following a vegan diet requires very careful planning, said ADA spokesperson Allison Boomer, R.D. Otherwise, you're likely to be deficient in essential nutrients, particularly vitamin B12 and vitamin D. "I don't advocate a vegan diet. When you start eliminating food groups, you narrow your possibilities for meeting the spectrum of necessary nutrients. Following such a restrictive diet, everything you eat needs to count—it must be a jewel!"

The Trouble with Animal Foods. Discussing the McDougall diet almost inevitably provokes an angry response: "You mean fish and poultry are bad, too?" Here's how McDougall explains some of his controversial ideas about diet.

Meat is dangerous to your health because it's high in fat and/or protein and deficient in carbohydrate and fiber—precisely the wrong proportion of nutrients. Animal fat, which is saturated fat, raises cholesterol levels and injures arteries, causing atherosclerosis, which leads to heart attacks and strokes.

The protein found in animal foods causes a tremendous loss of calcium through the kidneys. Meats are also high in purines, which break down into uric acid. This waste product causes kidney stones and gout in susceptible people.

Meats frequently contain organisms that cause hepatitis, salmonella, and trichinosis, and may even cause cancer. Meats also contain high levels of environmental contaminants such as fat-soluble pesticides, herbicides, and other chemical poisons.

Dairy products, the leading cause of food allergies, can cause colitis, asthma, skin rashes, and tonsillitis. In children, milk can cause ear infections, runny nose, or bedwetting. Dairy products have been linked to a cancer of the immune system called Hodgkin's disease and may contain unsafe amounts of environmental contaminants.

To prevent early bone loss, women are advised to consume 1,000 to 1,500 milligrams of calcium a day, a recommendation that runs contrary to scientific studies of worldwide populations. These show that osteoporosis is most common in the United States, England, Israel, Sweden, and Finland—countries in which people consume the largest quantities of dairy products and calcium supplements—but rare in Asian and African countries where only infants drink milk.

Eating large amounts of calcium is counterproductive since most of the mineral is blocked from absorption by the intestinal lining. Without the intestine's regulatory action, the kidneys, muscles, and other tissues would become calcified. When you eat lesser amounts of calcium, a larger percentage of the calcium is absorbed by the body, meeting your needs.

Protein has much more influence on bone health than calcium. Limiting protein-rich foods, such as chicken, fish, beef, eggs, cottage cheese, and skim milk, will result in more calcium staying in the body rather than being excreted by the kidneys into the urine. Another harmful effect of a high-protein diet is the tendency to develop calcium kidney stones. The calcium that ends up in the urine raises the level of calcium in the kidney system, causing these painful stones.

Eggs are high in protein and fat—both of which we consume in excess eating the American diet. (The yolk of an egg is 80 percent fat.) Even more significant, eggs contain one of the highest concentrations of cholesterol.

The Trouble with Fish.   Eating fish and fish oil is associated with lower risk of heart disease owing to the way fish oils affect the clotting mechanism in the arteries. Fish fat has a tendency to "thin" the blood by decreasing the stickiness of the blood-clotting elements called platelets, thus reducing the risk of the blood vessel's bursting. The other side of the coin is that this blood-thinning effect can cause serious bleeding problems. Eskimos, whose traditional diet is largely fish, are prone to nosebleeds. Another harmful effect of eating large amounts of fish is a change in the hormones called prostaglandins. In the Faulkes Islands, where half the diet is fish, women have a longer gestation period, produce bigger babies, and the infant mortality is double the usual figure.

In rare instances, people who consume all-vegetable diets for more than three years develop deficiencies in vitamin B12. To prevent this unlikely possibility, add a nonanimal source of B12 to your diet. These sources include fermented soybean products such as tempeh, some soyu-tamari sauces, nutritional yeast fortified with B12, and sea vegetables such as kombu and wakame. All these items can be found in a well-stocked health food store. Do not use vitamin pills to supply your requirements; stick to whole foods.

Bending the Rules

Is it necessary to totally eliminate all animal foods as McDougall advises? ("Even a tiny bit of fish or chicken teases the taste buds.") I asked our cooking teacher, Vicki Saunders, a dietician at St. Helena Hospital and Health Center, if she herself abided by this dictum. (Saunders is a Seventh Day Adventist who was raised on a vegan diet.) Saunders distinguished between the needs of sick people who participate in the McDougall Program and healthy individuals: "Healthy people can play around with small amounts of rich foods. I use a little olive oil in cooking, a tiny amount of butter here and there, small amounts of skimmed milk."

Assessing McDougall's Plan

As I warned earlier, I can see loopholes in some of McDougall's arguments. For example, in comparing older Orientals who have emigrated to the island of Hawaii, with their offspring, first generation Americans, he attributes the miserable condition of the younger people to the high-fat American diet. There's no mention of exercise, or lack of it, as a possible factor in the situation. In the 1920s and 1930s, Weston Price, a dentist, compared groups that had not been exposed to modern civilization with similar groups that had been. In each case he noted the deleterious effect of a "civilized" diet in terms of dental structure and teeth. But he also emphasized the physicial challenges that were part of the everyday lives of so-called primitive cultures. Swiss living in an isolated Alpine valley without trucks or any means of conveyance, for example, carried enormous loads on their backs up and down the mountainside.[18]

In regard to osteoporosis, it's encouraging to find that the American Dietetic Association agrees with McDougall that less protein in the diet may be beneficial. In the 1988 *ADA Reports,* they state, "Lower protein intake (found in vegetarian diets) . . . may be associated with a lower risk of osteoporosis in vegetarians."[19]

More convincing evidence (in my opinion) that a diet and exercise program can control and even reverse degenerative diseases comes from McDougall's examples of therapeutic diets that have stood the test of time. One is the rice diet, basically rice and fruit, devised by Dr. Walter Kempner of Duke University. In the 1940s Kempner began using this diet to treat patients critically ill with heart and kidney disease and hypertension, and restored them to health. At that time, physicians regarded those diseases as a death sentence, so when Kempner's findings appeared in a medical journal in 1944, they created tremendous interest.[20] In the ensuing years, however, as drug treatment edged out gentler methods of healing, doctors lost interest in dietary treatment. Nevertheless, the rice diet, the sole method of treatment at the Kempner Clinic in Durham, is still going strong. Kempner, vigorous at 85, continues to direct the program. For further information about the rice diet, write Kempner Clinic (Rice Diet), Duke University Medical Center, 1821 Green Street, Durham, NC 27705.

Another enduring therapeutic diet is the Swank low-fat diet devised by Dr. Roy Swank of the University of Oregon. For the past thirty-five years, Swank has treated thousands of multiple sclerosis (MS) patients with his diet, which restricts red meat and dairy products. Swank reports that this low-fat diet reduces the number and severity of recurrences in MS patients. For a detailed account of the diet, see *The Multiple Sclerosis Diet Book* that Swank coauthored (New York: Doubleday & Co., 1987).

Scientists Look at the Therapeutic Diet

More recently, researchers with impressive academic affiliations have reported studies using dietary treatment. One is Dr. Dean Ornish of the University of California. In the mid-1970s, Ornish, an internist, conducted a study in which he treated a group of patients with advanced heart disease with a diet almost devoid of animal fats along with stress management techniques and exercise. In a preliminary report published in 1977, Ornish showed that these life-style changes could improve the heart's function. For more information about Ornish's program, see his book, *Stress, Diet and Your Heart* (New York: Holt, Rinehart, and Winston, 1982).

Ten years later, a team of scientists from the University of Southern California made front-page news when they reported (*JAMA*, June 19, 1987) that reducing blood cholesterol could slow and in some cases reverse the formation and growth of fatty deposits in arteries. This was the first measurable evidence that an "aggressive" cholesterol-lowering treatment could shrink fatty deposits in the coronary arteries of critically ill heart patients. Treatment consisted of diet combined with a cholesterol-lowering drug.[21]

One year prior to the publication of this landmark study, McDougall wrote in *The McDougall Newsletter* (January/February 1986) that he had changed his mind about the best way to treat patients with elevated cholesterol. Previously he had used diet alone to lower cholesterol, but now, "If my patients fail to lower their cholesterol below 180 milligrams with diet alone, I start them on cholesterol-lowering drugs."

Results

McDougall's twelve-day crash course in a healthy life-style, which includes daily talks by a minister and psychologist, achieves results. Based on before and after measurements of 30 McDougall participants, the average drop in cholesterol is 44 points (a 17-percent decrease); triglycerides drop 14 percent; blood pressure comes down 8 percent for systolic, 11 percent for diastolic; average weight loss is 3.1 pounds.

Do participants stick to this regime of diet and exercise for any length of time? Since a survey that addresses this question is only in the planning stage one year after my visit to the St. Helena Health Center, I contacted the four McDougall participants I mentioned earlier.

Catherine, computer specialist, formerly obese with high blood pressure and diabetes, has kept to the diet the entire time, she said. "I feel great. I've lost fifty pounds. My dress size was 20 to 22; I'm now a 12 to 14." Other before and after statistics she related were cholesterol formerly 238 milligrams, now 150 milligrams; blood sugar down from 340 to 140; blood pressure, which had been 145/95, now varies between 115/75 and 120/75. She exercises every day. "Five days a week I do aerobic dancing at the Y, weekends I follow exercise tapes at home. The McDougall program has changed my life."

I wasn't surprised to learn from Stan's wife, Mary, that Stan (the retired college professor with a heart condition) had stayed on the program "religiously"; the couple had eaten a near vegetarian diet before McDougall's. In fact, Mary worries that her husband is overzealous about the program. "He's afraid of eating any fat because of his arteries—he got terribly thin at one time." Walking at a fast clip, he takes a daily two-mile hike over hilly terrain. Mary said that the McDougall Plan may have saved her husband's life. "Both of his brothers died in their 50s of a heart attack."

Dorothy, who had been sick all of her life with multiple health problems, has never deviated from the program and has reaped all kinds of benefits, including "no stomach pains since I left the McDougall center." She still has a touch of arthritis but her exercise program—pool exercises at the Y and walking on alternate days—has relieved the aching. Her weight has dropped from 200 to 170 pounds ("I still need to lose another 20"). A blood test two months ago showed that her cholesterol, 357 when she began the program, was now 141. Triglycerides, formerly 219, were 95. Prior to her stay at McDougall's, Dorothy had recurrent precancerous skin tumors that her dermatologist removed with a cautery from time to time. "My last visit, no tumors had appeared." Another bonus is the improvement in her skin. "All my life I've had rough, dry skin. Now it's satin smooth all over."

Carl, who had been considerably overweight, said that a stressful episode during the past year (acting as caretaker for a friend dying of lung cancer) had caused him to revert to his old pattern of using food as a stress reliever. But having recently attended a class reunion at the McDougall Center, he had freshly resolved to stick to the diet. ("You should have seen Cathy and Dorothy. You wouldn't believe how good they looked!")

Do physicians today agree with McDougall that a program of diet and exercise can control and reverse degenerative diseases?

Said Dr. Robert G. Wones, director of the Division of General Internal Medicine at the University of Cincinnati Medical Center, "If you're talking about adult-onset diabetes, the answer is yes. The majority of adult diabetics are overweight and can treat their problem with diet and weight loss measures and achieve success. In treating coronary heart disease, we believe that appropriate diet, to lower cholesterol levels, for example, can stabilize the patient's condition and keep it from progressing further. But it's debatable whether you can actually achieve regression of coronary heart disease."

MACROBIOTICS

The word *macrobiotics* comes from the Greek *macro,* meaning "large or great" and *bios* meaning "life." Its literal translation is "great life." The term *macrobiotics* was first used in the late 1950s by the Japanese philosopher George Ohsawa to describe an Oriental view of the universe and a diet. Ohsawa as a young man had cured himself of tuberculosis with diet. After Ohsawa's death in the mid-1960s, Michio Kushi, who began lecturing on world peace and diet here in the 1950s, assumed command of the macrobiotic movement.

Today Kushi and his wife, Aveline, head the Kushi Institute and Foundation based in Brookline and Becket, Massachusetts. There are eight major centers in the United States, each of which has spawned satellite centers, and there are centers or some kind of representation in twenty-three countries.

Macrobiotics, as a well-designed Kushi Institute brochure states, "is more than brown rice; it is a way of life." In macrobiotic literature, a description of the diet is generally accompanied by Kushi's "way of life" suggestions. These range from "Live each day happily without being preoccupied with your health" to "Sing a happy song every day."

Principles of the Macrobiotic Diet

Despite the unlimited scope of macrobiotics as "the universal way of health, happinesss and peace," diet is its centerpiece. "We are what we eat," Kushi says. "We are an image of what we take in. . . . When we have difficulties, we should seek the cause in what we eat. . . ."[22]

The macrobiotic diet consists of grains, beans, vegetables, soy products (a key item is miso soup), cooked fruit, and a small portion of fish (white meat) once or twice a week. Forbidden foods include meat, eggs, poultry, dairy products, fruit juices, canned or frozen foods, coffee or commercial tea, and refined sweeteners. Other foods that should be eliminated are the nightshade vegetables (among them tomatoes, potatoes, eggplant, and peppers).

Recommended foods must be eaten in correct proportions. Every meal should consist of at least 50 percent whole cereal grains. The prescribed daily intake is 20 to 30 percent vegetables, 5 to 10 percent beans and sea vegetables, and 5 percent fruit grown locally.

Despite the inclusion of such exotic items as sea vegetables (seaweed) and Japanese condiments, the macrobiotic diet is the diet of "ordinary people through history," Kushi writes. Like Pritikin and McDougall, Kushi contends that a grain-centered diet has been the mainstay of human beings since the beginning of time. "By eating grains, human consciousness developed and is evolving toward the heavens."[23]

A Sample Meal

To refresh myself on the taste of macrobiotic food, I attended a cooking class given by Gale Howe, who has taught macrobiotic cooking in Cincinnati for four years. Eight of us, seated in Howe's old-style kitchen, notebooks on our laps, watched Howe, homey-looking, a trifle plump, glasses slipping down her nose, prepare a dinner that utilized end-of-the-summer ingredients. One and a half hours later, carrying our bridge chairs to the dining room table, we began our meal with three-mushroom soup, pleasantly chewy and flavorful, cooked with two strips of kombu (seaweed) and white miso (fermented soybean paste). The main course dishes had been chosen for their contrasting colors and flavors, Howe said. One, pan-fried millet croquettes, was made with grated carrot and chopped scallions, which gave it a sweet-sharp flavor. The croquettes were served with a shoyu (tamari) sauce. Other dishes were chickpeas with corn (also cooked with kombu for nourishment and flavor), steamed turnip greens (crisp and slightly bitter), and a condiment of roasted red peppers. (Although red peppers are a member of the nightshade family, not recommended to be eaten on a daily basis, occasional use of such foods is acceptable, Howe said.) Dessert was a peach cobbler, made with rolled oats and sweetened with yinnie (rice) syrup. This meal, which Howe described as well balanced, left me pleasantly satiated but not stuffed.

Yin and Yang

What distinguishes macrobiotics from other traditional diets is the philosophy of yin and yang—"a carefully thought-out system of dealing with opposites," according to Annemarie Colbin, author of *Food and Healing* (New York: Ballantine Books, 1986). Yin originally meant "the shady side of the hill" and yang stood for "the sunny side of the hill," she writes. Thus, yin represents the cool dark element and yang, the hot light element. Ohsawa, founder of macrobiotics, classified foods in terms of expansive (more yin) and contractive (more yang).

Foods are classified in this manner as a means of developing a balanced diet. All foods have both yin and yang qualities, and various criteria are used to determine how a particular food is classified. One factor is the food's structure. According to Kushi, "Foods that are condensed and grow below ground such as burdock, carrot, and other root vegetables are yang, those that are expanded and grow on the ground such as onion and squash are more balanced, and those that grow above ground such as kale are yin."[24]

Another factor that determines whether a food is yin or yang is the part of the world where it originates. Foods grown in a tropical climate are more yin, and foods from more northern climates are more yang. For a full description of this complex subject, see Kushi's *The Book of Macrobiotics* (New York: Japan Publications, 1987).

Applying Yin and Yang

How do the principles of yin and yang work in real life? Here's how an experienced macrobiotic counselor, Robert Carr, director of the East West Center of Cleveland, describes the process:

> I use the concept of yin and yang when I first evaluate a person's health, and secondly, when I recommend foods that are appropriate for that person's condition. For example, last week, a man in his 40s, a dynamic businessman named Henry, came to me complaining of stomach problems. In the course of the interview, Henry told me that he disliked hot weather and liked cold weather. This preference tells me

that his overall condition is yang. Since our goal is to balance the individual, avoiding both extremes of yin and yang, I recommended a balanced diet that included grains that are more yin—medium or large grain brown rice, barley, and corn.

Martha, a bookkeeper in her 50s, who consulted me recently, represents the opposite type. Martha, who suffers from eczema, hates cold weather—she's always chilly—and loves hot weather. Martha is very yin. I recommended that she eat grains that are more yang such as millet, short grain brown rice, and buckwheat.

Other clues that reveal the balance of yin and yang come from people's faces, Carr said:

Henry's features were very tense and tight; we call that a yang or more contracted condition. In addition to the yin-type grains, I recommended increasing the proportion of more expansive vegetables such as celery, green beans, kale—vegetables that grow above the ground. Carrots and other root vegetables that grow below ground are more yang. I included them in his diet but suggested he eat only moderate amounts.

In devising a diet, a macrobiotic counselor also considers the individual's ethnic origins, Carr said.

If I'm recommending a yin vegetable to a person who is Italian-American, I'll include dandelion greens. All Italians know that those greens are good for you. If the person is from Japan or China, I might recommend a daikon radish; that food is as familiar to an Oriental as a carrot to Americans. Eating seaweed seems strange to many Americans, but if you're of Irish descent and familiar with the eating habits of your ancestors, you'll find an old friend, Irish moss, among the sea vegetables. The point is that the foods we recommend are traditional foods—strange to many Americans but foods that are part of other cultures.

Not all counselors use the terms *yin* and *yang*. "There has been a move to Americanize macrobiotics," said Neil Stapleton, a counselor at the Macrobiotic Center of New York. "We're more apt to describe foods in terms of acid and alkaline, or hot and cold. We want people to be as comfortable as possible with the philosophy."

Despite all the rules, which govern every phase of a macrobiotic diet including the order in which various dishes are eaten, Kushi describes macrobiotics as a flexible dietary approach, not a set diet. Our aim is to eat in a way that brings our condition into harmony with the environment around us, says Kushi's wife, Aveline Kushi. To do so, she gives the following advice in the *Changing Seasons Macrobiotic Cookbook* (Wayne, N.J.: Avery Publishing Group, 1985). First rely on foods that are grown in a climate similar to the one in which you live. (If you live in a temperate zone, eat a pear rather than an orange.) Second, eat according to the seasons. In summer, you crave cooling fruits and salads; when the weather turns cold you want to warm up with heartier, richer dishes such as vegetarian bean stews and sautéed vegetables.

A Sick Society

Like other proponents of a therapeutic diet, Kushi presents evidence that we Americans are experiencing a health crisis: 40 million people suffer from cardiovascular disorders, 3 million from cancer, over 30 million from some form of arthritis, 32 million from mental disorders, 6 million from alcoholism, 20 to 30 million from some form of sexually transmitted disease.[25] The high rate of divorce, crime, and drug abuse are evidence of the moral decay in our society.

Our poor state of emotional, spiritual, and physical health is due to improper diet and life-style, says Kushi. "In the past, most people appreciated the simple, natural taste and texture of brown bread, brown rice, and other natural foods [but today] we have created a totally artificial way of life and have moved further and further from our origins in the natural world."[26] To recover from our present-day disorders, "we need a more comprehensive approach to life," which is provided by macrobiotics.[27]

Macrobiotics Against Disease

Cancer. Thus far, Kushi's message, despite its lofty language, is similar to that of Pritikin and McDougall: you're sick and my diet/life-style program can cure you. But, whereas Pritikin and McDougall claim that their diets can reverse circulatory diseases—heart, hypertension, diabetes, and other disorders related to atherosclerosis—they do not make any claims about cancer. Here Kushi parts company with the two Westerners. Since cancer, like all degenerative disease, is "the product of our own daily behavior," including our way of eating, cancer can be relieved naturally "by centering the diet." Elsewhere he writes that persons considered "medically terminal" have a better chance of recovery through practicing macrobiotics than those who have been treated with radiation, chemotherapy, surgery, or some other form of treatment.

These sentiments are naturally anathema to the American Cancer Society, which places the macrobiotic diet on its list of Unproven Methods of Cancer Management.[28] There is no evidence that any diet "will influence the course of cancer once it starts," says Arthur Holleb, M.D., chief medical officer of the American Cancer Society. "You can improve your quality of life with a proper diet. You can reduce the risk of cancer. But it is dangerous to think that you can *cure* cancer with a diet."[29]

Macrobiotic literature abounds with case histories of cancer patients who recovered following a macrobiotic diet. A corporate executive who developed pancreatic cancer (a type of cancer that doctors consider incurable) discontinued chemotherapy in favor of macrobiotics. Two years after the diagnosis, he's playing vigorous singles tennis matches.[30] A 56-year-old mother and R.N. was found to have malignant melanoma (another fatal type of cancer) and told she had six months to live. After one year on the macrobiotic diet, tests show that she no longer has cancer in her body.

Macrobiotics' widespread reputation as a cancer cure can be largely attributed to a best-seller, *Recalled by Life: The Story of a Recovery from Cancer* (Boston: Houghton Mifflin, 1982). Its author, Anthony J. Sattilaro, M.D., president of Philadelphia's Methodist Hospital, described how after adopting the macrobiotic diet out of desperation he recovered from Stage IV prostatic cancer. (Sattilaro died of cancer in August 1989.) Two lesser known but also convincing accounts of cancer cures are Elaine Nussbaum's *Recovery: From Cancer to Health through Macrobiotics* (New York: Japan Publishers, 1986) and *Confessions of a Kamikaze Cowboy* by actor Dirk Benedict (North Hollywood, Calif.: New Castle Publications, 1987). (More about macrobiotics and cancer in chapter 1.)

AIDS.   Macrobiotics isn't afraid to tackle AIDS either. Beginning in 1984, 20 men who practiced macrobiotics and had been diagnosed with Kaposi's sarcoma lesions (a rare type of skin cancer that frequently occurs in AIDS) took part in a three-year study in New York City to test the effect of a macrobiotic diet on AIDS patients. (From time to time, other AIDS patients have been added to the group.) Participating in the study were two immunologists from Boston University's Department of Microbiology and a New York physician.

According to one of the two immunologists, Eleanor Levy, Ph.D., "Results are encouraging. All the men felt better, had fewer symptoms. T-cells and lymphocytes were stabilized in half of the group." (In people with Kaposi's sarcoma lesions, the general pattern is a steady decline in both T-cells and lymphocytes, she said.) Levy concludes that macrobiotics appears to prolong survival in AIDS patients: "Seven out of the nine men lived at least three years. Six are still alive and doing well. The rest are just OK." (Average life expectancy with Kaposi's sarcoma is twenty-two months.)

Tailoring Diet to Disease

One of the basic premises of macrobiotics is that each type of disease is caused by a particular wrong way of eating. As William Spear of Bantam, Connecticut, a senior macrobiotics counselor, explained, "Skin cancers and breast cancer that occur on the upper part of the body and toward its surface are caused by an excess of oils and sugar. Bone cancer and pancreatic cancer, which occur in the deep part of the body, are more often caused by animal foods and carcinogens produced by barbecuing meats, as well as an excess of salt and overcooked vegetables that lack vitality." A sick person therefore requires the services of a macrobiotic counselor who can prescribe an individualized diet.

What Takes Place in a Counseling Session.   A counseling session, said Spear, begins with a client filling out a form describing complaints and customary diet. During the interview, while a secretary takes notes, Spear probes further into the client's condition and life-style. At the same time, Spear learns a great deal about the client by employing the art of Oriental diagnosis—studying the client's face and other parts of the body. Using this tool, it's possible to detect disease before symptoms manifest themselves, he said. "For example, a person whose heart is struggling to pump enough blood, as evidenced by high blood pressure or an EKG, often has a nose which is swollen and purplish. A deep vertical crease in an earlobe frequently occurs in people with coronary heart disease." (Physicians are beginning to take note of the earlobe crease and other physical features as indicators of disease, according to a *New York Times Magazine* article (Feb. 14, 1988).

"After the interview I recommend a diet and discuss other aspects of the client's life-style. In some cases, I recommend a complementary therapy such as acupuncture or colonic irrigation, a type of yoga or psychotherapy. If the client has been diagnosed with a so-called incurable cancer, I may refer him to a supportive physician who will monitor his condition—regular examinations, blood tests, etc. My role is somewhat like a general practitioner who refers a patient to a specialist." Spear's consultation, which includes unlimited follow-up telephone calls, costs $150.

Results.   I asked Spear about his results treating cancer patients in terms of recovery or extended survival:

> I can't give you figures because every case is individual. Success depends on several factors—the accuracy of my assessment of the problem, how strictly the person adheres to the diet I recommend, the patient's support system. Elaine Nussbaum [the author of *Recovery,* who was a client of Spear's] had widespread bone cancer. At one point, she was encased in a full body cast—she had to sleep propped up in a chair. I don't think she could have made it without her husband and children's support.

Another factor that contributes to success or failure, he said, is whether an individual has been subjected to invasive cancer treatment. "Chemotherapy drugs destroy a person's sense of taste, affect the entire digestive system. Radioactive drugs used in radiation treatment severely weaken an individual."

The unique aspect of macrobiotics, he said, "is that this system demands that the person confront the origin of his illness—whether it's a relationship with a parent or spouse, job stress, or diet. By determining the cause of your illness, you can then begin to eliminate that unhealthy element from your life, and ask your consciousness to undo the harm that has been done."

Aside from the AIDS project, no scientific studies have been done showing the effect of macrobiotics in cancer or any other disease. Major cancer research groups have shown little interest in funding such studies. Two studies that deal with the relation of a low-fat diet to cancer are in the works, however. One is under the direction of Lawrence Kushi, Michio Kushi's son, at the Fred Hutchinson Cancer Prevention Research Unit in Seattle. Another is the Breast Cancer Prevention Program being conducted at the Wayne State University School of Medicine, which involves women at high risk of developing breast cancer.

Testimonials Aplenty

There's no shortage of "anecdotal evidence" from counselors and their clients. As I've discovered attending macrobiotic gatherings—cooking classes and pot luck suppers—stories about "how I overcame my health problem" are as plentiful as brown rice and greens. Here are a few from my collection:

Jeannie, 56, began practicing macrobiotics ten years ago. "I was gaining weight for no reason, feeling stiff in the joints, and had developed sinus headaches." She also suffered from chronic constipation. After a month on the new diet, she regained normal bowel function, her sinuses starting draining—"constant nose-blowing, coughing up globs of mucus"—after which her headaches ceased. Within a few months, she lost fifteen pounds "and the flab around my middle melted away."

Suzanne, 33, a registered dietician, not convinced that a diet based on the four basic food groups was sure to be a nutritious one, began investigating macrobiotics six years ago. At the time, "I had severe menstrual cramps and bloating; my doctor had found several cysts on my ovaries; every winter I had one or more bouts with flu." One evening she attended a lecture on Oriental diagnosis given by a macrobiotic counselor and volunteered to take part in the demonstration. The counselor studied her face a few seconds, then said, "This young lady eats lots of dairy (she was then a lacto-ovo vegetarian), her lungs are full of mucus, and she has ovarian cysts." The first winter she practiced macrobiotics, she had no problem with flu and menstrual problems. After one and one-half years, "I discharged most of the ovarian cysts."

Adrienne, mother of three school-age children, embarked on macrobiotics four years ago. Prior to adopting the new diet, "I had no energy, was always tired, but the doctor told me there was nothing wrong." She also had painful hemorrhoids and severe menstrual cramps. Learning a new way of cooking wasn't easy—Adrienne's specialty was pies and cakes—but before long, hemorrhoids and cramps were no longer a problem.

Kathy is the mother of three children under 7 and expecting her fourth. Prior to the birth of her second child, Audrey, now 5, "We ate what I considered a superior diet—organic vegetables, fruit and yogurt, lots of pasta dishes with tomato sauce. I baked my own bread." As a newborn, Audrey developed a skin rash. "I was nursing her so was very careful about my diet—no chocolate, no coffee—but the rash persisted." On the advice of a friend, Kathy consulted a nutritionist. Much to her dismay, he told her to eliminate most of the foods she was eating and follow a balanced diet, which turned out to be macrobiotic. "Try it for thirty days," he suggested. Reluctantly, she agreed. "In two weeks, the baby's rash was gone." Today, Kathy's children eat no dairy and few processed foods, she said. "It's not easy for them to eat differently from all of their friends, but when they deviate from the diet, Audrey gets a pimply rash and my son's cough comes back."

I've met or talked by phone to a great many vegan parents whose children appear to thrive on a vegan diet. One couple is George Eisman, a registered dietician in Miami, Florida, and his wife, Shelly. The Eismans' son, Thomas, at 11 months, was eating the same vegetarian fare as his parents and was given no vitamin supplements. Thus far, Thomas, who is 4, has been free of colds, ear infections, and other childhood ailments, his father said.

The Eismans are one of twenty-four families featured in *Pregnancy, Children, and the Vegan Diet,* by Michael Klaper, M.D. Klaper is a vegan physician who is also the author of *Vegan Nutrition, Pure and Simple.* To obtain a copy of either of these books, write to Michael Klaper, M.D., P.O. Box 1402, Eustis, FL 32727.

A word of caution: Several scientific studies, according to Jane E. Brody, *New York Times* health columnist, "show that a strict vegan diet (no animal foods or dairy) can be risky for young children unless it is carefully planned."[31] One of the studies that she cites was conducted by nutritionist Dr. Johanna Dwyer, professor of medicine at Tufts Medical School, in 1979. "Dr. Dwyer, who studied 32 Boston children who were on a macrobiotic diet, found that the children who were fed no supplements and only tiny amounts of animal foods frequently suffered from rickets. . . ."

In both its 1980 and 1988 *A.D.A. Reports,* the American Dietetic Association cautions that "vegan diets must be carefully planned to meet nutrient and energy needs of infants and children." Since a poorly planned vegan diet may be deficient in vitamins D and B12 and riboflavin, they recommend the use of a properly fortified soy milk. Another potential problem, they say, is that since vegan diets tend to be high in bulk, it's difficult for children with small stomachs to eat enough to meet energy needs.

Doubts about Macrobiotics

If you're over 40, you may have the uneasy sense that there's something unsavory about macrobiotics. Didn't you read somewhere that some young people starved themselves to death following the macrobiotic diet? Macrobiotics' image problem has its roots in the 1960s. At that time, George Ohsawa was promulgating his Zen macrobiotics system, which included the infamous diet No. 7. In his two books, *Zen Macrobiotics* and the *Philosophy of Oriental Medicine,* Ohsawa advised his followers to progress from one level of the diet to another, each level successively reduced in variety of foods, until they reached the highest level—Diet No. 7. This level, which represents the "purest" diet, is 100-percent grains, chiefly brown rice, and small amounts of herb tea. Fluids are restricted in order not to overwork the kidneys.

Repercussions of this starvation diet soon became known. In a March 1967 issue of the *Journal of the American Medical Association,* two physicians described a woman who was admitted to New York Hospital, "bedridden and near death," with classic signs of scurvy (bleeding gums, swollen joints, and severe malnutrition). The patient had been a healthy 125 pounder until she embarked on Zen macrobiotics and ultimately progressed to the seventh diet, which she adhered to for eight months, until she required hospitalization. "This rigid diet is a threat to life and should be condemned," the authors wrote.[32] The following year, 24-year-old Beth Ann Simon of New Jersey, who had followed the Zen diet for nine months, died of a heart attack. Her death inspired a spate of articles in the popular press. One that appeared in *Ladies Home Journal* (October 1971) was titled "The Diet that's Killing Our Young People."

What possessed the founder of macrobiotics to recommend such a dangerous diet? I've asked several counselors this question and received a variety of answers; for example, "Ohsawa wasn't accustomed to Americans who take things literally. The diet was designed for Japanese monks." Whatever the explanation, macrobiotics has had a hard time disassociating itself from this ugly phase of its history. As late as 1982, a spokesperson for the American Dietetic Association warned me about the Zen diet, which "leads to serious nutritional deficiencies and downright emaciation and starvation." This conversation occurred two years after the ADA recognized that "well-planned vegetarian diets are consistent with good nutritional studies."[33]

Objections Remain

Today, some experts still take a dim view of macrobiotics. Said Dr. Richard C. Bozian, director of the Division of Nutrition at the University of Cincinnati College of Medicine, "When you embark on a diet that's foreign to your culture, you run into difficulties. With the legumes and fish allowed on this diet, you probably get enough vitamin B12, but you'd be low in calcium. Furthermore, in view of the large amounts of grains, vegetables, and beans, the excessive amounts of fiber might interfere with your absorption of trace minerals, such as iron." Fredrick J. Stare, M.D., Ph.D., professor emeritus and founder of Harvard University's Department of Nutrition, describes the macrobiotic diet as "unnecessarily restrictive . . . the omission of meat, eggs, milk, and cheese could result in serious nutritional deficiencies. The elimination of all processed foods is quite impractical in today's world. . . ."[34]

But with scientists recognizing diet as a primary cause of degenerative diseases, the macrobiotic diet has gained recognition among some members of the scientific community. In 1984 a Congressional subcommittee, chaired by Congressman Claude Pepper, investigated various holistic diets and concluded that the "macrobiotic diet appears to be nutritionally adequate. The diet would also be consistent with the recently released dietary guidelines of the National Academy of Sciences and the American Cancer Society in regard to possible reduction of cancer risks."[35] Another macrobiotics supporter is William P. Castelli, M.D., director of laboratories for the Framingham Heart Study, started in 1948. In commenting on the study, Castelli noted that in people following a macrobiotic diet the ratio of total cholesterol to HDL was 2.5, even lower than that of Boston marathon runners (3.4). Coronary heart disease is rarely, if ever, seen in persons with such low ratios, he said.[36]

Bye-Bye Macrobiotics

Even some of the most gung ho advocates of macrobiotics find the regime too confining. One of these defectors is Barbara Lenhardt, a Cincinnati caterer known for her Viennese torte and other confections. Six years ago, I interviewed Lenhardt, then a recent convert to macrobiotics, about this change of life-style. Lenhardt extolled her new diet as a "miracle cure." After suffering from sinus trouble all her life, she had been free of symptoms for two months, she said. "I still have asthma, but I'm cutting down on medication. Before, I was using two inhalers and a bronchial dilator." She had also lost ten unwanted pounds and her allergies were better, she said.

Contacting Lenhardt recently, I learned that she was no longer practicing macrobiotics. "I was getting such pressure from macrobiotic people; they expected me to tell my customers not to eat rich desserts. I found myself referring to my business as 'gourmet death.'" Convinced at the time that macrobiotics was an instant cure, she had discontinued taking her asthma medication. "I landed in the hospital with a severe asthmatic attack; I was there for ten days and ended up having to increase my medication." She concluded, "I haven't completely given up the diet. When I want something wholesome I cook rice; I do sea vegetables and miso. But if I get a craving for meat I have it. I'm a much happier person than when I was on the diet."

For several years, prior to the mid-1980s, Natalie Hale taught macrobiotic cooking in Cincinnati:

> I became involved in macrobiotics both to heal myself and to lend support to my husband, Kelly, who had kidney stones. We both derived enormous benefit from

macrobiotics. Before going on the diet, I had a long list of ailments—chronic constipation, debilitating menstrual cramps, arthritis in the fingers. All these ailments vanished very rapidly. We also lost weight. I'm five foot five inches and went from 112 to 93 pounds. My husband's family were alarmed at our appearance; besides the weight loss, we were extremely pale.

Gradually certain things bothered me about macrobiotics—the fanaticism, splitting hairs over yin and yang, the arrogance of counselors who presume to know everything about you based on Oriental diagnosis. One major obstacle to practicing macrobiotics is the amount of time it takes to prepare an appetizing meal according to macrobiotic principles. When I was cooking for my husband following Michio Kushi's directions for healing his kidney stones, I spent an average of four hours each day preparing meals.

Another problem with macrobiotics is that you alienate yourself from most of the world, she said. "You can't eat the food at family dinners, go out to a restaurant with friends, or eat at a friend's house who is not macrobiotic."

At this time, when both Hale and her husband felt a growing need to expand their horizons, they went to Europe on a four-month sabbatical.

We brought along a portable stove, cooked two meals a day, and explored all the macrobiotic restaurants we could find. In Paris, much to our surprise, the macrobiotic restaurant was terrible; the food had been cooked to death—it was gray and lifeless. Everyone in that place looked miserable. We looked at each other—what is the point in taking the joy out of life? We walked out, found a marvelous bakery, and bought a bag of delicious pastries.

My belief is that adhering to a strict macrobiotic diet can be a great blessing for those who are very ill. But what I don't subscribe to is following a healing diet as a way of life. If you're the kind of person who tends to be rigid, then adopting this diet may tend to compound the rigidity. One issue I could never resolve was—why should we Americans eat Japanese food three times a day?

LOOKING AHEAD

It's pretty well agreed, as Annemarie Colbin, author of *Food and Healing,* writes, that these therapeutic diets accomplish what their name suggests: help heal people suffering from obesity, heart disease, hardening of the arteries, high blood pressure, and other degenerative diseases. But the question is, are these diets a good "maintenance" or lifetime diet as their proponents suggest? In discussing the Pritikin diet, one of the popular diets that Colbin evaluates in her excellent book, she says, "If adhered to . . . past the point where it balances original excesses," the total lack of fat in what is mostly a vegetarian diet can cause chilliness. Unless a person lives in a warm climate, or in overheated surroundings, this chilliness can extend to the emotions. "Many people on long-term very low-fat diets are notably irritable, fidgety, nervous, and depressed."[37]

Colbin also says that a no-salt, no-fat approach has particularly negative results when followed in a vegan diet. After several days of vegan meals with absolutely no salt or oil, people are apt to binge on foods containing these two missing elements, she says. (Of the three therapeutic diets in this chapter, only the McDougall diet is vegan.)

Colbin considers macrobiotics "the only truly holistic approach" because the diet is tailored to the individual and the individual's environment. ("An Eskimo eating whale meat and a Jamaican eating fried plantains are both 'macrobiotic.'") Colbin acknowledges, however, that "For many people the standard macrobiotic regime is too restrictive, too high in grains, and too alien culturally."

Undoubtedly, legions of Pritikin-McDougall-macrobiotic devotees will object to Colbin's assessment. But her differentiation between therapeutic and maintenance is worth considering if you're embarking on one of these diets.

8

Treating Disease with Vitamins and Minerals

"A revolutionary new form of vitamin C. . . . A nutritional breakthrough in the quest for life and longevity. . . . Antiaging rejuvenation formula for improvement in hypertension, relief from migraine headaches, increase in libido. . . . Testimonial letters credit our product with promoting a more positive mental outlook, higher overall energy levels, even rejuvenated sex lives. . . ." You've read these claims in nutrition company promotional brochures, health magazines, and books. There's no question that this kind of nutrition hype is widespread, and a great many health practitioners and people in the industry are unhappy about it.

"The nutrition industry has turned into a money-grabbing, hustling, lying, cheating scam," said the sales rep of an extremely reputable nutrition company. "Only 3 percent of nutrition companies manufacture their own product." (The rep's company, which sells only to health professionals, is one of these.) Other companies "slap on a private label," which in many cases contains incorrect information, and their marketing people make "misleading and simplistic claims."

Instead of taking massive amounts of supplements, people should eat plenty of good fresh food (many are malnourished because they're dieting) and take a multivitamin/mineral supplement, he said.

Let me assure you that the subject of this chapter bears no relation to the kind of hit-or-miss self-prescribing that is so prevalent today. Instead you'll become acquainted with the use of meganutrients, as prescribed by a medical doctor. I'm all for doctoring yourself when you have an acute health problem—plenty of vitamin C for a cold, for instance—but if you've been

208

diagnosed with a chronic ailment, you need a doctor who's knowledgeable about the biochemistry of food and nutritional supplements.

Arlene Paulson, a 46-year-old hair stylist in Manhasset, New York, recalls that she could never "think straight." "In school, the teacher would give us a homework assignment. Ten seconds later I couldn't remember it." But there were no major problems until age 26 when her mother died. "I went into a deep depression. I stopped eating and looked anorexic. I heard voices, had visual distortions. I'd walk through a room and think that objects were falling behind me. I told people we had ghosts."

Eventually Paulson sought psychiatric treatment but it didn't help: "The worst part was the drugs [an antidepressant]. I couldn't function. Driving to work I'd come to a red light and almost fall asleep."

Gradually the depression lifted. "I got married, had a baby. Then wham—I was hit with postpartum depression and I went to pieces. I can understand child abuse. There were times when I had to restrain myself from doing something violent. I made life miserable for my husband—accused him of being unfaithful."

During this period, Paulson attended a lecture given by Dr. Mollie Shriftman, executive director of the North Nassau Mental Health Center. The Center, founded in 1958, is an outpatient psychiatric facility that has pioneered in the biochemical approach to mental illness. "The doctor talked about hypoglycemia [low blood sugar]—the mood swings, the craziness—I felt as if she were describing me."

Desperate to be well, Paulson went to the Center for treatment. There, she spent an entire day undergoing extensive laboratory tests. These tests can detect imbalances in body chemistry that often cause severe mental disorders. One of these tests is the five-hour glucose tolerance test. Taking the test, "At first I got high as if I had drunk three glasses of wine," Paulson recalled. "Then I became suspicious and accused the doctor of trying to poison me. Finally I went out like a light." Paulson's diagnosis was severe hypoglycemia.

The treatment prescribed was a low-carbohydrate, high-protein diet, which restricted refined sugar and sugar products, plus daily megadoses of four vitamins: niacinamide (vitamin B3), ascorbic acid (vitamin C), pyridoxine (vitamin B6), and vitamin E.

Today, six years later, Paulson says she's fine as long as she follows the diet and vitamin regime. "But on our last vacation, I wasn't so careful about my diet and ate a lot of sweets. I paid for it. By the fourth day, I had visions of someone breaking in the room, hitting me on the head. But as soon as I got back on the diet, my thinking straightened out."

The diet and megadose therapy that Paulson received can help a number of medical problems. In this chapter, we'll talk about schizophrenia, depression, arthritis, hyperactivity in children, cancer, AIDS, autism, and carpal tunnel syndrome.

To understand why the nutritional approach works for Paulson and for patients with such diverse medical problems, let me describe what orthomolecular medicine is all about.

PRINCIPLES OF ORTHOMOLECULAR MEDICINE

The term *orthomolecular medicine* was coined by two-time Nobel Prize winner Linus Pauling in 1968. *Ortho* comes from the Greek word "to correct." Here Pauling refers to correcting the body's metabolism by prescribing the right combination of nutrients—vitamins, minerals, amino acids, enzymes, and others. All of these nutrients, about forty in all, are normally present in the human body.

In combating disease, orthomolecular physicians use nutrients, which are nature's biological weapons. These nutrients constitute a defense system that has been successful for millions of years in the battle against all forms of disease.[1] When these nutrients are provided in the amounts that the individual requires, then healing can begin at the cellular level.

In contrast to orthomolecular medicine, standard medicine uses drugs that are not normally found in the body. Orthomolecular doctors regard these drugs as "alien chemicals," which have no connection with the disease process.[2] For example, Ritalin is an amphetaminelike drug widely prescribed to control the behavior of hyperactive children. According to CIBA's package insert, Ritalin can "frequently" cause loss of appetite, abdominal pain, weight loss, and tachycardia (rapid heartbeat), but other adverse reactions (the list includes blood pressure and pulse changes and angina) "may also occur."

Dr. Bernard Rimland, leading authority on childhood autism, coined the term *toximolecular medicine* to define "the process of trying to bring about health by providing sublethal doses of toxic substances." He says, "Drugs in common use are nontoxic only because they are given in a dose small enough not to kill the patient."

Other beliefs shared by orthomolecular physicians include the following.

Recommended Dietary Allowances (RDAs) Are Far Too Low

RDAs are defined as meeting the nutritional needs of practically all healthy persons, and are based on age and sex. The RDAs were established by the National Research Council's Food and Nutrition Board in 1943 and are reviewed and published approximately every five years.

To confuse the issue, in 1963, the Food and Drug Administration promulgated minimum daily requirements, now known as U.S. RDAs. The U.S. RDA does not vary with age or sex and is a single standard used by food manufacturers to give nutritional information about their products.

These official recommendations reflect levels needed to prevent well-defined deficiency diseases like scurvy, pellagra, and beriberi. Although these diseases in their classical form are no longer a problem in our society, doctors continue to think in terms of small doses of vitamins. For example, the U.S. RDA for vitamin C is 60 milligrams. This amount is more than enough to prevent scurvy, the disease that decimated the ranks of seamen deprived of fresh food on eighteenth-century voyages. In fact, 10 milligrams of ascorbic acid will do the job. But 60 milligrams of vitamin C is not sufficient for optimal health. Vitamin pills aren't even dispensed in this small amount. Linus Pauling contends that everyone needs a maintenance dose of 6 to 18 *grams* of vitamin C per day (a gram contains 1,000 milligrams).

As you might suspect, determining RDAs involves much more than a scientific decision. As the authors of a University of North Carolina publication point out, "The RDAs have become powerful tools in shaping public policy."[3] Said Senator William Proxmire in 1974, "It is in the narrow economic interest of the industry to establish low official RDAs because the lower the RDAs the more nutritional their food products appear." The Food and Nutrition Board, Proxmire said, was "heavily financed by the food industry."[4]

Orthomolecular physicians are not alone in criticizing the low levels of vitamins and minerals established by the RDAs. When the RDAs were last reviewed in 1986, committee members proposed reducing them even further for certain minerals and vitamins. Scientists who reviewed these suggestions protested. As a *New York Times* news report described the conflict, "Instead of the narrower view of the past, in which the vitamin and mineral allowances were set to avoid deficiencies that might lead to diseases—like scurvy from too little vitamin C—scientists hope now to establish the RDAs for optimum health."[5]

No Two People Are Alike

Each of us is different and has different nutritional needs. For that reason, the standard dose— "Take two aspirin" or "Take two acromycin three or four times a day for ten days"—has no place in orthomolecular medicine. Dr. Roger J. Williams, who discovered pantothenic acid (one of the B vitamins) and folic acid, described the uniqueness that distinguishes each human being as "biochemical individuality." Early in his career as a pioneer in vitamin research, Williams found striking biochemical differences among inbred animals, which are supposed to have a very similar heredity. Some laboratory rats, for example, appeared to need about forty times as much vitamin A as others.[6] We humans are the same, Williams says; each individual has his or her own pattern of needs.

Stress Affects Biochemistry

In addition to each person's unique biochemical makeup, an individual's nutritional needs can change under stress. As Dr. Abram Hoffer, cofounder of orthomolecular medicine, points out, an extreme example of environmental stress is the prisoner of war incarcerated on a near starvation diet for a long period of time. But stress that creates a need for high doses of nutrients can occur in more usual circumstances. Let's say you're a single working mother who is so overwhelmed by the demands on your time that your diet consists mainly of fast foods. After some time subsisting on this deficient diet, you have a gallbladder attack and require surgery; complications develop—not unusual for someone in a depleted condition—and you end up spending close to three weeks in the hospital. This sojourn doesn't help your nutritional condition. (A medical director of a New York hospital described hospitals as "malnutrition centers."[7]) By the time you're discharged, your vitamin and mineral levels will be severely depleted.

The American Diet Kills

As I've mentioned—perhaps ad nauseam—the American diet is unhealthy because it consists largely (an estimated 70 percent) of processed or factory-made foods. These processed foods, according to Dr. Donald O. Rudin, author of *The Omega-3 Phenomenon: The Nutrition Breakthrough of the 80s,* "are hydrogenated, defibered, degerminated, defatted, refatted"—manipulated in countless ways by the food industry. We Americans eat what Rudin calls "the Great American Experimental Diet."[8]

Disease statistics reflect results of the experiment. Coronary artery disease accounts for nearly half the deaths in the United States. Hypertension occurs in 50 percent of individuals over the age of 40. One out of three people develops cancer. Sixteen million Americans are diabetic. One in ten Americans is mentally ill. Feed a colony of young monkeys the American supermarket diet, and within a few years these monkeys will develop all the modern diseases, Rudin says.

While it's agreed that the American diet creates widespread nutritional deficiencies, which deficiency is most critical may depend on the particular bent of the observer. The late Irwin Stone, author of *The Healing Factor* (Grosset and Dunlap, 1972) who introduced Linus Pauling to vitamin C, says that most people are deficient in ascorbic acid, the scientific term for vitamin C. (If you're always tired and catch colds and flu easily, then you may be suffering from "subclinical scurvy.") Dr. Derrick Lonsdale, thiamine (vitamin B1) authority, is concerned about—naturally—thiamine deficiency. He found that one third of his new patients were deficient in this vitamin. Dr. Alan Gaby, whose specialty is vitamin B6, says that we're witnessing an "epidemic" of B6 deficiency.

More recently, Dr. Donald O. Rudin has contended that our "experimental diet" produces widespread deficiency in *all* the B vitamins. These deficiencies, he says, are responsible for the entire gamut of modern diseases — irritable bowel syndrome (which tops the list of diseases treated by gastroenterologists), heart disease, depression, schizophrenia, and such common conditions as dry skin and dandruff. (Rudin points to the plethora of moisturizers and dandruff products being marketed today.) His solution is to provide omega-3 essential fatty acids in the form of linseed oil supplements.[9]

Dr. Mildred E. Seelig, magnesium authority, says that magnesium deficiency, coupled with an increase in vitamin D and phosphate, is the missing link in heart disease deaths and sudden infant death.

National surveys give some inkling of the deficiencies in our diet. A government survey known as the HANES (Health and Nutrition Examination Survey) of 1971–72 showed that up to 50 percent of the general population received less than the recommended daily amounts (U.S. RDAs) of some vitamins and minerals.[10] A preliminary report of the Department of Agriculture's Nationwide Food Consumption Survey of 1977–78 revealed that adolescents and young adults were most severely deficient in nutrients.[11] But these surveys seldom indicate how critical the problem is since the RDAs, which serve as the yardstick, are set so low.

ORTHOMOLECULAR MEDICINE AND MENTAL DISORDERS

Help for Schizophrenics

Orthomolecular medicine, or more accurately, orthomolecular psychiatry, began in 1952 when two psychiatrists, Drs. Abram Hoffer and Humphrey Osmond, in Saskatchewan, Canada, conducted a double-blind study with schizophrenic patients. At that time, schizophrenia was considered incurable and patients were incarcerated for life in a "snake pit" mental hospital where treatment consisted of drugs, shock treatment (which frequently caused broken bones), the straitjacket, and water hoses. The two psychiatrists had been searching for a way to help these unfortunates. After many years, they developed a theory that a biochemical abnormality in the schizophrenic causes an excess of a chemical called adrenochrome, which produces hallucinations.

One of the clues that led the two to theorize that large doses of nicotinic acid or niacin (both forms of vitamin B3) might prevent formation of hallucinogenic substances in the brains of schizophrenics was their knowledge of pellagra. Pellagra, which is caused by a vitamin B3 deficiency, produces symptoms of schizophrenia. Giving small amounts of of vitamin B3 virtually wiped out classic pellagra. In proper scientific fashion, Hoffer and Osmond gave vitamin B3 (3 grams per day for thirty days) to one group of recently admitted schizophrenics and a placebo to another group, which served as a control. The experiment showed that megadoses of vitamin B3 doubled their patients' recovery rate.[12]

The first patient in the study was a 21-year-old man who was catatonic. He had failed to respond to standard treatment and was dying. As Hoffer writes, when he and Osmond learned about the patient's condition, "We promptly went to the ward, inserted a stomach tube and poured in a solution containing a large amount of these two vitamins [nicotinic acid and ascorbic acid]. The second day he was able to sit up and drink the vitamin solution. After thirty days he was well. He was still well when seen many years later."[13] Later they added pyridoxine (vitamin B6) and ascorbic acid (vitamin C) to the regimen.

Dramatic results achieved by orthomolecular treatment were beginning to appear in professional journals in the 1950s when a development occurred that eclipsed this new approach: the introduction of a new group of drugs called phenothiazines, or tranquilizers. (Chlorpromazine, the first drug of this class, became available in 1954.) These drugs drastically changed the practice of mental health care. Pharmaceutical companies, quick to see the value and profit in such drugs, began testing and marketing them. The companies showed little interest in megavitamin treatment since vitamins cannot be patented and, furthermore, are inexpensive.

Ten years after the publication of Hoffer and Osmond's preliminary studies with schizophrenics, Dr. Linus Pauling stumbled upon a report about their work and was "astonished" that a substance as powerful as vitamin B3 was so low in toxicity. "A little pinch, 5 milligrams every day, is enough to keep a person from dying of pellagra, but it is so lacking in toxicity that ten thousand times as much can be taken without harm."[14] In his now famous article "Orthomolecular Psychiatry," Pauling defined orthomolecular treatment for mental disease.[15] This treatment provided "the optimum concentrations of substances normally present in the human body," or as it came to be known, "the right molecules in the right amounts." Pauling suggested that mental disease might result from low concentrations in the brain of specific vitamins. By carefully studying the patient, it should be possible to determine the optimum dose of nutrients the individual needs.

A world-famous scientist recommending orthomolecular treatment as the best way to treat mental disease naturally created tremendous interest in the subject. The American Psychiatric Association (APA), dismayed by the "considerable publicity" that Pauling's article created, issued *Task Force*

Report 7 in 1973.[16] This 54-page report, "Megavitamin and Orthomolecular Therapy in Psychiatry," was a scathing denunciation of the new treatment. The report criticized the proponents of megavitamin therapy for making "unsupported claims," presenting "anecdotal data," and for shifting their claims and theories over the years. It pointed to the possibly toxic effects of massive doses of nutrients and raised the "nagging question" of whether schizophrenics who benefited from orthomolecular treatment had been misdiagnosed. The report also included preliminary results of a study conducted by the Canadian Mental Health Association, in which Canadian psychiatrists concurred with their American colleagues that nicotinic acid or niacin "has no therapeutic effect and may have a negative effect" in schizophrenic patients.[17]

A rebuttal on the part of Hoffer and Osmond followed, and counter-rebuttals flew back and forth, but the damage was done; the APA's widely publicized report seriously undermined the credibility of megavitamin treatment. On the plus side, the report induced Pauling and a group of physicians trained in nutrition to form an orthomolecular medical society in 1976. Now called the American Association of Orthomolecular Medicine, or the Huxley Institute, it is based in Boca Raton, Florida.

What Is Schizophrenia?

To better understand the role of orthomolecular treatment in schizophrenia, it's helpful to know something more about the disease. According to the National Institute of Mental Health, schizophrenia is the most chronic and disabling of major mental diseases — the cancer of mental illness — afflicting 1 percent of the population. Each year 100,000 people are newly diagnosed. There are several different kinds of schizophrenia and no known single cause. Schizophrenia is a young peoples' disease; most develop the disease between the ages of 16 and 25, generally at a younger age in men. Symptoms of schizophrenia, which is characterized by the inability to distinguish between reality and fantasy, are hallucinations, delusions of persecution, inability to focus on any one thought, and displays of inappropriate emotion.

Standard Treatment for Schizophrenia

Again according to the National Institute of Mental Health, the best treatment now available is antipsychotic drugs, also called neuroleptics, which have been widely used since the mid-1950s. These drugs lessen symptoms such as hallucinations, delusions, and disordered thinking but are less effective in correcting lack of emotional expression, social isolation, and withdrawal. In addition, 20 percent of sufferers do not respond to antipsychotic drugs.[18] These drugs, the phenothiazines, cause adverse side effects that include drowsiness, muscle spasms, dry mouth, and blurring of vision. The most disturbing effect, according to Dr. Richard A. Kunin, orthomolecular psychiatrist, is "an incessant feeling of restlessness that keeps the patient in constant motion."[19]

The Thorazine Shuffle.   What is it like to be medicated with a tranquilizer? Here's how recovered patient Ronald Hazlett of New Haven, Connecticut, describes his experience: "One of the drugs they gave me was Thorazine. It slows you down. You get what we call the Thorazine shuffle. When I went out in public I could see people looking at me; my fingers were twitching, my jaw constantly moving." Finally, fed up with the way he was feeling—"I was never in control"—he told his doctor he wasn't taking any more drugs. "He refused to see me—it was scary." Hazlett, who acknowledges that tranquilizers worked fine for some of his friends, has been off all medication for five years. In his capacity as a consumer advocate for mental patients, Hazlett leads a support group at Fellowship House in New Haven, a center for people with long-term psychiatric illnesses, and serves on the advisory board of the Connecticut Valley Hospital, a state facility.

A Fearful Legacy.   A side effect of long-term use of antipsychotic drugs is a disorder called tardive dyskinesia (TD). This condition, which appears in 20 to 30 percent of those medicated for schizophrenia, produces uncontrollable movements of the tongue, lips, and hands and slow, writhing movements of the limbs and sometimes the trunk. "Dyskinesia does not always cease and may even be exacerbated when neuroleptic therapy is discontinued."[20]

Eleanor, a member of Fellowship House, has a severe case of TD. As Kate O'Connell, the center's executive director, described her, "Eleanor graduated from an Ivy League college; she had such potential. After her senior year, going through a difficult period in her life, she had a breakdown. She was hospitalized and given high doses of a drug called Trilafon" (an antipsychotic drug). Eleanor recovered from her mental illness—the breakdown was a phase—and she has since managed to live independently. But the drug she took has left her spastic. "She has continuous facial twitches, grimaces, her tongue darts in and out of her mouth; her hand twitches so badly she can't hold a cup. The terrible thing is that Eleanor and her family were never informed as to the possible side effects of the drug." According to Hazlett, this is not unusual. When he asked forty mental patients whether they had been fully informed of possible side effects of medication, only three answered yes.

Orthomolecular Treatment for Schizophrenia

Orthomolecular treatment today is basically the same that Hoffer and Osmond developed; it consists of vitamin B3 (either niacin or niacinamide), vitamin C, and vitamin B6. As described in Hoffer's *Common Questions on Schizophrenia and Their Answers,* niacin causes a flushing, tingling sensation; those patients who find this uncomfortable can take niacinamide. One advantage of niacin, however, is that it lowers cholesterol. Niacinamide does not.

Vitamins alone are not enough, Hoffer says. An orthomolecular prescription always includes a diet of whole foods—the opposite of processed junk foods. This diet, which human beings have thrived on for thousands of years, is low in fat and high in fiber.

In certain instances, Hoffer uses standard treatments such as tranquilizers, antidepressant drugs, and electroconvulsive therapy. But these conventional treatments take second place to nutrient therapy. Hoffer deplores the practice of psychiatrists who "keep their schizophrenic patients heavily and permanently tranquilized" as "cruel, ignorant, and inhumane treatment."[21] He claims that the program he and Osmond developed has been effective for 85 percent of schizophrenics, including both mild and severe cases.

In developing his megavitamin treatment for schizophrenia, Hoffer discovered that some of his "failures"—patients who were resistant to all therapy—were allergic to certain foods. This "cerebral allergy" produced symptoms of schizophrenia. The most accurate and cheapest way to track down a food that causes cerebral allergies is to use an elimination diet, Hoffer says, which involves fasting and then trying out foods one by one. For information on ways to determine multiple food allergies, see *Dr. Mandell's 5-Day Allergy Relief System* (New York: Pocket Books, 1980).

Treating TD. The first effective treatment to be reported for TD was devised by an orthomolecular psychiatrist, Dr. Richard A. Kunin of San Francisco. Early in the 1970s, Kunin discovered that TD occurs when, through a complex process, a tranquilizer binds with manganese creating a deficiency of the mineral. Treatment consists of 30 to 60 milligrams of manganese along with vitamins in which the patient is deficient. Since 1973 Kunin has treated 43 cases of TD "with outstanding results." In more than half of these patients with tremors of the extremities, symptoms cleared up within a day of taking manganese. Kunin reported his first 15 cases in the *Journal of Orthomolecular Psychiatry* in 1975[22] and additional ones in 1978 at the World Congress of Biological Psychiatry in Barcelona, Spain. Other orthomolecular physicians have confirmed the efficacy of manganese treatment for this drug-induced condition.

Preventing TD.   Megavitamin therapy can also prevent TD. Dr. David R. Hawkins, founder of the North Nassau Health Center, discovered this seren-dipitously when he realized that none of the patients at the Center, who had been treated with antipsychotic drugs and megavitamin therapy, had developed TD. Hawkins conducted a survey of the practices of 80 physicians, who treated a total of 58,000 patients with antipsychotic drugs combined with megadoses of vitamins over a period of ten years. Of this group of patients, only 26 developed TD.[23]

Judging by my conversations with schizophrenic patients and family members, orthomolecular psychiatry is little known to the public. (One mother said, "If there was any value in this treatment, my doctor would have told me about it.") According to one physician, psychiatrist Dr. Charles Enzer of Cincinnati, who specializes in schizophrenia, the "death knell" for orthomolecular treatment was the APA Task Force Report. "Since that time, the scientific world no longer considers niacin as a treatment for schizophrenia."

But dissatisfaction with psychiatric treatment for schizophrenia is growing. Before "rapid advances in brain imaging and biochemistry" that occurred in the early 1980s, "the grip of psychoanalytic theories of mental illnesses discouraged schizophrenia research," said Samuel Keith, head of the newly formed Schizophrenia Research Branch of the National Institute of Mental Health.[24] The National Alliance for the Mentally Ill, an organization of 66,000 families, is seeking "increased . . . funding for research on illnesses that currently have no cure."[25]

Acceptance of the biochemical basis for schizophrenia has even won a kind word for orthomolecular medicine from one of the standard psychiatrists I interviewed. Dr. Enzer acknowledged that this "unscientific" system had made one contribution—the hypothesis that psychiatric illnesses are due to biochemical abnormalities. "This theory has led the scientific community to look for biochemical pathways and reduced guilt and shame in family members of schizophrenic patients."

A Convert to Orthomolecular Psychiatry

What induces a standard psychiatrist to become an orthomolecular psychiatrist? Twenty-five years ago, Dr. Richard A. Kunin had little interest in nutrition. As a research fellow at Stanford University in the 1960s, he had devised an innovative brand of psychotherapy that combined hypnosis and behavioral therapy. (An article about his work appeared in *Time* magazine in December 1963.) But Kunin, who is board-certified in psychiatry, was dissatisfied with his results: "Psychotherapy worked reasonably well with 'healthy' patients, but those with schizophrenia, chronic depression, or addictions frequently suffered relapses," he said.

> Two patients changed my life. The first, Theresa, married to her third husband, regularly experienced schizoid episodes during which she heard the voices of her first two husbands heckling her. Her present husband, distraught over her condition, threatened to divorce her and regain custody of their four-year-old child. Treating her with psychotherapy worked while she was in the office, but once she left, the voices came back.

Then Kunin came across an article in a little-known journal that described the beneficial effects of niacinamide (vitamin B3) in psychotic patients. "I figured there was no danger in prescribing a vitamin with no known toxicity, and started her on a large dose of niacinamide. I was astounded by the results. In three days, she told me that the voices had subsided, and in a week, the hallucinations were gone."

The other patient who was instrumental in helping Kunin find a new direction was a professional singer. She was mildly depressed, subject to mood swings, and anxious to shed twenty-five excess pounds before her next performance.

> But after four visits, she had only lost a few pounds, and my hypnosis programming was not working. Some time later, not having heard from her, I called her up to see how she was doing.
>
> She chewed me out—told me I was incompetent! She had gone to another doctor who had diagnosed her condition as hypoglycemia and put her on a diet. She had already lost ten pounds and was no longer depressed.
>
> Now I had heard about hypoglycemia; according to a handful of maverick doctors, low blood sugar was widespread and caused a multitude of problems. I paid no attention to these claims. In those days I considered myself a pure scientist, and rejected any idea that hadn't been proved scientifically.

Reflecting on these two cases made Kunin realize that he was ignoring nutrition at his peril. "I developed a nutrition questionnaire that I gave to every patient, and discovered that my patients, well-educated people for the most part, ate a deplorable diet, myself included. At 35, I was having afternoon slumps and feeling old. Reading Adelle Davis, I realized that a great many essential foods were missing from my diet. The first time I ate liver, which I did not care for, I felt a veil lift from my mind."

After delving into the research of Abram Hoffer and other orthomolecular psychiatrists, "I learned to analyze a patient's diet with the use of computers. I was one of the first physicians in private practice to use hair analysis." (This laboratory test is used to detect the presence of toxic metals, such as lead and mercury, as well as the spectrum of essential trace minerals.)

Today, Kunin, 54, author of *Mega-Nutrition* and *Mega-Nutrition for Women* (New York: New American Library, 1980 and 1983), makes use of nutrition tests such as a vitamin and mineral profile, which gives levels for sixteen vitamins and thirty minerals. These laboratory tests can sometimes provide a quick answer to a problem, he writes:

> A patient named Joan, 24, suffered from excruciating headaches and was extremely depressed for several days before each menstrual period. Her gynecologist had assured her that her hormones were normal—"You have to live with this." A blood test showed low magnesium in the blood cells, a common cause of premenstrual symptoms. I prescribed 600 milligrams of magnesium per day, and by her next period her symptoms had diminished, and eventually disappeared.

Another patient, Marion, 54, had been plagued with recurrent bladder infection for years. "Antibiotics cleared up the infection for a few weeks, then her symptoms returned, and she was back on antibiotics. A vitamin profile showed her vitamin A levels were abnormally low." Vitamin A plays a key role in maintaining the health of epithelium tissue, which lines the bladder, lungs, and bowel. After improving her diet and supplementing with vitamin A, she has not had a bladder infection in several years.

Kunin concludes, "Without the benefit of these nutrition tests, it's unlikely that I could have detected these deficiencies. These tests take the guesswork out of analyzing nutritional deficiencies, but the average doctor is not taking advantage of this new technology."

Treating the Whole Person

Orthomolecular medicine, which began as a treatment for schizophrenia, makes no distinction between mental and physical disease; one or the other or both frequently result from a biochemical imbalance. This holistic point of view harkens back to the time before the era of specialization in medicine—and looks to the future. Said Dr. Sidney M. Baker, former executive director of the Gesell Institute of Human Development, "Medicine seems to be gradually reawakening to the old idea that mind and body are one and that we should not try to treat each apart."

Since the first crop of orthomolecular physicians were psychiatrists, they were naturally concerned with mental diseases. One of the diseases they treated was depression.

Standard Treatment for Depression

According to the National Mental Health Association, depression is one of the most prevalent mental illnesses: 25 percent of all women and 11.5 percent of all men in the United States will have a depressive episode during their lifetime. Every six months, 10 million children, teens, and adults experience depression. These episodes often recur. The causes of depression are not clear.

A poignant description of what clinical depression is like was given by William Styron, author of *Sophie's Choice,* in a *New York Times* article: "What had begun that summer as an off-and-on malaise and a vague, spooky restlessness had gained gradual momentum until my nights were without sleep and my days were pervaded by a gray drizzle of unrelenting horror. This horror is virtually indescribable since it bears no relation to normal experience."[26]

Treatment consists of medication or psychotherapy or both. Antidepressive drugs are tricyclic antidepressants, monoamine oxidase (MAO) inhibitors, and lithium. (Lithium is the treatment of choice for manic-depressive illness.) Common side effects of these drugs are dry mouth, constipation, bladder problems, sexual problems, blurred vision, dizziness, and drowsiness.

Orthomolecular Treatment for Depression

Dr. Harvey M. Ross, Los Angeles psychiatrist and author of *Fighting Depression,* was among the first to treat depression as a biochemical problem. An important finding that Ross and his colleagues made was that hypoglycemia (low blood sugar) is one of the causes of depression. This condition, which physicians still dismiss as "a fad," Ross says, requires a special diet— the high-protein, low-sugar diet developed by Dr. Seale Harris in the 1920s and later popularized by Dr. Robert C. Atkins. (For a description of the Atkins Diet, see page 67.) As Ross explained, the hypoglycemic diet is a temporary measure: "After four months you switch to a maintenance diet which is high in complex carbohydrates" (starches). The person who is hypoglycemic should eat small meals with frequent high-protein snacks, he said. Ross also prescribes nutritional supplements that supply vitamin B complex and essential minerals, but the basic treatment for hypoglycemia is diet.

One of Ross's patients, who complained of being tired and depressed all the time, was 27-year-old Georgette. Her symptoms were so severe she was unable to hold a job; prior to consulting Ross, she had attempted suicide. One of the tests Ross ordered for his patient was hair analysis, which revealed that she was deficient in manganese, potassium, and iron; consequently, Georgette's prescription included supplemental doses of these minerals. After three weeks, she was less depressed; in three months, she said she felt like her normal self. At this point, Ross felt that psychotherapy was in order, and after several psychotherapy sessions, Georgette went back to work.

This was seven years ago. Georgette has stayed well except for a few episodes when she strayed from the diet and vitamin program.

Georgette's case illustrates a point that needs clarifying: orthomolecular treatment for mental disorders does not preclude psychotherapy. "Both forms of therapy are needed," Ross said, but it is necessary to "balance" the patient's biochemistry before any benefit can result from psychotherapy.

More Help for Depressed People

A new generation of orthomolecular psychiatrists has contributed to the treatment of depression. One is Dr. Michael Lesser of Berkeley, California, author of *Nutrition and Vitamin Therapy* (Berkeley, Calif.: Nutritional Medicine, 1980). Lesser was trained to do classic psychotherapy and to prescribe drugs but soon realized the limitations of both treatments and, at the same time, became aware of the importance of diet and nutrients. In a phone conversation, I learned about one of Lesser's findings—that high doses of vitamin C can ameliorate the side effects of one antidepressant drug. "Lithium, which is used widely to treat manic depression, can depress the function of the thyroid, which slows down the metabolism," he said. "As a result, people start to balloon up and gain weight. Vitamin C appears to act as a diuretic; the patient loses water and doesn't gain all that weight."

Lesser also found that vitamin C helps addicts either withdraw from drugs or reduce their dosage:

> Susan, a 26-year-old secretary, had been addicted to large doses of Valium for several years. When she came to me she had just quit her job; she complained that she was always tired, couldn't concentrate. When we discussed her diet, I found that she often binged on sweets and junk food. All these symptoms are common side effects of tranquilizers.
>
> In the past, she had tried to lower the dosage of the drug but on several occasions wound up in the hospital experiencing hallucinations. I began treating her with megadoses of vitamin C (30 to 40 grams per day) several months ago. She has now reduced the dosage of her tranquilizer to the lowest level she has ever achieved, with no ill effects.

A Doctor Who Cured Herself

Dr. Priscilla Slagle, Los Angeles psychiatrist and author of *The Way Up from Down* (New York: Random House, 1987), has worked with depressed people for many years. When she spoke at a recent Huxley Institute conference, members of the audience paid rapt attention as she described her own bout with depression from the ages of 15 to 35. Five years of psychoanalysis plus other forms of therapy did little to relieve the condition. But once she became aware that her body chemistry affected her mental state, she began searching for a biochemical solution. The breakthrough was discovering certain nutrients that influence mood-elevating brain chemicals. For over a decade, Slagle has treated herself with these nutrients, and has remained free of depression. Prescribing the same nutritional program to her depressed patients, 70 percent have responded, she said.

Slagle's program involves the neurotransmitters, chemicals in the brain that regulate your moods, control your sleep, and perform many other functions. Probably the best-known neurotransmitters are endorphins, which are associated with a runner's "high." Neurotransmitters that pertain to depression are serotonin and norepinephrine. They belong to a chemical group called brain amines. Depressed individuals don't have enough of these brain amines; the function of antidepressant drugs is to increase their levels. But Slagle contends that precursor nutrients—vitamins, minerals, and amino acids—do a better job and without causing harmful side effects. Unlike other orthomolecular programs discussed in this chapter, Slagle's nutrient program for depression, which is described in detail in her book, does not require a physician's care unless you are severely depressed, she says.

VITAMINS

In the 1950s and 1960s, vitamins were the stars of orthomolecular medicine. One of the brightest was—and still is—vitamin C, or ascorbic acid.

Vitamin C

Think of vitamin C, and Linus Pauling comes to mind. In 1970 Pauling's *Vitamin C and the Common Cold* burst on the scene carrying the encouraging message that the common cold can be conquered! The public, grateful that someone (in this case, an award-winning scientist) cared about the misery of a cold, eagerly followed Pauling's advice and took megadoses of vitamin C to suppress cold symptoms. Pauling suggests, at the first sign of a cold, start taking 1 gram or more of vitamin C per hour throughout the waking hours of the day. For more information about the common cold, see Pauling's *How to Live Longer and Feel Better* (New York: W. H. Freeman and Co., 1986). An excellent discussion of the cold and other conditions that respond to vitamin C treatment appears in *The Vitamin C Connection, Getting Well and Staying Well with Vitamin C*, by Dr. Emanuel Cheraskin, W. Marshall Ringsdorf, Jr., and Emily L. Sisley (New York: Harper & Row, 1983).

Dr. Robert C. Cathcart III, a Los Altos, California physician, has extensive clinical experience with ascorbate. Over the past fifteen years, Cathcart has treated more than 11,000 patients with megadoses of vitamin C and reported his results in half a dozen medical articles. Cathcart first tried vitamin C on himself in 1969. At that time he had frequent colds and seasonal hay fever. Hearing Linus Pauling's claims that vitamin C could prevent the common cold, or lessen its severity (this was a year before the publication of Pauling's *Vitamin C and the Common Cold*), he followed Pauling's prescription—4 grams of vitamin C four times a day—and found that it worked. Vitamin C also relieved his hay fever.

On one rare occasion when he caught a cold, he stumbled on a crucial point in determining the right amount of vitamin C: "When you're well, a daily dose of 4 grams may be sufficient, but the sicker you are, the more vitamin C you need. At the first sign of illness, increase your maintenance dose until you reach 'bowel tolerance'—the onset of diarrhea."

More discoveries followed. In the early 1970s, Cathcart, then an orthopedic surgeon, was practicing in a ski resort town in the Lake Tahoe area. His patients, young athletes, were an ideal group for vitamin C therapy, he said. They were healthy, intent on staying that way, and when they developed an acute viral disease, able to tolerate the occasional discomfort of gas pains or diarrhea that sometimes accompanies large doses of vitamin C. "Those who had mononucleosis or other infectious diseases were back on the slopes in a week.

"Vitamin C is effective in treating infectious diseases because it's a free radical scavenger," Cathcart said. (Infectious diseases include colds, flu, viral pneumonia, measles, chicken pox, mumps, rubella, and infectious hepatitis.) "All acute viral diseases emit toxins in the form of free radicals; that's how these diseases suppress the immune system. Ascorbate neutralizes these toxins, which prevents the free radicals from harming the immune system."

Oscar G. Rasmussen, Ph.D., of the Department of Medicine and Nutrition at the American International Clinic in Zion, Illinois, confirms Cathcart's findings about vitamin C and mononucleosis. Rasmussen has treated half a dozen mononucleosis patients with megadoses of vitamin C, with excellent results. "By the end of the second day, the patient usually feels great," said Rasmussen. "Over a period of four days, we give 150 to 160 grams of ascorbate per day." Massive doses of vitamin C are best given intravenously to avoid digestive disturbances, and spaced throughout the day in equal amounts. "By the end of the fourth or fifth day, the patient is well enough to be discharged."

Cathcart has also achieved good results treating AIDS patients with vitamin C. "I give bowel tolerance doses of C almost every hour in conjunction with conventional treatment." Giving megadoses of C reduces the development of secondary infections, the most serious of which is pneumocystis pneumonia, which kills more than 50 percent of victims. "With good nutrition, exercise, and a proper attitude, AIDS patients can live a lot longer than ordinarily expected. Thus far, megadose vitamin C therapy appears to double life expectancy," he said.

Vitamin C and Infertility

If you're a man with infertility due to "sperm agglutination"—the tendency of sperm to clump together rather than move normally—1 gram of vitamin C per day can restore your fertility in just four days.

In a study conducted by Earl B. Dawson, Ph.D., and colleagues with the Department of Obstetrics and Gynecology at the University of Texas Medical Branch in Galveston, 35 male patients who could not impregnate their wives owing to this sperm disorder were given varying doses of vitamin C and told to come back for weekly visits. "At each visit, we measured changes in the sperm and their vitamin C levels to make sure they were taking the vitamin," Dawson said in a phone interview.

"At the very first visit, we found a tremendous increase in sperm activity and mobility. When all the data was in, we determined that men who took 1,000 milligrams of vitamin C could have been fertile by the third or fourth day of vitamin C supplementation." Men who took 200 milligrams per day took two weeks to reach the maximum effect, he said. Animal studies in the past have shown a relationship between vitamin C deficiency and male infertility, but Dawson's is the first to show the link in humans. The incidence of this sperm disorder in the male population is unknown.[27]

Dawson has received letters from individual clinicians in Europe and India who are using vitamin C with good results, but this simple solution for a distressing condition has been largely ignored outside of Dawson's institution. Dawson read me a letter he received from a woman who read about the study in a newspaper. She wrote, "After trying for five years to have a baby, my husband tried your vitamin C treatment. I am now pregnant and want to thank you."

"Brush, Floss, and Take Vitamin C." Scientists at the University of Southern California have made a discovery that may one day induce dentists to prescribe vitamin C to their patients for healthier gums. What they've found is that vitamin C normalizes a deficiency in collagen production that results from diabetes. (Collagen is a protein that gives structure and strength to skin, bone, gums, and other tissue.) Diabetics are known to heal poorly because they don't produce as much collagen as nondiabetics and, consequently, develop severe periodontal (gum) disease.

In experiments with diabetic rats, researchers led by Michael Schneir, Ph.D., head of biochemistry at the University of Southern California School of Dentistry, found that supplementing the animals' drinking water with megadoses of vitamin C (20 milligrams daily) improved the quantity and quality of their skin collagen.[28] Extrapolating data from the animal experiment, the dose that could be expected to improve gum tissue in humans would be 3,500 milligrams, or 3.5 grams per day.

Vitamin C and Cataracts.   For the past decade or more, researchers at several universities in this country have shown that humans and animals with cataracts have low levels of vitamin C in the aqueous humor (the fluid that surrounds and nourishes the lens of the eye). (For more about vitamin C and other nutrients at work in the eye, see chapter 9.)

Until recently, researchers were inclined either to dismiss vitamin C treatment or cite its potentially harmful effects. One adverse effect that's frequently mentioned is formation of kidney stones; another is risk of "rebound scurvy" when ascorbic acid is suddenly discontinued. Vitamin C is also claimed to destroy vitamin B12 in foods, increase iron absorption, and interfere with certain tests.

A sign that researchers have become impatient with such objections is a 1986 article by Mark Levine, M.D., of the National Institutes of Health. In this article, published in *The New England Journal of Medicine,* Levine describes these side effects associated with gram doses of ascorbic acid as "speculative." He cautions, however, that large doses of vitamin C, by increasing iron absorption, could be harmful in alcoholics and others with a rare disease that produces "iron overload."[29]

Thiamine (Vitamin B1)

Thiamine (vitamin B1) is best known as the vitamin that cured beriberi, a discovery that was made during the first decade of the 1900s. Talking to thiamine authority Dr. Derrick Lonsdale, I learned about some of its current uses.

Lonsdale, a 64-year-old British-born physician, was a latecomer to nutritional medicine. A member of the prestigious Cleveland Clinic, Lonsdale practiced standard pediatrics for twenty years until 1968, when fate brought him to the bedside of a 6-year-old boy named Tommy. The youngster had been hospitalized several times, and his case baffled Lonsdale's colleagues.

"Whenever Tommy became chilled or caught a cold, or encountered any kind of stress such as a routine inoculation, he developed a condition called 'cerebellar ataxia,' which caused him to behave as if he were drunk—his balance was poor, his speech slurred. These symptoms would gradually become worse over several days, then subside—until the next attack."

Analyzing Tommy's urine during one of these sieges,

> We found that it contained huge amounts of keto acids. Keto acids are a sign of faulty combustion. Tommy's system was like a car with a choked engine and black smoke coming from the exhaust pipe. Further studies showed that a component of his enzyme system that depended on thiamine was defective.
>
>   It suddenly struck me—these strange attacks were a symptom of beriberi. We gave him gradually increasing doses of thiamine until we observed a drop in urinary concentrations of keto acids. Tommy's problem was what Hans Selye called "a

disease of adaptation." When subject to stress, his body could not muster the energy to function normally. Today, twenty years later, Tom is free of attacks as long as he takes his thiamine. When he develops a cold or any infection, he doubles or triples his daily dose to abort neurological symptoms.

After this unusual case, Lonsdale began testing the urine of other children on the neurology ward and frequently found the same telltale keto acids. "These children had been diagnosed as cerebral palsy or cerebellar ataxia or encephalitis, but the disease label is meaningless. What's important to understand is that in each case the problem was biochemical, and the particular disease was merely the expression of this biochemical defect." When Lonsdale treated these children with vitamin B1, many improved dramatically.

Researching the history of thiamine, Lonsdale learned that during the early years of vitamin research (1925 to 1940), thiamine had been tested in a multitude of diseases and found beneficial in most cases. Lonsdale smiled. "But any agent which appears to be a 'cure-all' is automatically suspect, and thiamine fell out of favor."

While Lonsdale was reading every scrap of information he could get his hands on about vitamin B1, another lesson came in the guise of a 6-month-old boy on the ward who had a series of mysterious attacks during which he stopped breathing. Such behavior naturally raised the specter of Sudden Infant Death Syndrome (SIDS). On the basis of laboratory findings, Lonsdale suspected that the symptoms were caused by infantile beriberi, and gave the baby large doses of thiamine. In less than a week, the attacks stopped.

Is it possible that thiamine deficiency is one of the causes of SIDS, Lonsdale wondered. He went back to the library and came across a landmark discovery about crib deaths by a British public health doctor named Lydia Fehily. In the 1940s, Fehily was sent to Hong Kong to investigate infant mortality rate among the Chinese—an astronomical figure of 350 deaths per 1,000 live births. The victims, most often 3 to 4 months old and generally the best-nourished males, died in their sleep. The situation resembled "cot death," the British term for crib death.

Fehily concluded that Chinese babies were dying of infantile beriberi because they were deficient in thiamine. This deficiency was due to their mothers' staple food, polished white rice. This rice was subject to the machine-rolling process, introduced in the late 1800s, which scraped off the outer husk to create clean white kernels. This white rice, unlike unprocessed brown rice, could be stored for months or years without deteriorating. But it was this discarded outer husk of rice material that contained most of the grain's vitamins and minerals, including thiamine.

"But there's one crucial part of the story that is often missed," Lonsdale said. "When the Japanese invaded Hong Kong before World War II, they imposed starvation rice rations on the Chinese. Although nursing mothers were severely malnourished, the crib deaths disappeared overnight. Two years later, when the Japanese invaders withdrew from Hong Kong and rice was plentiful again, crib deaths resumed."

Stumbling on an animal experiment published in 1936 that showed that the need for thiamine was linked to calorie intake,[30] Lonsdale found the answer to the puzzle: "When Chinese mothers were on a near-starvation diet, they consumed few calories and their requirement for thiamine decreased. But when they added calories in the form of thiamine-deficient rice, they increased their need for thiamine, and beriberi resulted.

"This Hong Kong incident has a message for us today. When we consume empty calories in the form of junk food and soda drinks, we increase our need for thiamine. That's one of the reasons why thiamine deficiency is so common today."

Lonsdale explains: "I'm not saying that all crib deaths are due to vitamin B1 deficiency, but I believe babies are dying today because of a brain stem defect related to lack of oxygen. The lack of oxygen is caused by a vitamin deficiency, which could be thiamine or any of the other vitamins. We could wipe out crib death if every pediatrician was familiar with vitamin deficiency symptoms, and on the lookout for them."

As described in chapter 5, Lonsdale relieved his wife Adele's severe arthritic pains with a form of vitamin B1 that is widely used in Japan. "Arthritis is a biochemical disease; all disease is biochemical. The trick is to find the biochemical key that fits the lock."

Vitamin B6

Equipped with an armory of "biological weapons," the orthomolecular physician treats all kinds of disease. In most cases, determining the nutrient that the patient needs is an exceedingly complex undertaking. This task is simplified when the patient has been diagnosed with a condition known to be caused by a specific nutritional deficiency.

Carpal Tunnel Syndrome.   One such condition is carpal tunnel syndrome (CTS), a painful and frequently disabling condition of the hands and wrists. The first symptoms are generally numbness or a feeling of pins and needles in the fingers. Standard treatment consists of wearing a wrist splint, taking anti-inflammatory drugs or injections of cortisone in the wrist to reduce the swelling, or hand surgery that entails cutting ligaments at the bottom of the wrist.

Dr. Karl Folkers, director of the Institute for Biomedical Research at the University of Texas in Austin, reported in the mid-1970s that people with carpal tunnel syndrome, from teenagers to the elderly, have a severe deficiency of vitamin B6. In over ten years of research, Folkers has demonstrated in scientific studies that people with CTS will recover in three months or less if given daily supplements of vitamin B6. Depending on the severity of the condition, the patient's age and body weight, and other factors, dosage is from 25 to 100 milligrams per day.[31]

Autism. Bernard Rimland, Ph.D., director of the Institute for Child Behavior Research in San Diego and author of *Infantile Autism,* published in 1964, says that autism involves a vitamin B6 deficiency.

According to the National Society for Autistic Children, the autistic child cannot communicate with others or relate to people in a normal manner. Autism occurs more frequently in males; about 4 in every 10,000 children are autistic. "There is as yet no cure, but a growing body of research points to biochemical error. . . ."[32] When I spoke with a Cincinnati child psychiatrist who specializes in autism, he said bluntly, "There is no treatment for autism."

Twenty years ago, Rimland's first son, Mark, was born autistic. I recall reading the comment, "Mark's affliction has become his father's life work." Rimland conducted a double-blind evaluation of vitamin B6 in a group of autistic children, which appeared in the *American Journal of Psychiatry* in 1978.[33] This study, like Rimland's 1973 study, showed that when autistic children were given a large daily supplement of vitamin B6 (pyridoxine), 30 to 40 percent of them improved significantly. Although vitamin B6 alone may produce favorable changes, optimum results are most likely to occur when other nutrients are provided, Rimland says. Magnesium is the most important of these supplementary nutrients. A megavitamin product that contains all the necessary vitamins and minerals to treat autism is available.

Despite Rimland's published studies and those of other researchers, (twelve studies in all), which show positive results with vitamin B6, very few practitioners use megavitamin treatment, Rimland says.

For information about Rimland's treatment for autism, contact the Institute for Child Behavior Research, 4182 Adams Avenue, San Diego, CA 92116.

Vitamins remain the brightest stars in the orthomolecular firmament, but in the last two decades other nutrients have entered the picture.

TRACE MINERALS

In the early 1970s, Carl C. Pfeiffer, M.D., Ph.D., demonstrated that sixteen essential trace minerals, then little known, could make the difference between sickness and health. Some of Pfeiffer's findings were that zinc and manganese may be deficient in patients with such diverse diseases as cancer and schizophrenia; copper overload results in depression and aggravates arthritis; and *excess* iron can affect the heart and other parts of the body. Dr.

Richard A. Kunin further demonstrated the power of trace minerals when he discovered that patients afflicted with tardive dyskinesia caused by antipsychotic drugs could be helped with manganese supplements.

According to Dr. John A. Myers, coauthor of *Metabolic Aspects of Health,* "Our population needs mineral elements more than any other nutritional constituent in their diet."[34]

Research done in the past decade confirms Myers' statement. Low levels of magnesium and selenium are both linked to heart disease. Copper and zinc, which interact with one another, constitute a delicate balancing act. Chromium deficiency can cause atherosclerosis. On a more positive note, a magnesium infusion can be a lifesaver for a critically ill heart patient. (For more about trace minerals, see chapter 3.)

FOOD ALLERGIES

In the early 1970s, psychiatrist Dr. William H. Philpott, working with allergist Dr. Marshall Mandell, helped write another chapter in the orthomolecular story. These two physicians showed that many mental symptoms and behavioral problems are caused by food allergies. As Philpott, author of *Brain Allergies,* writes, "The real breakthrough came when I demonstrated . . . that certain nutrients could stop neurotic and psychotic symptoms and that the results could be immediate."[35] Mandell has reported (and shown in videotapes of patients) that many so-called psychosomatic illnesses are triggered by allergic reactions to food and environmental chemicals. These hidden allergens can be favorite or hated foods, or foods treated with antibiotics and food colorings—any substance that you encounter with some regularity.[36]

ENVIRONMENTAL TOXINS

An understanding of food allergies led physicians into the controversial area of environmental chemicals and their harmful effect on our health. Kunin, one of the pioneers in orthomolecular medicine mentioned earlier, is concerned about a growing list of toxins, including insecticides sprayed in restaurants to kill roaches and such. "When it gets warm in the room, the pesticide turns into gas and you inhale it," Kunin said. These insecticides lower the level of an enzyme called cholinesterase in the blood cells, which can cause nervous disorders. Kunin discovered the harmful effects of insecticides when one of his patients, a waitress, exhibited bizarre symptoms—her handwriting became barely legible, she lost her temper with customers, and she developed a tremor. Kunin also contends that fluoride in the water is linked to thyroid disease and other chronic ailments, and that using fluoridated water in aluminum cookware increases the amount of aluminum that leaches from the utensils.[37] The orthomolecular physician who detects the presence of one of these toxins by doing a biochemical evaluation of a patient has to play detective to find the source of the chemical in the patient's surroundings.

AMINO ACIDS

Amino acids are the "end product" of protein; most proteins are broken down into amino acids before being absorbed. Today doctors practicing nutritional/ preventive medicine are using expressions like "new frontier" to describe certain amino acids.

Dr. Eric R. Braverman, coauthor of *The Healing Nutrients Within,* a landmark book about amino acids, has been measuring plasma amino acids in hundreds of patients since 1972. Depending on the patient's individual amino acid levels and needs, Braverman uses one or a combination of amino acids to treat herpes, memory loss, depression, arthritis, heart disease, insomnia, alcoholism, baldness, and many other conditions.

The body normally uses amino acids to promote health and fight disease, Braverman says. "By using amino acid therapy, we are using the body's natural medicine."[38]

ESSENTIAL FATTY ACIDS

The role of essential fatty acids (EFAs) is a chapter in orthomolecular medicine that is still being written. These essential fats are a different breed than saturated (animal) fats and processed oils, which raise serum cholesterol levels. One of the two major types of essential fats is omega-3 oils from fish and other marine life. As I mentioned earlier, Dr. Donald O. Rudin contends that widespread omega-3 deficiency in the population is causing the current epidemic of degenerative disease. The other type of essential fat is omega-6 oil from plant and botanical sources. One of these sources is evening primrose oil. Since the early 1970s, Dr. David Horrobin has shown that evening primrose oil (EPO) lowers blood cholesterol, improves eczema, relieves arthritis, and eliminates premenstrual symptoms, among other conditions. (More about EPO in chapter 5.)

Hyperactivity

As I've learned from researching orthomolecular medicine, the "neat fit" that we've observed in carpal tunnel syndrome and autism, both caused by B6 vitamin deficiency, is the exception. More often, finding Lonsdale's "biochemical key that fits the lock" is a long, arduous search. Hyperactivity is one of the conditions that in most cases requires such a search.

According to Lonsdale:

> Hyperactive children tend to fall into two categories. The child who's typical of the first type sleeps fitfully, sweats at night, and eats too much sugar. That kind is relatively easy to treat; remove the sugar and give B vitamins. But the vast majority of hyperactive children have an overly sensitive computer, which releases neurotransmitters (brain chemicals) much too easily. This second condition is much more difficult to treat because any number of factors can interfere with the delicate workings which constitute brain balance.

Johnny, 10, typified this second type of hyperactive child:

> Sitting in my office, Johnny was all over the place, fiddling with the paperclips on my desk, playing with the telephone, generally making a nuisance of himself. Johnny's mother was distraught. "He can't sit still in class; his teacher wants to put him in a slow learners' group." One of the questions I asked her was if Johnny had a stuffy nose most of the time. "Yes, he must be allergic to something—he has hay fever."
>
> Johnny's case history was typical of the hyperactive child. He was a colicky baby who "cried all night." His mother couldn't hold him—he was so squiggly. He had recurrent ear infections, was repeatedly treated with antibiotics, and was given ear tubes (to drain the inner ear) at age 3.
>
> Johnny has had problems since birth because he was born with a biochemical defect; hyperactivity is only the most recent expression of this defect. In taking a history, you look for clues. Is Johnny unusually thirsty? "Yes, he's always drinking water," his mother says. Dry skin? "Yes, particularly in winter." This symptom tells me that Johnny may have a fatty acid deficiency, so I gave him evening primrose oil, then waited a month for Johnny's mother to report any change. (Johnny's lips were no longer so badly chapped.)
>
> Nutrition therapy is slow in its effect. It took me almost two years to solve Johnny's problem, but when I did, he became a normal child, and the change will be lasting.

It's difficult to estimate the number of orthomolecular physicians in this country. A scant three hundred physicians are members of the American Association of Orthomolecular Medicine based in Boca Raton, Florida, but the kind of rugged individualists who practice nutritional medicine are not apt to be joiners. Another factor that deters physicians from joining any society that advocates nutritional medicine is the fear of reprisal from orthodox colleagues. Resistance to new ideas on the part of the medical establishment, along with harassment of physicians who practice nutritional medicine, induces physicians to be "closet" orthomolecular specialists. The American Association, also called the Huxley Institute, has a mailing list of 8,500 physicians and laypeople, serves as a clearinghouse and referral service, holds twice-a-year conferences, and distributes literature and tapes about orthomolecular medicine.

To contact the Association, write to the Huxley Institute, 900 N. Federal Highway, Suite 330, Boca Raton, FL 33432, (407) 393–6167. For names of other societies whose members practice nutritional/preventive medicine, see Resources at the back of this book.

AN EXPLOSION OF NEW KNOWLEDGE

Paradoxically, while the medical establishment shows little interest in nutritional treatment, an explosion is taking place in vitamin research. At an international conference devoted to vitamin E, held in November 1988 in New York City, scientists from the United States, Canada, Europe, and Japan reported that megadoses of vitamin E produced a variety of responses; these included enhancing the immune response in healthy elderly people; reducing the incidence of infectious diseases; preventing cataracts when taken with vitamin C; and reducing the severity of Parkinson's symptoms and delaying the need for drug therapy when taken at an early stage of the disease.

Supplementation of vitamin E is necessary, said experts at the conference, "because it is impossible to get either protective or therapeutic effects of vitamin E from diet alone." One pointed out that the average American diet provides only 10 to 15 international units (IUs) daily, a minuscule amount compared to the hundreds of IUs taken daily by people participating in the reported studies.

Much of this research is described in the December 1988 issue of *Health Facts,* available from Center for Medical Consumers, 237 Thompson Street, New York, NY 10012. Proceedings of the vitamin E conference appear in the annals of the conference, published by the New York Academy of Medicine, which sponsored the conference. Contact the Marketing Department, New York Academy of Medicine, 2 East 63rd Street, New York, NY 10021.

Some academic researchers advocate using nutrients as drugs. One is Dr. Richard J. Wurtman of the Massachusetts Institute of Technology in Cambridge, Massachusetts. In 1978 Wurtman reported that lecithin, a choline-containing compound, or choline itself, can significantly diminish the involuntary movements of tardive dyskinesia.[39] Lecithin is more palatable than choline, which can cause diarrhea and produces an unpleasant "fishy" body odor, Wurtman says.[40]

Jean Lud Cadet of the Columbia University College of Physicians and Surgeons, one of the presenters at the vitamin E conference, reported that vitamin E reduced symptoms of TD in 13 of 15 patients treated with the vitamin for four weeks.[41]

The vitamin that doctors now regard as a heart drug is niacin. "Niacin has become the establishment's favorite vitamin," said Abram Hoffer at a recent Huxley Institute conference. In 1987 a California researcher, Dr.

David Blankenhorn, of the University of Southern California, made headlines when he showed that niacin along with a cholesterol-lowering drug can reverse arteriosclerotic lesions in heart patients. (More about niacin in chapter 3.)

LOOKING AHEAD

So it appears that many of the ideas generated by orthomolecular physicians are gradually seeping into establishment practice. In his book, *The Body Electric,* Dr. Robert O. Becker, who pioneered the use of electrical currents in bone fractures, reflects on the political struggle between the revolutionary in science and the old guard: "Sometime during or after the battle, it generally becomes obvious that the iconoclast was right. The counterattack then shifts toward historical revision. Establishment members publish papers claiming the new ideas for themselves and omitting all references to the true originator."[42]

That final stage may be at hand for orthomolecular medicine. In a 1987 scientific article by researchers at St. Elizabeth Hospital in Washington, D.C., the authors postulate that schizophrenia is caused by a chemical change in the brain, and thus "the use of antioxidants may significantly alter the course of this debilitating illness."[43] According to Dr. Hoffer, this is essentially the same adrenochrome hypothesis that he and his colleagues published in 1954.[44] So with vitamins proposed as a treatment for schizophrenia, it looks as if mainstream medicine, after more than thirty years, may be coming full circle in its treatment of that condition.

9

Cataract Surgery— Another Unnecessary Operation?

A cataract (from the Greek word meaning "to break down," or, if you prefer, the Latin word for "waterfall"), is a clouding of the normally clear and transparent lens of the eye. "When a cataract develops, the lens becomes as cloudy as a frosted window."[1] The most common symptom is blurred vision; some patients experience double vision or greater sensitivity to light and glare, making night driving difficult.

Recently, a friend, Phyllis, who's in her mid-60s, told me that she had a cataract in her left eye. "I knew something was wrong—things looked blurry with that eye," she said. "The doctor said I would probably need surgery in six months."

Meddler that I am, I asked, "What does he recommend in the meantime?" Phyllis looked surprised. "Nothing. He said, 'Let me know when the cataract interferes with your vision, and we'll remove it.'"

The advice that my friend received from her ophthalmologist—let the cataract ripen until it bothers you—is standard thinking in this country. According to the American Academy of Ophthalmology, the type of cataract found predominantly in older people, which they call by the unpleasant name "senile" cataract, is part of "the normal process of aging." A cataract surgeon in Honolulu, who has performed over 4,000 lens implants, calls cataracts "as inevitable as gray hair."[2]

It's true that cataracts, which impair the vision of 3.3 million persons in the United States, are associated with aging. Cataracts occur in only 4.5

percent of people aged 52 to 64, but one half of all people between the ages of 65 and 74 have cataracts, and this incidence increases to about 70 percent for those over 75. Medicare pays for more than one million cataract procedures each year, making cataract surgery the most frequently performed operation in people over 65.[3]

Aging Isn't the Whole Story   But a leading German eye researcher, Dr. Otto Hockwin, director of experimental ophthalmology at the University of Bonn, says that just because cataracts occur more often in older people does not mean that the cataract is only age-induced.[4] If this were true, then the majority of older people would have deteriorating vision, which is not the case, he says. According to Hockwin, who is one of the prime movers of EURAGE, an international agency that supports research on the causes of the senile cataract, aging is only one of many risk factors for cataracts. Other factors are ultraviolet radiation, deficient diet, chronic diseases such as diabetes, and the medications used for these diseases. For example, even small doses of cortisone can result in a cataract.[5]

Spare the Knife   Consequently, eye specialists overseas who are familiar with EURAGE research tell their patients how to prevent cataracts by reducing or eliminating these risk factors. In the event that a cataract has already developed, they treat their patients with a nutritional supplement or eye drop (or both) to prevent the cataract from developing further.

The one-world concept doesn't seem to operate in ophthalmology. When I asked a leading eye researcher at Tufts University if he was familiar with Hockwin's research, he said no. Very little international eye research, including Hockwin's sixty scientific studies on the cataract, has appeared in American ophthalmology journals, and the two eye specialists you'll meet later in this chapter, who offer nonsurgical treatment for cataracts, are rarities.

But take heart. If you have early signs of a cataract, or want to avoid developing one, you'll learn a great deal about nutritional treatment for cataracts from these physicians and other authorities that you can safely follow on your own.

If you have a cataract, you will, of course, be under the care of an ophthalmologist. In that case, you may want to discuss nutritional treatment with him or her. If your ophthalmologist is not acquainted with this treatment, the scientific references you'll find throughout this chapter will be enlightening.

PROBING THE CAUSES OF CATARACT

For the past twenty years, researchers at major medical centers in the United States have studied what causes a cataract and published their findings in scientific journals. This research identifies two factors as the main culprits in cataract formation: ultraviolet light and poor nutrition.

Light

Just as direct sunlight can fade your carpets, so ultraviolet light can damage your eyes. Ultraviolet light is not only produced by sunlight but is also emitted by many artificial lighting systems.[6] Prolonged exposure to ultraviolet light has been shown in laboratory animals to damage the lens and the retina.[7] This damage is caused by an excess of free radicals in the lens of the eye. (Free radicals, those bad guys that are implicated in all manner of disease as well as aging, are highly reactive chemicals that are generated by a normal chemical process in the body called oxidation.)

To protect itself against free radical damage, the lens is equipped with a brigade of antioxidants, the good guys of the body, which function as free radical scavengers; these antioxidants are vitamins C and E, zinc, selenium, and glutathione. (Glutathione, an enzyme system, is made up of three amino acids, glutamic acid, cysteine, and glycine.) Shortly before a cataract begins to form, the lens's defense brigade is depleted. Vitamin C concentrations within the eye (normally thirty times as high as in the blood) are severely reduced, as is the amount of glutathione normally present in the lens. This depletion of antioxidants initiates a series of biochemical changes which contribute to the formation of a cataract.

Current understanding of cataracts is largely based on a considerable number of animal studies; I've described a few in the following section. If studies of laboratory rats and guinea pigs bore you, then skip this section. But as a medical consumer accustomed to questioning medical pronouncements, you may want to know the scientific basis for alternative treatment of cataracts.

Vitamin C

Cataract authority Shambhu D. Varma, Ph.D., of the department of ophthalmology at the University of Maryland Medical School, has focused attention on the role of vitamin C in cataract formation. In a series of test tube experiments, Varma and his colleagues maintained rat lenses in a fluid that generated free radicals when exposed to light. He found that the lenses lost their transparency (as occurs in cataract). But when these lenses, maintained in the same mixture, were fortified with vitamin C, they were protected from free radical damage.[8]

Varma concluded that vitamin C is a powerful anticataract agent, but that human nutritional studies are necessary to tell us exactly how much vitamin C we should take to prevent a cataract. Meanwhile, Varma, in an unpublished article, advises 500 milligrams to 1 gram of ascorbic acid per day.[9]

An experiment with guinea pigs (which develop cataracts as readily as humans) performed in 1985 by optometrist Roy H. Rengstorff, O.D., Ph.D., a retired U.S. Army colonel, showed that levels of vitamin C in the aqueous humor, the fluid that surrounds and nourishes the lens of the eye, reflect the condition of the lens.[10] In this experiment, a small amount of a solvent called acetone (a solvent used in nail polish remover and other products) was applied to the backs of 40 young guinea pigs over a six-week period. (A control group received only saline on their backs.)

Use of acetone was based on a 1972 experiment that Rengstorff and coworkers conducted which revealed the startling finding that acetone, as well as dimethyl sulfoxide (DMSO), can induce cataracts in guinea pigs.

Three months after acetone treatment was concluded, 12 of the 40 guinea pigs had developed cataracts, and their vitamin C level, as measured in their aqueous humor, had dropped significantly. Vitamin C levels in the 10 control animals steadily increased during this period.[11]

This experiment not only adds to our understanding of vitamin C's role in cataract but illustrates a possible danger to humans who handle solvents. "A solvent penetrates the fatty layer of the skin," Rengstorff said, as illustrated by laboratory technicians whose fingers turn white. Others who use acetone routinely are manicurists and technicians who administer EEG.

The importance of vitamin C in preventing cataracts was demonstrated in another study performed by researchers at Tufts University's Laboratory for Nutrition and Cataract Research in Boston. Principal investigator Allen Taylor treated cultured lens tissue with ultraviolet light to cause oxidation. As reported in a June 28, 1986, issue of *Science News,* "He found that the more ascorbic acid present, the longer it took cataracts to form." The researchers also found that giving large amounts of vitamin C to guinea pigs led to a buildup of ascorbic acid in the eye.

Vitamin E

Varma's research shows that vitamin E also protects against cataracts. As described in *Prevention* (March, 1985), Varma and associates studied a strain of mice that has a tendency to develop cataracts. When given vitamin E, the mice developed fewer cataracts than expected.

Glutathione

According to William B. Rathbun, Ph.D., of the University of Minnesota School of Medicine, "glutathione is the prime defense mechanism of the lens against oxidation [natural damage that accelerates with age]."[12] Glutathione is a compound called a peptide containing the amino acid cysteine, which is in short supply in humans, says Rathbun, who has been researching glutathione for twenty-five years. "We're trying to find ways to get cysteine into the lens in aging people." Until Rathbun finds "the perfect compound," the best way to bolster the glutathione system, he says, is to maintain high levels of antioxidants vitamins E and C and selenium in the diet. In additions to a multivitamin, Rathbun takes a daily dose of 400 IUs of vitamin E, 1 gram of vitamin C, and "a small amount" of selenium.

Treating People With Nutritional Supplements

The message conveyed in these animal studies—that the cataract can be prevented and treated with certain nutrients—is also demonstrated in a human study. This study, whose investigators represent such institutions as the Human Nutrition Research Center on Aging at Tufts University and Harvard Medical School, shows that persons with high levels of at least two of three vitamins (vitamin E, vitamin C, and catenoid) are less likely to develop cataracts than those with low levels of one or more of these vitamins.[13]

Other human studies show that another so-called aging eye disease, macular degeneration, can also be effectively treated with nutritional supplements. In a study conducted at the Eye Center, Louisiana State University School of Medicine in New Orleans, principal investigator Dr. David A. Newsome found that daily zinc supplements can retard severe visual loss from macular degeneration (the leading cause of vision loss in people over the age of 55).[14] Despite these favorable results, Newsome warned against "widespread use of zinc in macular degeneration," theorizing that giving high doses of zinc might cause toxic effects and other complications. Such concerns are unfounded, according to a team of Ann Arbor, Michigan, researchers, Vilma Yuzbasiyan-Gurkan, Ph.D., and George J. Brewer, M.D., with twenty years' experience treating macular degeneration patients, and others, with zinc. To offset the effect of high doses of zinc, which, the authors say, induces copper deficiency in patients within a few months, Yuzbasiyan-Gurkan and Brewer give their patients 1 milligram of copper each day. None have experienced any adverse effects from zinc therapy.[15]

Caution: If you've been diagnosed with macular degeneration, don't reach for the copper and the zinc. Patients receiving zinc therapy should be under the care of a physician who will monitor zinc and copper levels, the Ann Arbor authors say. What you can do is discuss these zinc studies with your ophthalmologist. You might also mention a zinc-copper medication, ZCC (100 milligrams of zinc, 1 milligram of copper), developed by Long Beach, California, pharmacist Robert Nickell, whose Homelink Pharmacy specializes in compounding custom-made prescription medications. For further information about ZCC, call (1/800) 272-4767 (outside California) or (1/800) 332-4767 (within California).

STANDARD CATARACT TREATMENT

Given this impressive body of animal and human scientific studies by American investigators showing the value of nutritional treatment in eye disease, why isn't your ophthalmologist talking nutrition? A recent policy statement issued by the San Francisco-based American Academy of Ophthalmology, which sets guidelines on how to practice ophthalmology, tells the story. There is not one mention of nutrition in the 12-page document, which is sent to every ophthalmologist in this country. Quality of Care Committee members state, "Currently there is no medical treatment to prevent formation and progress of cataract in the otherwise healthy adult eye."[16]

According to the American Academy of Ophthalmology, "Surgery is the only effective way to remove the cloudy lens. . . . Eye drops, ointments, pills, diet or eye exercises have not been proven to dissolve or reduce a cataract. . . ."

Once the cloudy natural lens of the eye is surgically removed, the eye requires a substitute lens. Substitutes are glasses, contact lenses, and intraocular lens implants. The intraocular lens (IOL) is clearly the favorite; in 1987 it was used in 97 percent of cataract surgeries.[17] Other substitute lenses are cataract glasses, which are thicker than most ordinary glasses, and various types of contact lenses.

Cataract surgery takes about one-half hour to perform and, in most cases, is done under local anesthesia. "Over 90 percent of patients who undergo surgery regain useful vision."[18] However . . . sight . . . threatening complications following modern cataract surgery are not uncommon."[19] The national average charge for cataract surgery is $1,664, 80 percent of which is paid by Medicare.[20] During 1988, 1.25 million cataract operations were performed in the United States.[21]

On the front page of his newsletter, Gerald D. Faulkner, M.D., founder/director of the Faulkner Institute in Honolulu, writes, "As the cause of most cataracts is not known, there are few preventive measures." But on the back page of the same newsletter, Faulkner contradicts this gloomy statement with a news item that begins, "A study of 350 people suggests daily doses of vitamin E and C may help prevent cataracts, a leading cause of blindness in the elderly." (This study, reported in a UPI news story dated November 30, 1986, took place at the University of Western Ontario.)

Why the blind spot concerning nutrition on the part of policymakers in ophthalmology? A cataract surgeon who, for the past decade, has been quietly treating his cataract patients with a nutritional program, said the reason is economic. "Cataract surgery is big business. A cataract surgeon who does twenty-five to thirty-five operations a week makes millions." He has found nutritional treatment to be so effective that, "I've gone from one thousand cataract operations a year to one hundred and fifty," he said. This ophthalmologist, who does not wish to be identified for fear of losing prestigious positions in his medical society ("I'd be tarred and feathered"), also pointed out that owing to Medicare cuts in cataract fees (a 25-percent reduction of fees enacted from 1985 to 1987) there's an incentive to do more cataract operations.

ALTERNATIVE TREATMENT

In this section, you'll meet two intrepid eye specialists: one, an ophthalmologist, Dr. Gary Price Todd, author of *Nutrition, Health and Disease;* the other, an ear, nose, and throat specialist, Dr. Stuart Kemeny, coauthor of *Cataract Breakthrough.* For the past ten years, each has offered his patients an alternative to cataract surgery. In doing so, they not only forego some of the financial rewards of cataract surgery but have been subject to punitive measures on the part of medical societies.

As Dr. Gary Price Todd writes, "I was the golden-haired boy with the world by the tail in 1979, until I accidentally discovered that cataracts could be reversed nutritionally in a high percentage of cases." Following this discovery, "My office partner immediately left, then attempted to force me out of practice." Persisting in his conviction that many eye diseases and other conditions could be reversed or prevented with nutrition, his troubles with colleagues continued, finally culminating in an effort by the American Academy of Ophthalmology in concert with the North Carolina Board of Medical Examiners, and two other societies to revoke his medical license. Charges made against Todd were later shown to be fraudulent in court.

Gary Price Todd, M.D.

Early in his medical training, Todd, who practices ophthalmology in Waynesville, North Carolina, became convinced that the American diet was inadequate.[22] "As a resident in surgery I was the only doctor who prescribed supplements to surgical patients before and after their operation." It was during a stint in Ethiopia in 1974 with the International Eye Foundation that he arrived at a startling conclusion concerning the cause of eye disease. "Ethiopia was a land of blind people," Todd writes. "Almost everyone over 40 had cataracts, glaucoma was widespread and eye disease was common in children." People ate few vegetables even though they were available, and the staple food was a peppery sauce over bread. If, as he observed, a severely deficient diet caused eye disease in a third world population, was it possible that the American diet, also deficient but to a much lesser degree, might also be a factor in cataract and macular degeneration, so-called aging eye diseases?

Returning to private practice, he prescribed a multivitamin to all patients with such diseases, but saw no improvement in their vision until he tried a new product that contained a small amount of zinc. The first patient he treated with this zinc-containing multivitamin was a man with cataracts who was legally blind (20/100 vision) in both eyes. After Todd removed one of the cataracts, which restored sight in that eye, he gave his patient this new vitamin product to hasten healing in that eye, and told him to come back in six weeks for surgery on the other eye. When the patient returned, much to Todd's surprise, his sight was improved to the degree that he was able with some difficulty to read a newspaper. Todd advised the patient to postpone surgery and continue taking the supplement. "At the end of six months, my patient's vision was 20/25" (meaning he could see at 25 feet what a normal person sees at 20 feet). When other cataract patients who were given this multivitamin also had improved vision, Todd realized that they must be severely deficient in zinc. Later he discovered that they were also deficient in other trace minerals, such as copper, manganese, and selenium.

Here's how Todd describes his program for cataract patients as well as those with macular degeneration and diabetic retinopathy (a disorder that can cause partial loss of vision):

> First, I send a sample of the patient's hair to a lab for hair analysis. This relatively inexpensive test reveals any evidence of heavy metal poisoning, which we find in close to 35 percent of patients, and deficiencies in trace minerals. I then attempt to balance the patient's mineral levels by supplementing with those minerals in which he is deficient. ("Balancing" takes into account the way in which two minerals, such as copper and zinc, interact with one another.)
>
> Thirdly, I supplement with certain vitamins, which include betacarotene, vitamin E, bioflavonoids, B complex vitamins, and the enzyme glutathione. [Todd's Basic Prevention formula, if taken three times a day, contains 1,200 mg. vitamin C, 400 I.U. vitamin E and 20 mg. zinc.] Lastly, I evaluate the patient's thyroid function using the Dr. Broda Barnes method [see page 113]. If a patient's body temperature, when taken first thing in the morning, is below 97.8 and he has certain symptoms associated with hypothyroidism, such as lack of energy, depression, muscle cramps, dry skin, then I prescribe a thyroid extract.

Using this "eclectic" approach, "51 percent of patients who come to me for cataract surgery and are willing to try nutritional treatment no longer need surgery," he said. In a recently conducted two-year study of 50 patients, 88 percent showed improved vision. In a recent two-year study of 18 blind patients who had macular degeneration and/or cataracts, 54 percent had their sight restored.

One of the blind patients was a 45-year-old woman, Todd recalled. She was told at age 13 that she was congenitally blind and would never see again. She had never seen color. Ophthalmologists she consulted at Emory University, which specializes in eye research, and two other major medical centers, offered no hope. "We began treating her six weeks ago. Her vision is 20/100, which I expect to improve, and she is seeing color for the first time."

Todd agrees with standard ophthalmologists that the majority of patients (85 percent) who undergo cataract surgery have "superb" results, but not all, he says. "Four percent end up with vision that's worse than before. One-half to 1 percent have disastrous results and lose most of the sight in that eye. A patient who chooses cataract surgery should be aware that there is a risk of losing his eyesight. In my opinion, failure on the doctor's part to discuss nutritional treatment with a cataract patient is grounds for malpractice."

To prevent cataracts, Todd has designed a nutritional formula called Nutraplex. If you have early signs of cataract, Todd recommends a formula called Basic Prevention. For information about these two products, contact Bio-Zoe, Inc., P.O. Box 49, 112 Academy Street, Waynesville, NC 28786-0049, (1/800) 426-7581 (outside of North Carolina). This investor-owned co-op, under Todd's direction, also distributes Todd's tapes and his book, *Nutrition, Health and Disease.*

Since effective cataract treatment, Todd says, depends on "bringing minerals into balance," he urges persons with signs of cataract to consult an ophthalmologist trained in nutrition. If this is not possible, he suggests that you take the initiative in obtaining a hair analysis. You can do so by calling Bio-Zoe, Inc., or ask your physician to order a hair analysis from Omega Tech, P.O. Box 1, Troutdale, VA 24378, (1/800) 437-8888. "Listening to my tapes about cataracts will enable you or your physician to set up a treatment plan."

Stuart Kemeny, M.D.

Dr. Stuart Kemeny of Anaheim has treated an astonishing 7,000 cataract patients with nutrition. An eye, ear, nose, and throat specialist, his training includes optometry and ophthalmology.

In a remarkable book, *Cataract Breakthrough* by Dr. Alex Duarte, an optometrist, Kemeny's name appears as the author of the foreword. But a little detective work revealed that Kemeny actually coauthored the book. When I asked Kemeny, who has an unmistakably retiring manner, his reason for remaining anonymous, he cited the necessity for a physician "to keep a low profile." (His coauthor no longer practices his specialty.)

Ten years ago, Kemeny, dissatisfied with standard treatment of cataracts, traveled to Europe with Duarte after learning that eye treatment there was more progressive. The two conferred with numerous eye specialists in France and Germany, one of whom was Professor Otto Hockwin. Returning from his "grand tour," Kemeny (then a member of the International Cataract Clinic in Tijuana, Mexico, which closed its doors in 1987) devised a program to prevent and treat cataracts that was modeled on European practices.

Kemeny's multifaceted treatment for cataracts, which he describes in *Cataract Breakthrough,* consists of:

1. A supplement called DEOX CAG (formerly named C-Thru) that contains glutathione plus a great many vitamins and trace minerals. (A complete list of ingredients appears on page 54 of *Cataract Breakthrough.*)
2. Ultraviolet-light–absorbing glasses.
3. Eye drops containing phenoxazine carboxylic acid and glutathione.
4. Daily intake of the following:

   500 milligrams of vitamin C with bioflavonoids, two or three times a day with meals.

   400 IUs of vitamin E, two or three times a day. (If you have high blood pressure, do not exceed 400 IUs per day.)

   100 micrograms of selenium twice a day.

   100 milligrams of vitamin B complex, taken after breakfast. (If you have cancer, omit the vitamin B complex.)

   30,000 units of vitamin A with zinc.

In Kemeny's first clinical study, conducted in 1980 at the International Cataract Clinic in Mexico, 54 percent of patients treated with nutritional therapy had improved vision. Ophthalmoscopic examination showed a decrease in density of the cataract. Patients reported that images were less gray and the halo effect seen around lights was less pronounced.

A study completed in 1982 showed that 85 percent of patients had improved vision. As might be expected, patients who derived least benefit from treatment were those with far-advanced cataracts. (Kemeny's results are identical to those reported by Hockwin.)

All these nutrients as well as the book *Cataract Breakthrough* can be ordered from Stuart Kemeny, M.D., 3400 W. Ball Road, Suite 100, Anaheim, CA 92804.

Assessing the Alternatives

In examining these alternative treatments, two questions come to mind: First, is there enough evidence to warrant prescribing nutrients to people? Research showing that certain nutrients can prevent cataracts and arrest their development is based largely on animal studies, with only a handful of recent human studies. As I mentioned, David A. Newsome, M.D., author of a study showing that patients with macular degeneration benefited from zinc therapy, cautioned against "widespread use" of zinc in macular degeneration. But as I learned talking to Newsome by phone, this cautious researcher advises all his patients to take certain nutrients. Newsome's nutritional formula consists of 500 milligrams of vitamin C, 200 IUs of vitamin E, and 50 milligrams of zinc.

Second: Why don't these experts come up with the same nutritional formula? I asked optometrist Roy H. Rengstorff, whose study of vitamin C in guinea pigs with cataracts was mentioned, about this. Rengstorff, author of 132 scientific studies relating to nutrition and eye disease, said that until good human studies are done, it's difficult to prescribe exact amounts. "They're all on the right track because it's obvious that we're not getting the nutrients we need in our diet," he said. He confided that he needed a fishing tackle box to store his vitamins and minerals until he found a multivitamin he liked. His choice: Bronson Pharmaceutical's formula 130, which he said contains most of the antioxidants plus trace minerals. This formula, however, does not contain glutathione. For further information about Bronson supplements, call (1/800) 521-3322.

What Happened to Carrots?

Food for the eyes need not come in a bottle. In a course that Rengstorff gives to eye care practitioners, he advises them to tell their patients to eat foods that contain generous amounts of the "four aces," that is, vitamin A, vitamin C, vitamin E, and selenium. Among foods high in vitamin A, liver heads the list, with red peppers runner-up. Red peppers are also number one among foods that are rich sources of vitamin C, followed by kale, turnip greens, green peppers, and collards. Nuts and oils are high in vitamin E. The best sources of selenium are shrimp, smelts, lobster, and scallops— considering the cost of these luxury foods, hardly a practical way to offset the effect of selenium-poor soil.

For a complete list of foods containing high levels of vitamins A, C, E, and selenium, see John O. Kirschmann's *Nutrition Almanac* (New York: McGraw-Hill, 1984).

LOOKING AHEAD

When can you expect your ophthalmologist to talk nutrition? As soon as doctors who control the American Academy of Ophthalmology are honest enough to acknowledge more than twenty years of cataract research which shows that nutrition can prevent and arrest cataracts. They must then be willing to forego income from patients no longer requiring cataract surgery.

This would seem unlikely to occur except for growing concern on the part of government and insurance planners over the $3 billion-a-year cost of cataract care. (As evidence of this concern, they've been cutting fees from cataract surgery since 1983.) Scientists engaged in cataract research are well aware of the financial benefits of nutritional treatment. A leading researcher at Tufts' USDA Human Nutrition Research Center on Aging, who has successfully used vitamins C and E to prevent cataracts, remarked, "If you could delay cataract formation by just ten years, you would eliminate the need for half of the cataract extractions.[23]

10

Energy Medicine

A Las Vegas physician, one of the pioneers in a method called electrodiagnosis (ED), says that ED enables him to diagnose disease at any stage in its development, even before physical signs appear. Equally startling, using this technique, which involves electronic instruments, he can effectively treat existing disease or prevent emerging disease from developing.

A Los Gatos dentist says that using the latest electrodiagnostic instrument he can reverse gum disease in record time. Using electrodiagnosis, he can also identify dental materials that the patient is sensitive to, which could cause problems ranging from a sensitive tooth to trigeminal neuralgia.

An Oklahoma City physician uses magnets in conjunction with other therapies to treat pain, allergies—almost every type of medical problem. He also teaches his patients how to use magnets to treat simple ailments.

A Chatham, New Jersey, pediatrician reports excellent results using acupuncture of the ear to treat learning disabled children and those with cerebral palsy.

An internationally known pain control specialist in Springfield, Missouri, confers regularly with a clairvoyant in another locale who is skilled in "intuitive diagnosis."

A New York psychiatrist successfully treats patients who suffer from phobias with Bach Flower Remedies.

All of these practitioners are employing some form of energy medicine, and as high-tech as some of the treatments sound, all are based on principles that are hundreds, even thousands of years old.

LIFE FORCE

The concept of energy as a life force is found in all the ancient cultures. The Chinese call it *ch'i* (pronounced chee). In India it's called *prana*. The German physician Samuel H. Hahnemann, who founded a system of medicine called homeopathy in the early 1800s, used the term *vital force*. All these terms refer to a fundamental force that relates to healing."

Until very recently, there was little interest on the part of American physicians in this nebulous "force." But starting in the mid-1980s, the concept of energy medicine, which had been simmering for some time, exploded on the scientific scene. In the past few years, there has been an outpouring of scientific papers and books on the subject. The first international conference about energy medicine, which was held in Madras, India, in March 1987, attracted several hundred scientists and practitioners. The $190 million Fetzer Foundation in Kalamazoo, Michigan, supports energy medicine research at Harvard University, Princeton University, and the Menninger Foundation.

What Is Energy Medicine?

Definitions of energy medicine abound, but I think the one given by Dr. Richard Gerber, author of *Vibrational Medicine: New Choices for Healing Ourselves* (Santa Fe, N.M.: Bear & Co., 1988), best fits our needs. Gerber defines energy, or vibrational, medicine as "the emerging science of utilizing various forms of energy for diagnosis and healing." According to Dr. Harvey Grady, director of the Center for Human Potential in Phoenix, some of these forms are "subtle energies" that at present cannot be measured. This category includes those energies involved in psychic healing, prayer, meditation, hope, faith, the will to live. Other forms of energy can be measured. These are such physical energies as magnetism, electricity, heat, sound, light, gravity, and motion.

Why concern ourselves with such an elephant of a subject, which I can only give you inklings of in the confines of a chapter? Energy medicine deserves our attention because it offers tangible ways in which to improve our health and well-being.

The Energy Medicine Practitioner

Why the sudden excitement about the age-old subject of energy medicine? Some of the same reasons, I suspect, that ushered in the holistic revolution in the early 1970s. Dissatisfaction with the way medicine is practiced, its narrow focus on drugs and surgery, and its skyrocketing cost (an estimated $1 billion a day).[1]

Another factor is the influence of modern physics. The Newtonian model of the world as an intricate machine has given way to the Einsteinian view, in which "mass is nothing but a form of energy." (For the reader like myself, who lacks any background in physics, Fritjof Capra, author of *The Tao of Physics* [Berkeley, Calif.: Shambala Publications, 1975], presents an intelligible explanation of how the two basic theories of modern physics—quantum theory and relativity theory—shattered the Newtonian model of the universe.)

But standard medicine hasn't kept pace with modern physics, says Gerber. Stuck in the Newtonian Age, "Present-day physicians still see the human body as a complex machine. In approaching a problem such as atherosclerosis, doctors act like a high-tech plumber trying to fix a clogged drain. They use chemicals to increase blood flow past cholesterol blockages, and when that fails, they use a balloon plunger or even a laser beam to blast away the dysfunctional debris. More commonly, a new pipe is carefully stitched in place to bypass the old clogged artery."[2] Reading about the array of materials and devices—artificial hips, knees, shunts, pacemakers, breast and dental implants—used as "spare parts," you, too, may have pictured the physician as a mechanic.

The new breed of health practitioner who practices energy medicine looks at living organisms as an Eastern mystic might. (This comparison is the theme of Capra's *The Tao of Physics*.) Energy medicine "doctors" see their patients as living creatures surrounded by energy fields, or etheric bodies. "We all wear an invisible garment, an electromagnetic cloak that shields us from head to toe."[3] Or: "We walk around in an electromagnetic envelope which serves as a communication link [with] bioelectromagnetic fields."[4] To better understand this new concept of the individual as an energy system, let's look at the oldest form of energy, the spiritual or "subtle" energies.

MIND AND SPIRIT

Subtle energies are the elusive butterflies of energy medicine. Since standard medicine, like Elmer Green's definition of the left brain, "cannot tolerate anything it does not understand," physicians and scientists have ignored this form of energy.[5]

The holistic movement, a giant wave that crashed on the California shores in the early 1970s, carried with it Eastern concepts of health. One of these concepts, the power of the mind to control the body, inspired interest in yogis, who perform what seem like superhuman feats. As Dr. Herbert Benson, who journeyed to remote areas of the Himalayas, observed, a neophyte Tibetan monk, sitting cross-legged in the chill night air, wraps a sheet that has been dipped in icy water around his shoulders, then raises his skin temperature to dry the sheet. Another wet sheet is draped around him and the process continues until dawn.[6] Dr. Elmer Green, director of the Menninger Foundation, tested an American, Jack Schwartz, who displayed equally astonishing feats of mind control. When Schwartz pushed a sailmaker's needle through his biceps or placed a lighted cigarette against his arm so the skin sizzled, he was able to control bleeding and felt no pain.

The medical profession was slow to accept any evidence that the body didn't run the show, but for ordinary people with no investment in medical dogma, the message that the mind controls the body was a familiar one. Popular sayings give a clue to this innate wisdom: "Worry can make you sick" or "She gives me a pain in the neck." At this time, when awareness of the power of the mind was taking hold, Norman Cousins's *Anatomy of an Illness,* an account of his bout with a crippling and possibly life-threatening disease, appeared and became a best-seller. Cousins, then a magazine editor, described how he restored himself to health by moving into cheerful surroundings and devising a health-producing program that included vitamin C and laughter. By the mid-1980s, physicians could not ignore scientific evidence that linked a patient's mental state with the immune system. This recognition of the mind-body connection has created a new specialty called psychoneuroimmunology.

The Mind

Energy medicine provides further evidence of the power of the mind. "A thought has energy," writes Marcel Vogel, Ph.D., a senior scientist with IBM for twenty-seven years, who is researching crystals. "In our laboratory experiments we have found that the act of thinking releases an energy which we can store in the lattice system of a cut quartz crystal. These patterns of thought vibrations are stored and oscillate like a magnetic field. . . . When one pulses one's thought, that energy . . . has the power of a laser."

According to Vogel, crystals can be used to relieve pain and suffering and reverse catastrophic illness. For further information about Vogel's research with crystals, contact Psychic Research, Inc., 1725 Little Orchard Street, Unit C, San Jose, CA 95125, (408) 279-2291.

Dramatic illustrations of the power of the mind appear in *Encounter with Qi* by Dr. David Eisenberg (New York: W. W. Norton, 1985). Eisenberg, then a clinical research fellow at Harvard University, described the exploits of Qi Gong masters in China. (Qi Gong is one of the oldest of the martial arts.) Performing one form of Qi Gong called "external" Qi Gong, they have reportedly split stones with their foreheads and survived having trucks driven over them. Eisenberg relates an encounter with a Qi Gong master who claimed that he could conduct electricity: "I allowed the Qi Gong master to touch me for a split second, long enough to feel the live current emanating from his forefinger."

If you use a relaxation exercise to help you sleep, or visualize yourself hitting a winning serve before a tennis match, you are tapping into subtle energies. Cancer patients use visualization exercises to shrink tumors, a method pioneered by Dr. O. Carl Simonton. Dr. C. Norman Shealy, pain specialist, advises his patients to use positive affirmations, another form of mind-body interaction.

The Spirit

If you pray or meditate, you are tapping into what Gerber calls "higher dimensional energy systems"—the subtle energies of the human spirit or soul. "It is the endowing power of spirit that moves, inspires, and breathes life into that vehicle we perceive as the physical body," he writes.[7] If you feel uncomfortable using the word *spirit,* an Indian philosopher suggests that you substitute the words *subtlest form of matter.* If you are familiar with new physics, you may think of spirit in terms of subatomic particles.[8]

Spirit, banished from the sick room during this century while wonder drugs and surgery held sway, was rescued by holistic practitioners. Meadowlark, the first holistic health center in this country, founded by Dr. Evarts B. Loomis, is called "a spiritual and growth center." When I spent a week at Meadowlark some years ago, Loomis's mother, Amy (now deceased), held a weekly prayer session for guests. In the book that Loomis coauthored with a clergyman, *Healing for Everyone: Medicine of the Whole Person* (Hawthorn Books, 1975), Loomis says that for genuine healing to take place, patients must realize their "oneness" with God.

Here and there a few signs appear that spirituality is seeping into standard medicine. As reported in a 1986 issue of *Medical News & International Report,* a study conducted by a San Francisco cardiologist, Dr. Randy Byrd, showed that patients whose doctors prayed for them (Byrd recruited two other cardiologists) did better than patients who were not prayed for.[9]

In diagnosing a mentally ill patient, University of Louisville psychiatrist Dr. Clifford Kuhn includes a "spiritual inventory" as part of his examination of patients. Asking well-designed questions that reveal how his patients view their illness, their belief system, and their capacity to give and receive love, Kuhn assesses the state of health of their spirit. He concludes that "to be healthy is to be whole" and urges physicians to take a critical look at their own spiritual well-being.[10]

Healing with the Hands

Doris Krieger, R.N., now a tenured professor at New York University, has devised an updated version of the laying on of hands, called therapeutic touch. Since the early 1970s, Krieger has introduced therapeutic touch into nurses' training programs and hospitals (therapeutic touch is an accredited course at New York Hospital), and estimates that she has instructed over 18,000 health professionals.

Unlike the laying on of hands, therapeutic touch does not require actual contact with the physical body; holding her hands at a distance of four to six inches from the patient's body, the therapist scans the patient's energy field for blockages. According to Krieger, therapeutic touch elicits a rapid relaxation response, which helps alleviate or eliminate pain, accelerates healing of bones, is successful with certain types of emotional illness (manic depression but not schizophrenia), helps reduce fever and restlessness in AIDS patients, and exerts a calming effect in Parkinson's and Alzheimer's patients.[11]

Krieger attributes the acceptance of therapeutic touch by the medical establishment to her willingness to conduct careful scientific research. This research consists of measuring patients' hemoglobin values before and after a healing session. Tests revealed a significant increase in oxygen-carrying red blood cells.

For further information about therapeutic touch, see Krieger's latest book, *Living the Therapeutic Touch* (New York: Dodd Mead, 1987). To find a nurse trained in therapeutic touch, contact Nurse Healers Professional Associates Cooperative, Inc., 175 Fifth Avenue, Suite 3399, New York, NY 10010.

Studies conducted by Dr. John Zimmerman suggest that healers emit magnetic energies. While assistant professor of psychiatry at the University of Colorado School of Medicine in Denver, Zimmerman studied the magnetic fields of healers practicing therapeutic touch. Using the most sensitive type of magnetic field detector, he recorded magnetic patterns during healing that were different from those before the session or those of a nonhealer.[12]

Medical Center of the Future

Although we've incorporated these subtle energies into our lives, we know very little about "the nature and character of these subtle energy fields," says William A. Tiller, Ph.D., professor in the Department of Material Sciences and Engineering at Stanford University.[13] What is needed, says Gerber, is "a kind of Mayo Clinic of healing research which could study the many dimensions of healing phenomena within an academic research setting." Here, "medical personnel from all fields of study . . . could design experiments to measure the subtle energies of human function and observe how they are affected by different modalities of healing. . . ." In this healing center, anticipated by the ancient Greeks, key modalities would be acupuncture and homeopathy along with Bach Flower Remedies and psychic diagnosis. In this clinic, healers would use crystals and gem elixirs, color and sound and sunlight — all the "vibrational gifts of Nature" — along with existing technologies.

Bach Flower Remedies

In the early 1930s, a British physician, Dr. Edward Bach, devised a system of medicine based on "treating the patient's personality, not his disease." Bach, an esteemed bacteriologist, became aware that many of his patients' ills were related to anxiety, worry, fear, and other negative states of mind. Forsaking the laboratory for nature, Bach roamed the Welsh countryside in search of healing plants.

The legacy of his six-year wanderings are thirty-eight flower essences, prepared by a method that he devised to eliminate toxicity. Among the remedies are Mimilus for known fears, Aspen for unknown fears and anxiety, Willow for resentment, Wild Rose for apathy, Holly for jealousy, and Larch for lack of confidence. Most widely used of the Bach Flower Remedies is the Rescue Remedy, a combination of five flower essences used to treat mental and physical shock.

Bach flower remedies are included in the U.S. *Homeopathic Pharmacopoeia* and are sold over the counter. They are nontoxic, are not habit-forming, have no side effects, and will not interfere with other medical treatment.

Dr. Herbert Fill, psychiatrist and former New York City commissioner of mental health, has treated patients with Bach flower remedies for ten years. "The remedies are very effective for people with phobias," he said. "A businessman with a fear of flying, whose work required him to fly, did not respond to psychotherapy, but after being treated with the appropriate remedy, no longer has a problem." Fill said he uses the flower remedies instead of tranquilizers and psychotropics and gets excellent results.

Another New York psychiatrist, Dr. John L. Bolling, recently conducted a study with 40 of his patients who were experiencing emotional and psychological stress. "After three to six months of treatment with Bach flower remedies, 80 percent of the group experienced significant improvement."

For information about Bach flower remedies, or to obtain remedies or books, contact Ellon Bach USA, Inc., 644 Merrick Road, Lynbrook, NY 11563-9815, (1/800) 433-7523 or (516) 593-2206. Ellon Bach USA, Inc., is the sole authorized distributor in the United States and Canada.

Psychic Diagnosis

Here and there, practitioners are using some of these healing modalities. Dr. Harvey Grady, psychologist, director of the Center for Human Potential in Phoenix, reads a patient's aura (energy field or etheric body) in making a diagnosis. "A patient named Joan, a teacher in her early 40s, came in with a frazzled looking aura—I could see the stress lines. Questioning her, she told me that she had been in a recent automobile accident. Studying her aura, her low back looked out of alignment. I advised her to see a chiropractor, which she did, and my diagnosis was correct." Grady attributes much of his success as a counselor to his ability to read auras. "I can tell what emotions a person is holding inside." But he never looks at a person's aura without asking permission. "It's too much of an invasion of privacy."

Grady has firsthand knowledge of auras — "I've seen them since I was a kid." Viewing one of the levels in the auric field — "There are seven or more" — is like finding a channel on your television set, he says. "First you scan all the levels, then tune into the one you want."

The ability to see auras can be learned, he said. "When I teach a group of people how to see auras, in two hours, 80 percent of the class will begin to see auras in their peripheral vision." Grady conducts ongoing classes.

Science is beginning to confirm the validity of these auras. In one study, Valerie Hunt, Ph.D., and associates at UCLA electronically recorded data from subjects before and after rolfing (a type of body work) and meditation. At the same time, Rosalyn Bruyere, a psychic, recorded a description of the subjects' auric fields. Color changes that Bruyere saw occurring within an auric field correlated exactly with electronic printouts, Hunt reported.[14]

Since 1970, Dr. C. Norman Shealy, M.D., Ph.D., neurosurgeon and director of the Shealy Institute for Comprehensive Pain and Health Care in Springfield, Missouri, has worked closely with several psychics who provide intuitive diagnosis. Beginning in 1985, Caroline Myss, a psychic, has done readings on several hundred patients of Shealy's. Many of these case histories appear in *The Creation of Health* (Walpole, N.H.: Stillpoint Publishing, 1988), coauthored by Shealy and Myss. Myss's data indicates that she is 93 percent accurate, "a fantastic accomplishment," Shealy says.

The Parapsychology Sources of Information Center (PSI Center or PSIC) maintains an extensive collection of books, journals, and newsletters on parapsychology and PSI research. One of its services is the PsiLine, a computerized database covering parapsychological literature from the earliest times to date. This unusual service is directed by parapsychologist-librarian Rhea A. White, who founded the PSI Center in 1983. Contact PSI Center, 2 Plane Tree Lane, Dix Hills, NY 11746.

PHYSICAL ENERGIES

Magnetic

Magnetic treatment was popularized by a Viennese healer, Franz Anton Mesmer, who practiced in Paris beginning in the late 1770s. Early in his career, Mesmer discovered that placing a magnet over a diseased area of the body would often improve the patient's condition. Magnets, he theorized, were conductors of subtle healing energies, which he called "animal magnetism." He later concluded that the human body is the best source of such energy, and reportedly achieved miraculous cures by laying on of hands. Since there was no way of measuring animal magnetism, scientists at the time dismissed Mesmer as merely a good hypnotist, hence the term *mesmerize.*

Using Magnetism for Diagnosis There was a long hiatus between Mesmer and current research in "biological magnetism." In the early 1980s, scientists began to explore the body's magnetic fields and found that humans do, indeed, emit a very weak form of magnetic energy. Dr. David Cohen of the Massachusetts Institute of Technology reported on a diagnostic tool that employs the body's magnetic energy—a device called a magnetoencephalograph (MEG). The MEG provides more precise information about the electrical activity of the brain than the electroencephalograph (EEG), Cohen said.[15]

It's still on the drawing board, but Dr. John T. Zimmerman, president of the Bio-Electro-Magnetics Institute (BEMI) in Reno, is convinced that his "bio magnetic imager" (BMI) will outperform the MEG, and unlike other diagnostic devices that utilize the body's magnetic field, it is noninvasive. The BMI, which will cost several million dollars, utilizes 60,000 SQUIDS (Superconducting Quantum Interference Devices), each smaller than a shirt button, hooked to its own computer. The technology is already in use, Zimmerman said. "Imagine stepping inside a chamber electromagnetically shielded and having 64,000 soda straws (sensors) gently reach out towards every square inch of the body but stopping short of physical contact." The purpose of the BMI is to display the "dynamically changing patterns of magnetic field energy surrounding a living organism like an aura." The biomagnetic "picture" produced by the BMI will make it possible to diagnose cancer, Alzheimer's disease, arthritis, and other medical conditions at a much earlier stage than can be done today, Zimmerman predicted.

For a complimentary newsletter of the Bio-Electro-Magnetics Institute, write BEMI, 2490 W. Moana Lane, Reno, NV 89509.

Using Magnets for Treatment In 1974, researchers Albert Roy Davis and Walter C. Rawls, Jr., based in Green Cove Springs, Florida, published their findings about "biomagnetism" in a popular book, *Magnetism and Its Effects on the Living System* (Hicksville, N.Y.: Exposition Press, 1974). These findings, based on hundreds of experiments treating large and small animals with magnets, describe favorable results in such conditions as arthritis, cancer, glaucoma, infertility, and aging. Applying the north pole (negative energy) of a magnet to a cancer site arrests tumor development, they say. Conversely, applying the south pole (positive energy) of a magnet to a cancer accelerates its growth. (The magnets Davis and Rawls used were designed, constructed, and treated according to a patented process.)

For thirty years, Davis and Rawls tried to interest the scientific community in their research, without success. Their goal appears to be in sight. In July 1989, Rawls presented a paper at a meeting of the National Medical Association (NMA). The paper, to be published in a forthcoming issue of the NMA journal, contains the finding that "in 96 hours, magnets can kill cancer cells." Since 1986, magnetic research, based on Davis and Rawls's work, has taken place at Columbia University, Rutgers University, and others. Magnetic technology for both diagnosis and treatment is being developed by Bio-Magnetics Systems, Inc., of Newark, New Jersey, in conjunction with the Enterprise Development Center of the New Jersey Institute of Technology.

Researchers who want information about Davis and Rawls' scientific papers and books, write Davis Research Laboratory, P.O. Box 655, Green Cove Springs, FL 32043.

Dr. W. H. Philpott, author of *Brain Allergies* and *Victory over Diabetes,* treats many of his patients with magnets. Magnetic energy is not a cure-all, he says, but used along with nutrition and other therapies is surprisingly helpful for pain, inflammation, allergies, infections, and chronic diseases.

Philpott depicts the body's efforts to attain good health and stay that way as a struggle between north pole magnetic energy (the good defense system) and south pole energy (the bad invaders). "Any time magnetic south pole energy gains a foothold and overpowers north pole energy, you are ill and symptoms develop," he said. The solution is for the individual "to recognize a problem before it develops into a serious disease and then to accurately apply sufficient north pole magnetic energy to correct the problem and overcome the south pole magnetic invaders." In a booklet, "New Hope for Physical and Emotional Illnesses," one of the many case histories that Philpott presents is a 40-year-old woman who suffered from sinus headache and stuffy nose. She was diagnosed by an allergist as being allergic to molds and pollens, but immunization therapy failed to help her. One treatment with the magnets (here Philpott specifies strength needed and where to place them) and all of her symptoms disappeared. Continuing magnetic treatment on her own, she remains free of symptoms.

To obtain a copy of "New Hope" as well as medical magnets and information about Philpott's self-help seminars, write Enviro-Tech Products, 17171 S.E. 29th Street, Choctaw, OK 73020.

Electricity

The word *electricity* was coined by a young English physician, William Gilbert, whose monumental work about electricity and magnetism appeared in 1600. Although scientists during the next two centuries couldn't agree on the nature of electricity, by the mid-nineteenth century, "electrotherapeutics" had become very popular with doctors. In 1894, an observer wrote that 10,000 physicians in the United States were using it (and undoubtedly plenty of charlatans).

Partly due to the backlash created by the Flexner Report in 1910 (which endeavored to eliminate all "non-scientific" treatment), "electrotherapy became a scientifically insupportable technique and disappeared from medical practice. . . ."[16]

Electricity reappeared in medicine in the early 1960s with the work of Dr. Robert O. Becker, an orthopedic surgeon. Becker, delving into the mysteries of the regeneration process in animals, in particular the salamander, which can recreate destroyed body parts, made a major breakthrough with the discovery that electric currents exist in parts of the nervous system. Becker's research, which was rejected by the scientific establishment, has been a major influence in shaping the energy revolution.

Despite the profession's resistance to innovators, electricity has transformed certain areas of medicine. Electrical devices such as the electrocardiograph (EKG), electroencephalograph (EEG), X ray, CAT scan, and more recently, magnetic resonance imaging, known as MRI, are standard methods of diagnosis. One of the first electrical devices to control pain, the transcutaneous electrical nerve stimulator (TENS), has led to newer models such as the Acuscope and the Myopulse (both used to treat Olympic athletes and sports stars). Research into the effects of electricity and magnetism on the growth, repair, and regeneration of living tissue is taking place all over the world. A September 1989 conference of the Bioelectrical Repair and Growth Society, formed in 1980, included close to sixty presenters from over a dozen countries.[17] A researcher in the Veterinarian Department at Purdue University is using electrical fields to regenerate spinal-cord nerves in injured animals.[18]

One of the latest uses of electricity to treat sick people is reported by a Swedish radiologist, Dr. Bjorn Nordenstrom. Nordenstrom contends that disturbances in the individual's electrical network may be involved in the development of cancer and other diseases. To treat lung and breast tumors, he implants electrodes in the center of the tumor, with encouraging results. Thus far Nordenstrom's research, described in a monumental work, *Biologically Closed Electric Circuits*, has been ignored by the medical community.[19]

Electromagnetic Radiation   Electricity produces both electrical and magnetic fields, which are called electromagnetic fields. These are the price we pay for our dependence on electric power. "The environment is now thoroughly polluted by man-made sources of electromagnetic radiation," says Dr. Robert O. Becker.[20] One of these sources, high-voltage transmission lines, has been linked to cancer. Warnings issued by Becker, biophysicist

Andrew Marino, and a few other lone Cassandras beginning in the late 1960s about the harmful effects of electromagnetism created by small kitchen appliances, video display terminals, electric blankets, etc., appear to be well founded. A recent study reported by the Congressional Office of Technology Assessment finds that the greatest source of electromagnetic radiation is common household appliances and wiring.[21] (For a chilling account of the way the National Academy of Sciences and other organizations suppressed evidence about the harmful effects of electromagnetic energy, see the three-part series "Annals of Radiation," which appeared in *The New Yorker,* June 12, 19, and 26, 1989.)

Environmental Troubleshooter   Concern about electromagnetic fields has created a new occupation. "Environmental specialist" Vince Wiberg of Los Angeles makes house calls to check out sources of what he calls "electronic smog." These sources include dimmer switches, power lines, TV cables, telephones, gas lines, fluorescent lights, computer display terminals, burglar alarm systems, radon, and asbestos.

To check electronic smog in your home, Wiberg advises, "Take a portable AM radio, tune it to a spot where there is no station, turn the volume up high. Then walk around your house with the radio and see what happens when you get near the TV, the lights, the oven, all your different appliances. The loud buzzing noise that you hear coming from the radio is the sound of magnetic fields." As long as appliances are plugged in, you need not turn them on for this test; all the wires act as antennas, Wiberg says. In fact, all appliances act as antennas. They may be broadcasting electromagnetic fields from as far away as a neighbor's house at the end of the block.

If bedroom appliances—lamps, clocks, radio, telephone—give off a lot of noise, move them at least an arm's length from your head at night. To avoid close contact with wires at the back of your bed, move your bed six inches from the wall. Replace dimmer controls with on/off switches. (Dimmer control pulsations create electromagnetic fields.) Do not use an electric blanket or heating pad or sleep on a water bed. Do not sleep in a room that has a transformer outside the window.

To locate a qualified individual to check electronic fields in your home, contact the American Society of Dowsers, Inc., Danville, VT 05828-0024. Recent books dealing with electronic pollution are *Currents of Death* by Paul Brodeur (New York: Simon & Schuster, 1989) and *The Healthy House: How to Buy One, How to Build One and How to Cure a "Sick" One* by John Bower (Secaucus, N.J.: Carol Publishing Group, 1989).

ENERGY MEDICINE

Using age-old methods of diagnosis and treatment, practitioner/psychics can view or sense the individual's energy field, or etheric body. This ability is nothing new; for thousands of years clairvoyants have observed auras and claim that they can detect disease from changes that appear in the energy field. The resurgence of interest in auras and the like on the part of energy medicine practitioners springs from a basic premise of clairvoyant lore — that illness first manifests itself as a disturbance in the individual's energy field. Gerber writes, "If this is so, then signs of illness can be seen in the etheric body earlier than they can be detected in the physical body."

The prospect of detecting disease at its earliest stage is an alluring one; of all the criticisms being leveled at medicine today, a primary one is its inability to detect disease at a stage when the cancer can be cured, the heart attack prevented. Judging by the epidemic of degenerative diseases, it's generally agreed that preventive methods are not adequate. Breast cancer deaths increase year by year. Although experts say that close to 20 percent of the deaths attributed to breast cancer could be prevented if the patient had undergone mammography, detecting a tumor at what is considered an early stage does not insure recovery. According to the National Cancer Institute, in women with early stage breast cancer, "up to 30 percent or more have recurrence of the cancer."[22] Although heart disease is decreasing, one in four men with no previous signs of heart disease succumb to heart attacks. Another shortcoming of modern medicine is the plight of the patient who falls in the "gray zone" of disease: you go to the doctor complaining that you don't feel well, but after running a battery of tests, the doctor can't find anything wrong.

Electrodiagnosis

Reading auras and the like may work for certain individuals, but for the average energy medicine practitioner looking for a "window" on the patient's energy field, engaging a psychic or developing psychic skills is hardly a reasonable solution. Enter the electronic tools called electrodiagnostic (ED) instruments. They have been used in Europe since the early 1970s and were introduced to this country in the early 1980s. According to a Japanese researcher who invented one of the ED devices called the Apparatus for Measuring the Function of the Meridians and Corresponding Interval Organs (AMI), "by detecting disease tendencies, the AMI can catch some diseases before they blossom into pathological conditions requiring intensive medical care."[23] Other ED machines can do more than diagnose disease. In describing machines in use at his clinic, Dr. F. Fuller Royal, medical director of the Nevada Clinic in Las Vegas, says that these instruments "assist the doctor in diagnosing illness and in selecting the correct medication for the patient."

Electrodiagnosis (also known as bioenergetic medicine) holds out the promise of "lowering health care costs by providing a faster and cheaper method of diagnosis with an earlier warning system of impending problems before they fully manifest at the chemical level."[24] Can ED fulfill this promise? Let's take a look.

Bioenergetic medicine is based on two systems of medicine, acupuncture and homeopathy. Acupuncture provides the basis for the *diagnostic* function of electrodiagnosis; homeopathy is the mode of *therapy* that electrodiagnosis utilizes. To understand how electrodiagnosis works, here's a capsule description of these two systems:

Acupuncture   According to traditional Chinese medicine, a life force or energy called *ch'i* controls the workings of the body. *Ch'i* is present in every living creature and circulates along specific pathways in the body, called meridians. In a healthy person, *ch'i* flows freely along these pathways, but when the flow of *ch'i* is blocked for any reason, pain and disease result. By inserting acupuncture needles into the body to stimulate appropriate points along the meridians, the blocked energy is released and health is restored.

Americans first became aware of acupuncture at the time of President Nixon's visit to China in 1972. It was then that a *New York Times* journalist, James Reston, who was stricken with appendicitis, reported the astounding results of acupuncture in controlling pain. Western physician-researchers, unwilling to accept a technique whose mechanism could not be explained, finally hit on the theory that release of endorphins within the central nervous system causes an analgesic effect. Consequently, in this country acupuncture is used chiefly to treat pain. In Chinese medicine, however, acupuncture is a very complex system. A basic premise is that acupuncture points are linked to specific organs and organ systems. As I observed on a visit to China, acupuncture is widely used to treat a variety of conditions including gynecological problems, digestive disorders, asthma, and eye diseases.

Although the American Medical Association still classifies acupuncture as experimental, this ancient treatment is rapidly gaining acceptance. Thousands of doctors are trained in acupuncture. (No one has an exact count because no central clearinghouse exists.) In California, there are 2,000 to 3,000 licensed acupuncturists, which includes M.D.s and non-M.D.s.

To locate a medical doctor who practices acupuncture and has passed "exceedingly stiff requirements," contact the American Academy of Medical Acupuncture, 2520 Milvia Street, Berkeley, CA 94704, (415) 841–7600.

To locate a licensed acupuncturist, M.D. or non-M.D., contact Traditional Acupuncture Institute, American City Building, Suite 100, Columbia, MD 21044, (301) 997–4888.

Homeopathy Homeopathy is a therapeutic system of medicine developed by Dr. Samuel Hahnemann almost two hundred years ago in Germany. Hahnemann called the life force (*ch'i*) that animates the human body the *vital force*. This vital force, or defense mechanism, is always striving to keep the body healthy, or in balance.

The word *homeopathy* is derived from *homeo,* meaning "similar," and *pathos,* meaning "suffering." The fundamental law upon which homeopathy is based is the law of similars, or "like cures like." According to this law, a substance given in large, crude doses will produce specific symptoms, but when the same substance is given in a highly diluted form, it can stimulate the body's defense mechanism to remove those symptoms. Take ipecac, for example. If taken in large quantities, it produces vomiting, but taken in minute quantities, it stops vomiting.

The mysterious aspect of homeopathy is that the higher the degree of dilution (when prepared in a particular manner called "potentization"), the greater the potency of the medicine. A highly diluted potentized remedy may not contain even one molecule of the original substance. As you can imagine, the power of the infinitesimal dose, which runs counter to conventional thinking, has subjected homeopathy to ridicule by mainstream doctors (and puzzled homeopathic physicians as well).

Researching *Homeopathic Medicine at Home,* a book I coauthored almost a decade ago, I couldn't find anyone who could explain how homeopathy works until I approached Dr. William A. Tiller, Stanford University professor, who is an authority on "subtle energies." Tiller said, "Homeopathic remedies treat at the etheric level of substance." (*Etheric* refers to the energy field that surrounds the physical body.)

To locate a homeopathic physician in your area, call the National Center for Homeopathy, (202) 223–6182. To obtain a national directory of homeopathic physicians, send $5 to NCH, 1500 Massachusetts Avenue, N.W., Suite 41, Washington, DC 20005. The directory includes a list of homeopathic pharmacies and homeopathic study groups.

To obtain books about homeopathy, contact the Foundation for Homeopathic Education and Research, 5916 Chabot Crest, Oakland, CA 94618, (415) 420–8791.

Energy Machines The story of electrodiagnosis begins in the office of a German physician, Dr. Reinholdt Voll, in the early 1950s. Voll, who was also an acupuncturist, was naturally familiar with the concept of Chinese medicine that acupuncture points are related to specific organs and organ systems. Acupuncturists had observed for centuries that if a specific organ, say the large intestine, was not functioning properly, needling certain points grouped together along the large intestine meridian improved the condition. If this were the case, Voll speculated, it should be possible to use these same points for diagnostic purposes. So Voll and his coworkers painstakingly charted the relationship of acupuncture points to their corresponding organs. Applying a weak (approximately one-volt) electrical current to each acupuncture point, they measured the degree of electrical resistance at that point. To measure skin resistance, Voll, with the assistance of an electronics engineer, devised an instrument now called the Dermatron that is in use today. Voll found that a very high or low reading at points along the large intestine meridian indicated that the large intestine itself was not healthy. The pioneering work that led to the Dermatron is known as Electroacupuncture According to Voll (EAV).

The Dermatron has one other important function that Voll discovered serendipitously. While measuring a patient's acupuncture points with the Dermatron, he left the room for a few minutes and, when he returned, discovered that the patient's measurements were not the same. Questioning the patient, he discovered the cause; while out of the room, the patient had obtained a homeopathic remedy from the nurse and placed the bottle in his coat pocket. This incident led to the discovery of "substance testing"; a physician can test a patient's reaction to a particular homeopathic remedy by putting the remedy into the machine's test circuit.

Electrodiagnosis and Cancer

The messenger that was needed to spread the word about electrodiagnosis in the United States soon appeared. He was Floyd E. Weston of Salt Lake City, then president of the North West Life Insurance Company. The year was 1973, and Weston, then 52, had just learned that he had a particularly lethal form of colon cancer. After three operations within two and a half years, Weston's doctor told him he couldn't do anything more, and his only recourse was chemotherapy and radiation. "I knew I couldn't find any answers in this country, not with the health insurance payments I was making!" Having heard that doctors in Germany were using advanced methods, he went there and made the rounds of the well-known doctors looking for one who could correctly diagnose his condition and offer some hope of cure.

"At this point, I looked fine; there were no external signs of the terrible disease I was harboring." Weston was told by one doctor after another that he was in excellent health until he arrived at Voll's office:

Dr. Voll spoke no English. He checked me with his electronic machine, and within two or three minutes his secretary relayed the diagnosis: "This man has cancer of the colon. We can find the cause and eliminate it." Voll questioned me while playing the electronic machine as if it were an organ. "Have you ever had a tubercular skin test that caused a severe reaction?" Yes, my arm had swelled up when I was given one a few years ago. Said Voll, "The technician put the serum in your bloodstream instead of subdermally; it was live TB and went into your descending colon." Dr. Voll prescribed homeopathic tuberculinum to be given by injection for ten weeks, and I returned home. My energy started coming back and, after completing homeopathic treatment, I went back to my surgeon. Two and a half months after the original diagnosis, he could find no sign of cancer. "You've had a spontaneous remission," he said.

Weston resigned from the insurance company to devote his time to promoting electrodiagnosis, and is now president of Bio Path Systems, Inc., a computer-assisted evaluation system, in Reno, Nevada.

The Latest Machines

Voll's Dermatron has spawned several "new, improved" ED instruments, which include the Vegatest method, the Acupath 1000 and the Interro. These later models offer two new features: (1) The operator no longer has to manually test each homeopathic remedy, one by one. Instead, the magnetic blueprint of a remedy is stored in the instrument. (Each of these instruments stores more than 1,700 homeopathic remedies.) When the "right" homeopathic remedy is found, the reading on the instrument is "normal" indicating that the remedy "resonates in harmony with the body's energies." (2) By electronically measuring the reaction of the body to a suspected allergen (whose magnetic blueprint is stored in the machine), the physician can dispense with food sensitivity tests. These tests are extremely time-consuming and expose the patient to food allergens that can provoke unpleasant or dangerous reactions.

An Electronic Examination

To see electrodiagnosis in action, I made an appointment with Dr. F. Fuller Royal of the Nevada Clinic in Las Vegas one Saturday afternoon in March of 1989. Royal has practiced bioenergetic medicine since the clinic opened its doors in 1980.

Royal, a 55-year-old former general practitioner and U.S. Air Force flight surgeon, gave me a quick tour of the clinic's sleek suite of offices and described its operation. A new patient has the standard lab tests (blood and urine), but Royal does not review the patient's case history at the time of the initial evaluation. "I prefer the patient not to say anything. Every patient knows what's wrong with him, but this information is stored in the right brain. I can communicate with this part of the patient and obtain information through my electrical equipment." He also takes a Kirlian photo of fingers and toes "to show imbalances in the electrical system" (Kirlian photography is a technique practitioners claim can measure changes in the energy fields of living objects) and tests dental fillings in search of galvanic electrical currents, which can upset the body's electrical system. Using a Vi-tel ("the simplest electrodiagnostic instrument"), he then tests to see what nutrients will benefit the body.

Being tested with a Vi-tel, the size of a desk calculator, is a procedure similar to examination by other electrodiagnostic devices. I held a brass electrode in one hand, which serves as a ground for the current, while Royal applied a brass-tipped probe, which emits a current flow of approximately four volts of direct current, too little to feel, to acupuncture points on the other hand. He placed a vitamin on a metal plate on top of the Vi-tel. The dial showed a reading close to 100 (50, which is "normal," indicates that the substance would benefit the body). "No, you don't need that." He looked at me — "I would guess you need pancreatic enzymes" — and placed a bottle of the substance on the plate. The instrument registered near 50, an electronic yes. I asked him how he arrived at that conclusion. "You probably eat lots of raw food — carrots and such. They're good for you but difficult to assimilate." He made a note, "Take two after each meal."

The Interro, introduced in 1986, "the most advanced system of its kind," according to the Esion Corporation in Pleasant Grove, Utah, the firm that markets it, is kingpin of testing at the Nevada Clinic. The Interro consists of a standard computer attached to a matrix unit. I sat comfortably on an examining chair, an electrode in my left hand, while Royal, probe in hand, sat facing me. "I'm going to measure specific acupuncture points called CMPs (control measurement points). There are fifty CMPs we have to check. Normal on the computer scale is fifty. Readings above fifty indicate an inflammatory condition which may be chronic or acute. Low readings, below fifty, indicate a degenerative condition, the most serious being cancer."

He first placed the probe on the thumb of my right hand. The probe emitted a buzzing sound. "One hundred plus," he said, reading the number that appeared on the computer monitor screen. "Something is not right in your lymphatic system on the right side." He probed another point on the same thumb. "Lymphatic two is ninety-four — some blockage in the lymphatic tissue of the upper and lower jaw." (Here I reminded myself that he was describing blocked energy flow, not a physical condition.)

After probing the fingers of one hand ("Right side of heart, small intestine, allergy point, pancreas, liver") and the other hand, he applied the probe to each toe. Here he found a third problem area. "Fat control measurement point" was elevated above normal. "Something is blocking the energy." Although half an hour had passed by, his energy was unflagging. "Now let us go back and test the three problem areas — lymphatic, elevated endocrine system, trouble in the upper and lower jaw on the left side — and find the cause." The probe buzzing merrily, he hit on the culprits — three of them — responsible for the inflamed fat point within seconds. "It's a toxin, a pesticide and a defoliant." (I recalled a chemical lawn spray truck parked in front of a neighbor's house.) "Toxins are largely stored in the fat in the body, including nerve cells in the brain. This can cause people to forget things, suffer headaches and depression."

The next step, he said, was to recheck these points after placing homeopathic remedies in the system. He then interrupted the electronic testing with an old-fashioned practice—questioning the patient to elicit symptoms. (This procedure, called "repertorizing," is the mainstay of prescribing in "classical" homeopathy.)

Royal began with questions that pertained to the emotional sphere ("Do you get depressed, any fears or phobias, trouble getting to sleep?"). Next, the physical sphere ("Do you have any dizziness?"). Lastly, the mental ("Do you try to accomplish more than you can?"). Based on my answers, the machine spewed forth five remedies in seconds. "Now we'll go back to the acupuncture points and see if these five remedies are going to make you healthy."

More work remained to be done. The kidney control point on the right side was still high as was the fat point. "And you have a jaw problem that we need to address." This last point didn't surprise me. My jaw cracked occasionally and I frequently awakened with clenched jaw and a tension headache. "First I'll adjust your jaw, if you wish [I nodded], then give you an injection of a small amount of vitamin B12 that has been imprinted with the five homeopathic remedies you need." Noting a smallpox scar on my upper arm, "Vaccination scars contribute to chronic disease," he said. "First, the scar interferes with the natural electrical transmission of the body, and second, the viral influence is still present in the skin tissue." To eradicate these harmful effects, Royal injected the smallpox scar with vitamin B12.

Then, with the zest of a jigsaw puzzle buff, he said that we were still missing the "pieces" for three problem areas—endocrine on the left, kidney and fat on the right. More checking, the probe now sounding like a whine—then an inspiration. "Did you have your tonsils out as a child?" Inspecting the tonsil area, "Just as I thought. You have some pretty hefty scars back there. Many times these scars block the energy flow along certain acupuncture energy channels." Reaching for the syringe, "I'm going to inject a small amount of vitamin B12 into those two scars." After doing so, he rechecked the three problem points. The reading for each was near 50.

"You are now balanced and over a period of time will feel a greater sense of well-being." He wrote out a prescription for the five homeopathic remedies, to be taken for the next six weeks. These included a high-potency remedy "that works on the emotional and mental levels" and others "to clear out the pesticides." (The clinic has its own pharmacy, which provides nutritional supplements and homeopathic remedies.) "If you were a patient I'd suggest that you come back for a follow-up evaluation in six to eight weeks." Clearing out toxins, or any acute problem, is like peeling an onion, he said. "As you remove one layer, deeper problems may surface." "Will the pesticides come back?" I asked. "It's likely, living in the same environment, but balancing your system on a regular basis will help you develop resistance to pollutants. I encourage patients to come in at least once a year as a preventive." He smiled. "Most people wait till they have symptoms."

Since this "balancing" session, my jaw no longer cracks and early morning tension headaches have not recurred. But an ED examination (performed by Dr. Fred M. K. Lam of Honolulu) in April of 1990 showed that my system once again harbored several pesticides.

An Energy Physician's Story

Royal's encounter with electrodiagnosis in the mid-1970s represented the end of a lengthy search. (It was Weston, the recovered cancer patient, who introduced Royal to electrodiagnosis.) As a general practitioner in Eugene, Oregon, "I enjoyed my practice, but too many patients didn't get well and I couldn't find the cause. I'd send patients with chronic backache or headache to a specialist—back they came in worse shape from the side effects of drugs." Royal recalled an incident that occurred during his senior year of medical school that made an indelible impression:

> A woman was admitted to the hospital who was severely jaundiced. She had no real symptoms except extreme fatigue. During a meeting of the staff, doctors and students discussed her case. Did she have a gallstone, liver cancer, hepatitis? We couldn't reach a decision. The surgeon who was in charge of the meeting took a vote. "How many think she should be operated on?" The majority voted for surgery. The surgeon operated, and the woman died two days later from the trauma of surgery. No pathology was found other than a simple case of hepatitis.

Royal investigated different alternative methods—orthomolecular medicine, clinical ecology, then homeopathy. He was impressed with the results that homeopathy achieved but impatient with the way it was practiced. "Methods hadn't changed since Hahnemann's time, two hundred years ago." He went to Germany, studied with Voll, then trained and practiced with Dr. William Khoe in Las Vegas, founder of electrodiagnosis in the United States. (Royal ranks as number two). In 1980, the Nevada Clinic, under Royal's direction, opened its doors.

Royal relishes describing his successes using ED. "A couple brought their 3-month-old baby girl who was having seizures. They had gone to other doctors who treated the baby with drugs; the seizures continued. We tested the baby and found she was reacting to the pertussis in the diphtheria-pertussis-tetanus (DPT) vaccination. We treated her with homeopathic remedies to clear out the pertussis. She stopped having seizures. Once you find the cause, you have the treatment."

I asked about cancer. "Electrodiagnosis is not reliable in the diagnosis of some cancers, such as brain cancer. It's accurate in detecting colon cancer, lung cancer, not as accurate with prostate. Remember, ED is an adjunct to conventional testing. The patient still needs routine checkups, Pap smears, breast examination, a rectal." According to Dr. Julian N. Kenyon, British authority on bioelectronic regulatory (BER) techniques—another term for electrodiagnosis—one of the problems in diagnosing cancer with the BER system is that, given the presence of a malignancy, there is no way of knowing whether a tumor will take months or years to develop.[25]

Shingles, a disease that can cause agonizing pain, is easy to treat, Royal said. The right homeopathic remedies, as determined by ED, relieve the pain in minutes and dry up the lesions within two to three days.

ED can also reveal the unsuspected cause of a problem:

> Ken, a man in his 50s, had such severe angina he couldn't talk without chest pain. He had had two bypass operations; the doctors were advising him to have a third procedure. His family decided to remove him from the hospital, rent an oxygen tank, and bring him to the clinic. We tested him, found that he needed a dentist, not a doctor; the problem involved his left lower wisdom tooth. The dentist had filled the tooth with an amalgam material (containing mercury, silver, copper, and tin) some years earlier. This tooth was electrically blocking the body's own electrical energy flow along the small intestine energy channel. This channel passes through the area of the tooth. Furthermore, the small intestine channel receives its current from the left side of the heart through the heart energy channel. We sent him to a dentist who pulled the tooth. Later Ken told me, "It felt like an elephant jumped off my chest!" We gradually eliminated most of the fourteen drugs he was taking for control of his symptoms. Within six months he was walking four and a half miles a day without heart pain.

Even Royal's West Highland white terrier has benefited from ED:

> During a bad dust storm, she became ill, feverish, couldn't breathe. My wife took her to the vet, had blood tests, X ray. The vet said she had valley fever (coccidioidomycosis), which was incurable, and advised putting the dog to sleep. I told my wife to bring the dog to the clinic. I tested her, found her homeopathic remedy was Lachesis, snake venom. The dog recovered. I took her back to the vet. "I see you found another dog like the other one." He couldn't believe it was the same dog. But the vet wasn't interested in the treatment.

One of the great advantages of ED is that it can reveal inherited weaknesses, Royal said.

> Why does a person who has never smoked and who practices a healthy life-style develop cancer? He has probably inherited weaknesses from distant ancestors who had gonorrhea, syphilis, and tuberculosis. Hahnemann said miasms, hereditary weaknesses, are the basis of all disease. When you break health laws, the disease reverberates through the generations. Voll believed that every couple who plan to have children should have electrodiagnosis before doing so to discover and treat these miasms.

Electrodiagnosis in Dentistry

Dentists in this country have shown greater interest in electrodiagnosis than physicians, says Dr. Peter V. Madill in a 1980 medical article, and explains why. Imbued with the concept of holistic medicine—treating the patient as a whole person rather than, in this case, a jaw full of teeth—a great many dentists were seeking a wider role than "drilling and filling." (I've also detected resentment on the part of holistic dentists at being ignored by doctors.) Acupuncture according to Voll's system (EAV) offers dentists the opportunity they crave, to be a doctor to the whole body. One of the selling points of EAV for dentists is that Voll devised a systematic scheme that shows the relationship between certain teeth and various organs and tissues of the body. Another point: Voll provides a means of testing dental materials *before* the dentist places them in the patient's mouth. All of these materials have the potential to disrupt normal body functioning through their effect on the nervous system, Madill says.[26]

A Dentist's Story

One of the dentists who has incorporated electrodiagnosis in his practice is Dr. Philip A. Jenkins of Los Gatos, California. Before his introduction to ED, Jenkins, a general dentist, had developed a nonsurgical approach to gum disease ("Periodontists solve the problem by pulling the difficult teeth"). This approach involves taking a culture from the patient's dental pocket. Laboratory analysis reveals the type of bacteria causing the problem and the extent of gum disease. But nonsurgical treatment, which consists of regular prophylactic treatment (scaling, curettage, and root planing) and a hygienic home regimen, did not always produce satisfactory results. "For years I kept after patients to keep their teeth clean, but even some patients who followed all the instructions got worse."

Electrodiagnosis provides the missing link, Jenkins said. After the lab report identifies what type of anaerobic bacterium is the culprit, Jenkins places a homeopathic remedy prepared from that particular bacterium—let's call it "Bug Ana"—in the Interro's electronic circuit. The instrument then indicates how the patient responds to the energy of Bug Ana, and what potency (dosage) the patient requires. Armed with this information, Jenkins prescribes the homeopathic remedy that is the antidote to the problem. This remedy, called a nosode, is similar to the substance that an allergist gives to desensitize a patient. Results using this two-pronged treatment are amazing, Jenkins said. "In the most stubborn cases of periodontal disease, I've seen inflamed gums become free of disease in one month."

Another important use of the Interro is testing a patient's sensitivity to dental materials. If a patient has silver fillings and is experiencing any health problems, Jenkins tests for mercury, silver, and other metals used in silver amalgams. If he discovers a sensitivity to, say, mercury ("the worst offender"), and the patient opts to have the silver fillings removed, Jenkins prescribes homeopathic mercury. "The homeopathic remedy will protect the patient against exposure to any mercury that occurs during extraction of silver amalgams."

Prior to electrodiagnosis, Jenkins did a root canal on a patient who complained afterward that he felt a twinge every time he chewed on that tooth. Later, testing him electronically, Jenkins found that the patient was allergic to the cement used in the root canal. Giving him a homeopathic remedy eliminated the problem. Bell's palsy (which causes paralysis of facial muscles) and trigeminal neuralgia (severe pain on one side of the face from a damaged nerve) are both associated with sensitivity to silver, Jenkins said. In some cases, removing the source of silver combined with homeopathic treatment will eliminate the problem.

But Can You Prove that It Works?

There's plenty of anecdotal evidence about the benefits of electrodiagnosis but thus far only a few scientific studies testing the procedure. One, reported in 1985, was conducted by three physicians and a dentist at UCLA. Using the Dermatron, the investigators ran a blind test involving 4 subjects with confirmed lung cancer and 26 healthy individuals to see if measurements clearly identified the cancer patients. The authors conclude that "a significant level of agreement was found between the acupuncture measurement and traditional diagnosis."[27]

Four physicians at the University of Hawaii conducted a double-blind test in which they performed six diagnostic procedures for allergy on 30 volunteers; one of these procedures was EAV. Results of EAV were similar to results of the other five, particularly the food challenge test, the authors say.[28]

A Critical Look at Electrodiagnosis

Not all practitioners who use electrodiagnosis remain convinced of its value. In the 1970s, Dr. Madill, a physician in Sebastopol, California, became a fervent advocate of ED. In a 12-page medical article directed to dentists, Madill described EAV as "a novel, sensitive and efficient method" that represented acupuncture's "crowning achievement."[29]

But in a 1987 magazine article in which Madill discussed his views about EAV, it's obvious that his ardor has cooled. Madill says that until we do some "decent science," it's "too early to be making claims [about electrodiagnosis] both in terms of diagnosis and therapy."[30]

I asked Madill what happened during the intervening years to change his mind about electrodiagnosis. He replied that at the very beginning, when training with Voll in Germany, "I asked Dr. Voll if he had subjected his work to acceptable means of testing, and he assured me that he had done so. When I discovered that this was not the case, I realized that we had better do some research."

The experiment that Madill participated in (although his name does not appear as one of the four authors) was the UCLA study I mentioned earlier. Madill disagrees with the authors' favorable assessment of the results of the study. "I didn't feel that we were diagnosing these patients with any greater degree of accuracy than chance would afford."

This experiment was Madill's first clue that the operator influences the results of EAV, he said. To test his suspicion, he set up an experiment in which he tested a small group of people with the Dermatron two separate times; these testings took place within a few hours so that one would expect the measurements to be the same, he said. The second time, however, he turned the equipment in such a fashion that he was unable to see the dial. The second measurements were very different from the first measurements, he said.

Losing faith in electrodiagnosis was a blow to Madill. As one of its prime exponents, "I had a big practice—a six-month waiting list." Once convinced that ED was not a reliable diagnostic tool, he discontinued using the method. "I'm not saying that Voll's idea of measuring acupuncture points is not correct. But we need a device that will do the job objectively."

According to Dr. Albert E. Nehl, a naturopathic physician in Kingston, Georgia, who teaches the Vegatest method of electrodiagnosis, condemning this technique because it fails to eliminate the "observer effect" is a throwback to Newtonian mechanistic thinking. "Modern physics, quantum physics, describes the relationships of things and their interactions [and] the parts are themselves changed in some fashion as a result of interacting with each other."[31] Based on this new dynamic view of the world, the observer effect figures in any doctor-patient interaction and affects the outcome of the treatment, he says.

Dr. Robert Milne of Las Vegas, Nevada, who has had extensive experience with a number of ED devices, regards electrodiagnosis as an "adjunct" to other procedures: "I use the instrumentation to give me extra information once I already know the diagnosis." The most important part of the diagnostic process is a correct physical examination, he said. "But physicians aren't being trained in the basics of physiology, and without this grounding, the electrodiagnostic practitioner is merely a technocrat."

The Interro is not a diagnostic tool but a "communications device," says Howard Roy Curtin, Ph.D., president of the Esion Corporation, the company that developed the Interro. "Our bodies contain a great deal of information and knowledge that our conscious brain is not aware of. The Interro functions as an interface between a highly intelligent living being—the Body-Mind—and the computer."[32]

To locate a health practitioner who is trained to use the Interro, contact the Esion Corporation, 599 West Center, Pleasant Grove, UT 84062, (1/800) 367–7550 or (801) 785–1137. A source for practitioners trained in Vegatesting is Albert Nehl, N.D., P.O. Box 129, Kingston, GA 30145, (404) 448–4535.

Ear Acupuncture

This form of acupuncture, also known as auricular therapy (*auricular* refers to the external part of the ear), is used by pediatrician Dr. Catherine E. Spears of Chatham, New Jersey, to treat children who have learning problems. Acupuncture of the ear, known to the ancient Chinese, is based on the belief that the ear is a replica of the entire body—brain, torso, and extremities. (The ear somewhat resembles a fetus within the womb in an upside-down position.) The right ear corresponds to the right side of the body and the left ear to the left side.

Spears was trained at the Neurological Institute, a division of prestigious Columbia Presbyterian Hospital in New York City. Early in her career, she was engaged on behalf of juvenile court judges to examine adolescents on drugs for signs of brain damage. After the evaluation she referred the young people for psychotherapy. Inevitably they were back on drugs within the year, she said.

Puzzling over the thorny problem of drug addiction, she read a medical article by a Chinese doctor, who reported that acupuncture eliminated a craving for drugs in his patients. Spears set out to learn all she could about the subject, taking courses in Chinese acupuncture, Japanese pulse, and electroacupuncture (electrical stimulation of acupuncture points). Although she was convinced that acupuncture was a valid and effective medical treatment, a system that involved sticking needles in the patient had serious disadvantages for a pediatrician. She then learned that a physician in France, Dr. Paul Nogier, had devised a system of auricular therapy in which he placed tacks in the auricle of the ear. Spears trained with Nogier and became certified in the specialty. (Spears uses gold and silver pellets, her own discovery.)

The Case of Peter. One of the hundreds of learning disabled youngsters Spears has treated with ear acupuncture is 9-year-old Peter. "Peter wanted so badly to read and write like his classmates but it was such an effort for him—he couldn't recognize the letters." Peter's problem was typical of learning disabled youngsters, she said. "He was naturally left-handed but had been taught to use his right hand." (One of the best clues in determining Peter's natural bent was watching him write his name with each hand, she said.) Natural lefties are right brain dominant; this means that the right brain is their learning hemisphere. Information travels from the left hand to the right brain and goes into a memory bank that can be retrieved. But when natural lefties are made to use the right hand, all the information goes into the left brain and cannot be retrieved. It's like putting a valuable possession in a safe deposit box and losing the combination. Spears' treatment consists of placing several gold and silver ion pellets in the acupuncture points of both ears. Gold pellets are placed in acupuncture points that correspond to a part of the brain that connects the two cerebral hemispheres. (This connecting cable is called the corpus callosum.) Silver pellets are placed in points that direct the flow of information into the proper hemisphere.

After wearing the pellets for a little over two months, Peter went back to using his left hand, and is now right brain dominant. Reading and writing are no longer a chore. Using this combination of ear pellets is successful in 85 percent of children, Spears said. "After ear acupuncture has opened up the pathway to both the right and left brain, children can think better, read more easily, retain information." There's an extra bonus in this use of ear acupuncture. "Mothers often call me and report, 'Johnny has stopped wetting the bed.'"

Use in Cerebral Palsy.   Ear acupuncture can also help the individual with cerebral palsy, Spears says. As reported in *The American Journal of Acupuncture,* Spears treated five adolescent boys with spastic hemiplegia (paralysis of one side of the body). Despite extensive physical therapy over the years, the boys had limited function in the afflicted hands, arms, and legs. After the pellets had been inserted for twenty minutes, the spastic muscles in these areas relaxed and the boys could move these parts. In other children, who were more severely handicapped, using a silver ion pellet in the ear reduced and, in some cases, stopped their drooling. Ear acupuncture also improved the tongue-swallow movement in these children.[33]

In addition, placing gold pellets in the "eye" points of the ear can correct crossed eyes, Spears said.

Infrared Laser.   In the early 1980s, Spears began combining ear acupuncture with use of the infrared (cold) laser. "When I stimulate points in the ear to reduce spasticity, say in the patient's hand, I follow up by directing the laser beam on the hand itself." Adding the laser, "The hand stays open longer." Combining ear pellets and laser treatment also relieves sciatic pain that causes misery in back patients.

In some conditions Spears uses the laser alone. A 92-year-old woman with newly diagnosed shingles had excruciating pain in the lower leg and foot. Despite painkillers and steroids, she hadn't slept in a week. In the first of three laser treatments, "I treated the lesions — you could see them dry up. That night she slept ten hours, and the next night the same. When she came for her second treatment two days later, she was like a new person."

In a patient with rheumatoid arthritis (the most severe form of arthritis), the laser reduces swelling, Spears said. "With osteoarthritis, we work directly on the joints, and in most cases, the patient is pain-free without medication." Other conditions that Spears has treated successfully with the infrared laser include problems in the mouth (canker sores, gingivitis, toothache) and temporomandibular joint and neurological disorders (trigeminal neuralgia and tic douloureux).

Energy Medicine and AIDS

Philip S. Callahan, Ph.D., an entomologist affiliated with the Biocommunications Research Institute of the Olive W. Garvey Center for the Improvement of Human Functioning in Wichita, Kansas, advocates yet another energy treatment. Callahan proposes that the way to control and even cure certain diseases is by matching the type of energy wave to the particular organism—bacteria or virus—you want to destroy.

It's well established that energy waves (radiation) vary in length, from the very long radio wave to the shorter infrared wave to the still shorter ultraviolet and finally the X ray. Radio antennas also vary in shape and length. The enemy organism is like a radio antenna: it can only resonate to a particular wavelength. So to zap a virus—say, the AIDS virus—the trick is to match the frequency of the energy wave to the frequency of the virus.

Here's how Callahan describes his battle plan for curing AIDS: The AIDS virus attacks a host cell called the T-4 lymphocyte, a white blood cell that regulates the immune system, he says. "What the AIDS virus does is operate as a small communications satellite looking for a landing strip—the host T-4 lymphocyte." Callahan compares the AIDS communication system to the radio navigation system found at major air terminals, a circular structure with numerous little knoblike balls at the end of metal rods, called an omni range. When an aircraft approaches the air terminal in bad weather or at night, the omni range transmits high-frequency radio beams that the aircraft can pick up to guide the pilot home.

The AIDS virus looks like an omni range, Callahan says. It is a perfect sphere surrounding a core; projecting from the surface of the sphere are rodlike structures. By treating the AIDS virus like an unfriendly aircraft that we want to keep from landing on the T-4 lymphocyte, we can "jam" the AIDS virus with radiation tuned to the virus's wavelength and thus inactivate it, he says.[34]

Recently, Callahan has talked to several laser company representatives who say that the concept is feasible and only requires funding. Why laser companies, I asked. "Lasers, like radio, produce coherent (in-step tuneable) radiation. So a tuneable laser system could be utilized to jam the AIDS virus communication."

LOOKING AHEAD

Plans for Gerber's "Mayo Clinic of Alternative Medicine" are in the works. A Healing Research Center Fund is being created under the auspices of the World Research Foundation (WRF), a nonprofit organization in Sherman Oaks, California. WRF is in the process of creating an alternative medicine/ healing research database. The second step will be to create a computer network to facilitate networking among health practitioners who utilize alternative methods.

For further information about the Healing Research Center, contact the World Research Foundation, 15300 Ventura Boulevard, Sherman Oaks, CA 91403, (818) 907–5483.

Resources

LOCATING AN ALTERNATIVE PHYSICIAN

This may take some leg work—they're not listed as such in the classified section of your telephone book—but I'm convinced that it's worth the effort.

At the end of this section I've provided a list of medical societies whose members practice nutritional medicine and offer nontoxic treatments. The American Holistic Medical Association (AHMA), for example, will send you a list of physicians organized by state. Other societies charge a nominal fee for a membership directory.

If you live in a big city, you can probably find an alternative physician in your area; otherwise, you may have to go out of town. Once you're equipped with some names of alternative physicians, call their offices and learn as much as possible by talking to the office manager or secretary. Explain your interest in being a patient and ask what medical schools the doctors attended, how long they have been in practice, what diagnostic procedures and treatments they use, and what their fees are. If they have written medical articles or a book, ask for a reprint of the article or ask how to obtain the book. (Such questions, of course, should be standard procedure in interviewing any physician.)

Once you appear for your appointment, continue evaluating the physician. How do *you* respond to the practitioner's office and staff? For other considerations to keep in mind during the evaluation process, ask the AMHA for a copy of "How to Choose a Holistic Health Practitioner." For a comprehensive guide to choosing an alternative doctor, ask the People's Medical Society, 462 Walnut Street, Allentown, PA 19102 to send you their health bulletin, "How to Choose a Doctor."

From my own experience, you can also learn a lot about the doctor by talking to patients in the waiting room.

Within the United States

Academy of Orthomolecular Medicine
Huxley Institute
900 N. Federal Highway, Suite 330
Boca Raton, FL 33432
(1/800) 847–3802

American Academy of Advancement in Medicine (ACAM)
23121 Verdugo Drive, #204
Laguna Hills, CA 92653

American Academy of Environmental Medicine
P.O. Box 16106
Denver, CO 80216
(303) 622–9755

American Association of Naturopathic Physicians
P.O. Box 20386
Seattle, WA 98102
(206) 323–7610

American Holistic Medical Association
2727 Fairview Avenue E
Seattle, WA 98102
(206) 322–6842

Great Lakes Association of Clinical Medicine, Inc. (GLACM)
Jack Hank, Executive Director
70 W. Huron Street
Chicago, IL 60610
(312) 266–6246

International Academy of Nutrition and Preventive Medicine
P.O. Box 5832
Lincoln, NE 68505
(402) 467–2716

North Nassau Division of Nutritional and Preventive Medicine
1691 Northern Blvd.
Manhasset, NY 11030
(516) 627–7535

Nutrition for Optimal Health Association (NOHA)
P.O. Box 380
Winnetka, IL 60093

Price-Pottenger Nutrition Foundation
P.O. Box 2614
La Mesa, CA 92044-0702
(619) 582–4168

Rheumatoid Disease Foundation
5106 Old Harding Road
Franklin, TN 37064
(615) 646–1030

Outside the United States

SOMA
P.O. Box 180
Bondi Beach 2026
Australia

Health Action Network Society
5262 Rumble Street, Suite #202
Burnaby, British Columbia V5J2B6
Canada

Canadian Schizophrenia Foundation
7375 Kingsway
Burnaby, British Columbia V3N3B
Canada

Centre for the Study of Complementary Medicine
51 Bedford Place
Southampton
Hampshire S01 2DG
England

RECOMMENDED READING

Books

Brecher, Arline. *Bye-Bye Bypass*. Medex Press, P.O. Box 683, Herndon, VA 22070, (703) 471–4734. Can be ordered from your local bookstore, or contact publisher.

Carper, Jean. *The Food Pharmacy*. New York: Bantam Books, 1988.

Cheraskin, Emanuel, M.D., D.M.D., and W. M. Ringsdorf, Jr., D.M.D., with Arline Brecher. *Psychodietetics: Food as the Key to Emotional Health*. New York: Stein & Day, 1974.

Cousins, Eleanor. *Caring for the Healing Heart: An Eating Plan for Recovery from Heart Attack*. New York: W. W. Norton & Co., 1988.

Cranton, Elmer, M.D., and Arline Brecher. *Bypassing Bypass*, 1989. Can be ordered from American College of Advancement in Medicine (ACAM) (800) 532–3688.

Glassman, Judith. *The Cancer Survivors*. New York: Dial Press, 1983.

Hoffer, Abram, Ph.D., M.D., and Morton Walker, D.P.M. *Orthomolecular Nutrition: New Lifestyle for Super Good Health*. New Canaan, Conn.: Keats Publishing, 1978.

Hunter, Beatrice Trum. *Consumer Beware*. New York: Simon & Schuster, 1971.

Kunin, Richard A. *Mega-Nutrition*. New York: New American Library, 1980.

Moss, Ralph W. *The Cancer Industry: Unravelling the Politics*. Paragon House, 1989. Can be obtained from publisher (800) PARAGON or Project Cure (800) 552–CURE.

Price, Weston A., D.D.S. *Nutrition and Physical Degeneration*. Price-Pottenger Nutrition Foundation, P.O. Box 2614, La Mesa, CA 92044-0702.

Randolph, Theron G., M.D., and Ralph W. Moss, Ph.D. *An Alternative Approach to Allergies*. New York: Bantam Books, 1982.

Weil, Andrew, M.D. *Health and Healing*. Boston: Houghton Mifflin, 1983.

Werbach, Melvyn R. *Third Line Medicine: Modern Treatment for Persistent Symptoms*. New York: Arkana, 1986.

Williams, Roger J. *Nutrition Against Disease*. New York: Bantam Books, 1971.

Wright, Jonathan V., M.D. *Dr. Wright's Guide to Healing with Nutrition*. Emmaus, Penn.: Rodale Press, 1984.

Some of the older books are out of print but can be found at your public library.

Health Newsletters

Alternatives
Mountain Home Publishing
P.O. Box 829
Ingram, TX 78025

The Cancer Chronicles
161 West 61st Street, Suite 5B
New York, NY 10023

The Doctor's People Newsletter
1578 Sherman Avenue, Suite 318
Evanston, IL 60201

Healthfacts
Center for Medical Consumers
237 Thompson Street
New York, NY 10012

People's Medical Society Newsletter
462 Walnut Street
Allentown, PA 18102

Notes

INTRODUCTION

1. Lauren Chambliss and Sharon Reier, "How Doctors Have Ruined Health Care," *Financial World,* Jan. 9, 1990.
2. Robert H. Brook, "Practice Guidelines and Practicing Medicine, Are They Compatible?" *JAMA* 262 (Dec. 1, 1989).
3. Karen Southwick, "A Prescription for Trouble," *Health Freedom News,* June 1989.
4. Alan H. Nittler, *A New Breed of Doctor* (New York: Pyramid Books, 1975).
5. Melvyn R. Werbach, *Third Line Medicine* (New York: Arkana, 1986).
6. Ross McWhirter, "Valve of Simple Mastectomy and Radiotherapy in Treatment of Breast Cancer," *British Journal of Radiology* 21 (Dec. 1948): 599–610.
7. Henry J. Heimlich, "F.A.C.S.," *Annals of Surgery* 182 (Aug., 1975).
8. Elisabeth Rosenthal, "Innovations Intensify Glut of Surgeons," *New York Times,* Nov. 7, 1989.
9. J. Warren Salmon, ed., *Alternative Medicines* (New York: Tavistock Publications, 1984).

1. CANCER TREATMENTS DESIGNED TO STRENGTHEN THE IMMUNE SYSTEM

1. This analogy was made by Michael L. Culbert, editor of *The Choice,* at a talk in Washington, D.C., May 11, 1988.
2. John C. Bailor III, and Elaine M. Smith, "Progress Against Cancer?" *New England Journal of Medicine* 314 (May 8, 1986).
3. John Cairns, "The Treatment of Diseases and the War Against Cancer," *Scientific American,* Nov. 1985.
4. Haydn Bush, "Cure," *Science 84,* Sept. 1984, 34–35.
5. Robert K. Oye and Martin F. Shapiro, "Reporting Results from Chemotherapy Trials," *JAMA* (Nov. 16, 1984).
6. See note 2 above.
7. U.S. General Accounting Office, "Cancer Patient Survival: What Progress Has Been Made?" GAO/PEMD 87–13, March 1987.

8. American Cancer Society, "Unproven Methods of Cancer Management," Professional Education Publication, 1982.

9. C. Barber Mueller, "Surgery for Breast Cancer," *New England Journal of Medicine* 312 (March 14, 1985): 712–713.

10. Ralph W. Moss, *The Cancer Syndrome* (New York: Grove Press, 1980).

11. "Ten-Year Results of a Randomized Clinical Trial Comparing Radical Mastectomy and Total Mastectomy with or without Radiation," *New England Journal of Medicine* 312 (March 14, 1985).

12. "Five-Year Results of a Randomized Clinical Trial Comparing Total Mastectomy and Segmental Mastectomy with or without Radiation in the Treatment of Breast Cancer," *New England Journal of Medicine* 312 (March 14, 1985).

13. *Medical World News,* Jan. 21, 1980.

14. Pat McGrady, Sr., *The Savage Cell* (New York: Basic Books, 1964).

15. Thomas H. Maugh and Jean L. Marx, *Seeds of Destruction Cancer Syndrome,* 315.

16. Philip Rubin, ed., *Clinical Oncology for Medical Students and Physicians: A Multi-Disciplinary Approach,* 3rd ed. (University of Rochester, School of Medicine and Dentistry, and American Cancer Society, 1971).

17. American Cancer Society, "Modern Cancer Treatment," *Cancer Book* (Garden City, N.Y.: Doubleday & Co., 1986).

18. "Primary Treatment is Not Enough for Early Stage Breast Cancer," *Update,* National Cancer Institute, Office of Cancer Communications, May 18, 1988.

19. "Postoperative Radiation for Women with Cancer of the Breast and Positive Axillary Lymph Nodes," *New England Journal of Medicine* (Jan. 8, 1981).

20. American Cancer Society, *Cancer Book* (Garden City, N.Y.: Doubleday & Co. 1986).

21. Rochelle E. Curtis et al., "Risk of Leukemia Associated with the First Course of Cancer Treatment: An Analysis of the Surveillance, Epidemiology, and End Results Program Experience," JNCI 72 (March 1984).

22. See note 17 above.

23. See note 12 above.

24. See note 18 above.

25. Philip M. Boffey, "Breast Cancer Analysis Stirs a Debate at Parley," *New York Times,* Sept. 13, 1985.

26. "The Thrombogenic Effect of Anticancer Drug Therapy in Women with Stage II Breast Cancer," *New England Journal of Medicine* (Feb. 18, 1988).

27. Rose Kushner, "Is Aggressive Adjuvant Chemotherapy the Halstead Radical of the 80s," *CA-A-Cancer Journal for Clinicians* 34 (Nov./Dec. 1984).

28. Gina Kolata, "Breast Cancer Anguish, Mystery and Hope," *New York Times,* April 24, 1988.

29. Petr Skrabanek, "False Premises and False Promises of Breast Cancer Screening," *The Lancet* (Aug. 10, 1985).

30. William H. Redd, "Behavioral Approaches to Treatment-Related Distress," *CA-A-Cancer Journal for Clinicians* (May/June 1988):138–145.

31. American Cancer Society, "Principles of Cancer Therapy," *Cancer Book* (Garden City, N.Y.: Doubleday & Co. 1986).

32. Richard J. Whitley and Wilm Christ, "Management of Infections," *Pediatric Annals* 12 (June 1983):6.

33. See note 30 above.

34. Nancy Bruning, *Coping with Chemotherapy,* (Garden City, N.Y.: Dial Press, 1985).

35. See note 26 above.

36. See note 17 above.

37. See note 21 above.

38. Roy B. Jones et al, *California Journal of the American Cancer Society* 33, no. 5 (1983): 262–263.

39. Vincent T. Devita, *Principles and Practice of Oncology* (Philadelphia: J. B. Lippincott, 1982).

40. R. Weiss, "Cancer Therapy Risks Assessed," *Science News,* Sept. 12, 1987, 165.

41. T. J. Powles et al., "Failure of Chemotherapy to Prolong Survival in a Group of Patients with Metastatic Breast Cancer," *The Lancet* (March 15, 1980): 580.
42. Elizabeth Abernathy, "Biological Response Modifiers," *American Journal of Nursing* (April 1987).
43. Elizabeth Abernathy, "Biotherapy: An Introductory Overview" *Oncology Nursing Forum* 14, no. 6, (Nov./Dec. 1987, supplement): 13–15.
44. Joan O. C. Hamilton, "The New War on Cancer," *Business Week,* Sept. 22, 1986.
45. Charles G. Moertel, "On Lymphokines, Cytokines, and Breakthroughs," *JAMA* 256 (Dec. 12, 1986): 3141.
46. Linda Edwards Hood, "Interferon," *American Journal of Nursing* (April 1987):459–463.
47. Gene Bylinsky, "Science Scores a Cancer Breakthrough," *Fortune,* Nov. 25, 1985, 17–21.
48. See note 45 above.
49. Andrew Pollack, "The Next Wave of Diagnostics," *New York Times,* Aug. 28, 1989.
50. American Cancer Society, *Cancer Manual* (Boston: ACS Massachusetts Division, 1982).
51. Edward A. Patrick, "Pattern Recognition May Resolve Management of Breast Cancer: Limited Mastectomy versus Radical Mastectomy," *Science* 187 (Feb. 28, 1975): 764–765.
52. Ingrid Wickelgren, "Shedding Light on Cancer," *Science News* 135 (Jan. 14, 1989).
53. Maurice Natenberg, *The Cancer Blackout* (Los Angeles: Cancer Book House, 1959).
54. See note 10 above.
55. Allan Sonnenschein, "Warning: The American Cancer Society may be Hazardous to Your Health," *Penthouse,* May 1982.
56. See note 8 above.
57. Wil Jarvis, "Helping Your Patients Deal with Questionable Cancer Treatments," *CA-A-Cancer Journal for Clinicians.*
58. Michael S. Evers, "Report: Legal Constraints on the Availability of Unorthodox Cancer Treatments, Freedom of Choice Viewpoint," Congress of the United States, Office of Technology Assessment.
59. Stephen Barrett, *Health Robbers* (Philadelphia: George F. Stickley Co., 1980).
60. See note 10 above.
61. Herbert Bailey, *Krebiozen—Key to Cancer?* (New York: Hermitage House, 1955).
62. See note 58 above.
63. Herbert Bailey, *A Matter of Life or Death* (New York: G. P. Putnam's Sons, 1958).
64. See note 58 above.
65. Ibid.
66. Publication, Burzynski Research Institute, Inc., 6221 Corporate Drive, Houston, TX 77036.
67. See note 8 above.
68. Bruce Halstead, "The Halstead Cancer Battle," *Health Consciousness,* P. O. Box 550, Oviedo, FL 32765.
69. Tim Friend, "Cancer Fraud Lures Thousands," *USA Today,* March 17, 1988.
70. Susan Porter, "Health Fraud—When Magic Replaces Medicine," *The Ohio State Medical Journal* (Dec. 1986).
71. *Merck Manual,* 14th ed., 1982.
72. Judith Glassman, *The Cancer Survivors* (Garden City, N.Y.: Dial Press, 1983).
73. Bernie S. Siegel, *Love, Medicine & Miracles* (New York: Harper & Row, 1986).
74. Robert G. Houston, "Repression and Reform in the Evaluation of Alternative Cancer Therapies," I.A.T. Patient's Association, Inc., Box 10, Otho, IA 50569-0010.
75. Barrie R. Cassileth et al., "Contemporary Unorthodox Treatments in Cancer Medicine," *Annals of Internal Medicine* vol. 101, no. 1 (July 1984).
76. Gary Null, with Anne Pitrone, "Alternative Cancer Therapies," *Penthouse,* Nov. 1979.
77. Michael Lerner, *Integral Cancer Therapies* (Bolinas, Calif.: Commonweal).
78. Lisa Kreger, "Unorthodox Clinics Flourishing in Tijuana," *American Medical News,* August 9, 1985.
79. "Project on Unorthodox Cancer Treatments," Office of Technology Assessment, June 1988.

80. "Turning Point," *Project Cure,* Spring 1989.
81. See note 72 above.
82. See note 75 above.
83. Albert Marchetti, *Beating the Odds: Alternative Treatments That Have Worked Miracles Against Cancer* (Chicago: Contemporary Books, 1988).
84. I. Peterson, "Depression and Cancer: No Clear Connection," *Science News* 136 (Sept. 2, 1989).
85. Lawrence LeShan, *You Can Fight for Your Life* (New York: M. Evans & Co., 1977).
86. O. Carl Simonton, *Getting Well Again* (Los Angeles: J. P. Tarcher, 1978).
87. See note 73 above.
88. See note 86 above.
89. Ibid.
90. See note 77 above.
91. Gilda Radner, *It's Always Something* (New York: Simon & Schuster, 1989).
92. Harold H. Benjamin with Richard Trubo, *From Victim to Victor* (Los Angeles: Jeremy P. Tarcher, 1987).
93. See note 77 above.
94. Josef Issels, "Immunotherapy in Cancer," lecture given in New York, May 1987.
95. Gary Null and Leonard Steinman, "Suppression of Alternative Cancer Therapies: Dr. Joseph Issels," *Penthouse,* August 1980.
96. John Clark, *The Cell: A Small Wonder* (New York: Torstar Books, 1985).
97. Robert G. Houston, "Repression and Reform in the Evaluation of Alternative Cancer Therapies," I.A.T. Patients' Association, Inc., Box 10, Otho, IA 50569-0010.
98. Committee on Diet, Nutrition, and Cancer, Assembly of Life Sciences, and National Research Council, *Diet, Nutrition and Cancer* (Washington, D.C.: National Academy Press, 1982).
99. American Cancer Society, "Cancer Facts and Figures—1988."
100. Michio Kushi, with Alex Jack, *The Cancer Prevention Diet* (New York: St. Martin's Press, 1983).
101. Ted J. Kaptchuk, *The Web Is Not the Weaver* (New York: Congdon & Weed, 1983).
102. *Healing,* Gerson Institute, P. O. Box 430, Bonita, CA 92002, 1981.
103. Max Gerson, *A Cancer Therapy: Results of Fifty Cases* (New York: Whittier Books, 1959).
104. "Nutrition as a Treatment," *HealthFacts,* Jan. 1984, Center for Medical Consumers, 237 Thompson St., New York, NY 10012.
105. See note 8 above.
106. "Manner Metabolic Therapy," *Cancer Control Journal,* vol. 6, no. 1, 1982.
107. "Laetrile Used Properly Can Be Successful, M.D. Says," Letters, *American Medical News,* Jan. 15, 1982.
108. See note 72 above.
109. See note 10 above.
110. Ibid.
111. *New England Journal of Medicine* 306 (Jan. 28, 1982).
112. Mark Lockman, "Laetrile Proponents Flay Clinical Trials," *Public Scrutiny,* April 1982.
113. Evan Cameron and Linus Pauling, *Cancer and Vitamin C* (Linus Pauling Institute of Science and Medicine, 1979).
114. Charles G. Moertel et al., "High-Dose Vitamin C Versus Placebo in the Treatment of Patients with Advanced Cancer Who Have Had No Prior Chemotherapy," *New England Journal of Medicine* 312 (Jan. 17, 1985).
115. E. T. Creagan et al., "Failure of High-Dose Vitamin C (Ascorbic Acid) Therapy to Benefit Patients with Advanced Cancer: A Controlled Trial," *New England Journal of Medicine* 301:687–90.
116. Henry Dreher, *Your Defense Against Cancer* (New York: Harper & Row, 1988).
117. Mucos Pharma GmbH & Co., Alpenstr. 29 D-8192 Geretsried 1, Germany.
118. See note 75 above.
119. See note 72 above.
120. Ken Ausubel, "The Troubling Case of Harry Hoxsey," *New Age Journal,* July/Aug 1988, 43–86.

121. See note 10 above.

122. Virginia Livingston, *Food Alive: A Diet for Cancer and Chronic Diseases* (Livingston-Wheeler Medical Clinic, 1977).

123. See note 90 above.

124. Joseph Issels, "Immunotherapy in Progressive Metastatic Cancer: A Fifteen-Year Survival Follow-up," *Clinical Trials Journal* (London), vol. 7, no. 3 (1970): 357–366.

125. Philip M. Boffey, "Use of Fetal Tissue as Cure Debated," *New York Times*, Sept. 15, 1988.

126. Robert Langer, "Shark Cartilage Contains Inhibitors of Tumor Angiogenesis," *Science*, Sept. 16, 1983.

127. Otto Warburg, "On the Origin of Cancer Cells," *Science* 123 (1956): 309–315.

128. S. Rilling and R. Viebahn, *The Use of Ozone in Medicine* (Heidelberg, Germany: Karl F. Haug Publishers, 1987).

129. Gerard U. Sunnen, "Ozone in Medicine: Overview and Future Directions," *Journal of Advancement in Medicine*, in press.

130. Charles H. Farr, "The Therapeutic Use of Intravenous Hydrogen Peroxide," (Nov. 1986, rev. Jan. 1987).

131. James W. Finney et al. "Differential Localization of Isotopes in Tumors Through the Use of Intraarterial Hydrogen Peroxide," *American Journal of Roentgenology, Radium Therapy and Nuclear Medicine*, 94, vol. 4 (1965): 783–788.

132. Charles H. Farr, "Physiological and Biochemical Responses to Intravenous Hydrogen Peroxide in Man," *Journal of Advancement in Medicine* (Summer 1988).

133. Daniel McCabe et al., "Polar Solvents in the Chemoprevention of Dimethylbenzanthracene-Induced Rat Mammary Cancer," *Archives of Surgery* 121 (Dec. 1986).

134. Stanley W. Jacob and Robert Herschler, "Pharmacology of DMSO," *Cryogiology* 23 (1986): 14–27.

135. *Urology Times* (April 1987).

136. Joel Warren et al., "Potentiation of Antineoplastic Compounds by Oral Dimethyl Sulfoxide in Tumor-Bearing Rats," *Annals of the New York Academy of Sciences* 243 (Jan. 27, 1975).

137. Robert Gosselin, *Clinical Toxicology of Commercial Products*, 5th ed. (Baltimore: Williams & Wilkins, 1984).

138. Harris L. Coulter, *Divided Legacy, vol. III* (Wehawken Book Company, 4221-45th St., N.W., Washington, D.C. 20016).

2. TREATING HIGH BLOOD PRESSURE WITHOUT DRUGS

1. Department of Health and Human Services. Press Release, April 5, 1988.

2. Norman M. Kaplan, *Prevent Your Heart Attack* (New York: Charles Scribner's Sons, 1982).

3. The following account is largely based on the American Heart Association's "1988 Heart Facts."

4. Thomas G. Pickering, "How Common Is White Coat Hypertension?" *JAMA* 259 (Jan. 8, 1988).

5. National Institutes of Health, *1988 Report of the Joint National Committee on Detection, Evaluation, and Treatment of High Blood Pressure*, NIH Publication No. 88–1088, May 1988.

6. "Tackling High Blood Pressure," *Nutrition Action Healthletter*, May 1989.

7. "Report of the Joint National Committee on Detection, Evaluation, and Treatment of High Blood Pressure," *JAMA* 237 (Jan. 17, 1977).

8. "Five-Year Findings of the Hypertension Detection and Follow-Up Program," *JAMA* 242 (Dec. 7, 1979).

9. "Multiple Risk Factor Intervention Trial," *JAMA* 248 (Sept. 24, 1982).

10. Richard H. Grimm, Jr. "Effects of Thiazide Diuretics on Plasma Lipids and Lipoproteins in Mildly Hypertensive Patients," *Annals of Internal Medicine* 94 (1981): 7–11.

11. P. I. Whelton, "New Trial Tightens Link between Thiazides and Cardiac Arrythmia," *Medical World News*, Jan. 24, 1983.

12. Herbert G. Langford et al., "Dietary Therapy Slows the Return of Hypertension After Stopping Prolonged Medication," *JAMA* 253 (Feb. 1, 1985).
13. Rose Stamler et al., "Nutritional Therapy for High Blood Pressure," *JAMA* 257 (March 20, 1987).
14. Gina Kolata, "Link of Salt and Blood Pressure Becomes Cloudy," *New York Times,* Dec. 3, 1987.
15. David A. McCarron, "Calcium Metabolism and Hypertension," International Society of Nephrology, *Kidney International* 35 (1989).
16. David A. McCarron, "Is Calcium More Important than Sodium in the Pathogenesis of Essential Hypertension?" *Hypertension* 7 (July–Aug. 1985).
17. Norman M. Kaplan et al., "Potassium Supplementation in Hypersensitive Patients with Diuretic-induced Hypokalemia," *New England Journal of Medicine* 312 (March 21, 1985).
18. Norman M. Kaplan, "Non-Drug Treatment of Hypertension," *Annals of Internal Medicine* 102 (March 1985): 359–373.
19. O. Ophir et al., "Low Blood Pressure in Vegetarians: The Possible Role of Potassium," *American Journal of Clinical Nutrition* 37 (1983): 755–62.
20. See note 7 above.
21. J. Wikstrand et al., "Primary Prevention with Metoprolol in Patients with Hypertension," *JAMA* 259 (April 1, 1988): 1976–1982.
22. Sydney H. Croog et al., "The Effects of Antihypertensive Therapy on the Quality of Life," *New England Journal of Medicine* 314 (June 26, 1986).
23. Medical Research Council Working Party, "MRC Trial of Treatment of Mild Hypertension: Principal Results," *British Medical Journal* 291 (1985): 97–104.
24. "Hypertension: Is the Diagnosis Accurate?" *HealthFacts,* vol. XIII, no. 105, Feb., 1988.
25. Eileen M. Stuart et al., "Nonpharmacologic treatment of hypertension: A Multiple-Risk-Factor Approach," *Journal of Cardiovascular Nursing* (Aug. 1987).
26. *Journal of Cardiac Rehabilitation* 3 (Dec. 1983): 839–846.
27. H. A. Diehl and D. Mannerberg, "Regression of Hypertension" in *Western Diseases: Their Emergence and Prevention,* ed. H. C. Trowell and D. R. Burkitt (London: Arnold 1981), 392–410.
28. Robert A. Atkins, *Dr. Atkins' Diet Revolution* (New York: McKay, 1972).
29. Sharon J. Fahrion and Steve L. Fahrion, "Biofeedback in Physical Medicine," submitted to *American Journal of Occupational Therapy,* Aug. 1977.
30. Ibid.
31. Elmer E. Green et al., "Self-Regulation Training for Control of Hypertension," *Primary Cardiology* (March 1980).
32. Elmer E. Green and Alyce M. Green, "General and Specific Applications of Thermal Biofeedback," in *Biofeedback, Principles and Practice for Clinicians,* ed. John V. Basmajian (Baltimore: Williams & Wilkins, 1983).
33. See note 29 above.
34. See note 31 above.
35. Ibid.
36. Steven Fahrion et al., "Biobehavioral Treatment of Essential Hypertension: A Group Outcome Study," *Biofeedback and Self-Regulation* 11 (1986).
37. L. John Mason, *Guide to Stress Reduction* (Culver City, Calif.: Peace Press, 1980).
38. The following is based on Herbert Benson's *The Relaxation Response* (New York: William Morrow, 1975) and *Beyond the Relaxation Response* (New York: Times Books, 1984).
39. "Discover the Mind/Body Connection" (Boston: New England Deaconess Hospital, Behavioral Medicine Section).
40. Eileen M. Stuart et al., "Nonpharmacologic Treatment of Hypertension: A Multiple-Risk-Factor Approach," *Journal of Cardiovascular Nursing* (Aug. 1987).
41. Debora De Ping Lee et al., "Neurohumoral Mechanisms and Left Ventricular Hypertrophy: Effects of Hygienic Therapy," *Journal of Human Hypertension* 1 (1987): 147–151.
42. The following account is based on James J. Lynch's *Language of the Heart* (New York: Basic Books, 1985).

3. HOW TO PREVENT HEART DISEASE

1. "Progress in the Fight against Heart Disease," *Science News,* Jan. 28, /1989.
2. "Lowering Cholesterol," *JAMA* 253 (April 12, 1985).
3. *Your Heart* (People's Medical Society, 462 Walnut St., Allentown, PA 18102, 1985).
4. "Lowering Blood Cholesterol to Prevent Heart Disease," *JAMA* 253 (April 12, 1985).
5. Thomas H. Ainsworth, *Live or Die* (New York: Macmillan, 1983).
6. "U.S. Research Shows How Smoking Causes Cardiovascular Problems," Univ. of Southern California, U.S. News Service, PVW 205, Los Angeles, CA 90089-1227.
7. Cindy L. Jajich et al., "Smoking and Coronary Heart Disease Mortality in the Elderly," *JAMA* 252 (Nov. 23/30, 1984).
8. Ronald E. Vlietstra et al., "Effect of Cigarette Smoking on Survival of Patients with Angiographically Documented Coronary Artery Disease," *JAMA* 255 (Feb. 28, 1986).
9. William P. Castelli and Glen C. Griffin, "How to Help Patients Cut Down on Saturated Fat," *Postgraduate Medicine* 84 (Sept. 1, 1988).
10. "Coronary Disease among U.S. Soldiers Killed in Action in Korea," *JAMA* (July 18, 1953).
11. See note 4 above.
12. Roger J. Williams, *Nutrition Against Disease* (New York: Bantam Books, 1971).
13. Maria C. Linder, *Nutritional Biochemistry and Metabolism* (New York: Elsevier, 1985).
14. *Medical World News,* May 13, 1985.
15. Russell L. Smith, *Diet, Blood Cholesterol and Coronary Heart Disease: A Critical Review of the Literature* (Vector Enterprises, 1930–14th St. Santa Monica, CA 90404, Sept. 1988).
16. "The Lipid Research Clinics Coronary Primary Prevention Trial Results," *JAMA* 251 (Jan. 20, 1984).
17. Allan S. Brett, "Treating Hypercholesterolemia," *New England Journal of Medicine* 321 (Sept. 7, 1989): 676–679.
18. Thomas J. Moore, "The Cholesterol Myth," *The Atlantic,* Sept. 1989.
19. Ibid.
20. Alfred E. Harper, "Transitions in Health Status: Implications for Dietary Recommendations," *American Journal of Clinical Nutrition* 5 (1987): 1094–1107.
21. See note 18 above.
22. "Hold the Eggs and Butter," *Time,* March 26, 1984.
23. See note 4 above.
24. William C. Taylor et al., "Cholesterol Reduction and Life Expectancy: A Model Incorporating Multiple Risk Factors," *Annals of Internal Medicine* (April 1987).
25. D. Mark Hegsten, "Dietary Advice: The Individual Versus the Herd," *Journal of Applied Nutrition* 40 (1988).
26. "Dietary Cholesterol Still a Lively Discussion Topic," *JAMA* 259 (March 11, 1988).
27. H. Kaunitz, "Dietary Lipids and Arteriosclerosis," *Journal of the American Oil Chemistry Society* 52 (Aug. 1975).
28. E. H. Ahrens, Jr., "The Diet-Heart Question in 1985: Has It Really Been Settled?" *The Lancet* (May 11, 1985).
29. See note 13 above.
30. James E. Dalen, "Lowering Serum Cholesterol: It Is Time to Proceed," *Archives of Internal Medicine* 148 (Jan. 1988): 35.
31. See note 17 above.
32. Stephen C. Stinson, "Drug Industry Steps Up Fight against Heart Disease," *C & EN Northeast News Bureau,* Oct. 3, 1988.
33. Harold M. Schmeck, Jr., "Value of Daily Aspirin Disputed in British Study of Heart Attacks," *New York Times,* Jan. 30, 1988.
34. Annlia Paganini-Hill, *British Medical Journal* (Nov. 18, 1989).
35. "Improved Survival of Surgically Treated Patients with Triple Vessel Coronary Artery Disease

and Severe Angina Pectoris: Report from the Coronary Artery Surgery Study (CASS) Registry," *Journal of Thoracic and Cardiovascular Surgery* 97 (April, 1989).

36. Sandra Blakeslee, "Study Hints of Harm in Heart Operations," *New York Times,* Feb. 20, 1990.
37. National Center for Health Statistics, National Hospital Discharge Surgery, 1984.
38. See note 36 above.
39. Constance Monroe Winslow et al., "The Appropriateness of Performing Coronary Artery Bypass Surgery," *JAMA* 260 (July 22/29, 1988).
40. "Hospitals Get Most from Cardiovascular Surgery," *American Medical News,* Sept. 4, 1987.
41. Glenn Kramon, "A Few Medical Costs Are Focus of Campaign," *New York Times,* Feb. 18, 1988.
42. Robert Mendelsohn, "Coronary Bypass Surgery," *The People's Doctor,* vol. 2, no. 12.
43. "Timi II and the Role of Angioplasty in Acute Myocardial Infarction," *New England Journal of Medicine* 320 (March 9, 1989).
44. National Institutes of Health, Dept. of Health and Human Services.
45. "Hearts and Balloons," *Harvard Medical School Health Letter,* Nov. 1986.
46. "New Caution on the Heart Balloon," *U.S. News & World Report,* July 25, 1988.
47. James M. Seeger et al., "Initial Results of Laser Recanalization in Lower Extremity Arterial Reconstruction," *Journal of Vascular Surgery* 1 (Jan. 9, 1989): 10–17.
48. "The Expert Panel: Report of the National Cholesterol Education Program Expert Panel on Detection, Evaluation, and Treatment of High Blood Cholesterol in Adults," *Archives of Internal Medicine* 148 (Jan. 1988).
49. Ibid.
50. David H. Blankenhorn et al., "Beneficial Effects of Combined Colestipol-Niacin Therapy on Coronary Atherosclerosis and Coronary Venous Bypass Grafts," *JAMA* 257 (June 19, 1987).
51. Edward C. Lambert, M.D., *Modern Medical Mistakes* (Bloomington: Indiana University Press, 1978).
52. Lawrence K. Altman, "Study Finds a $2,200 Heart Drug No Better than One Costing $76," *New York Times,* March 9, 1990.
53. Thomas W. Nygaard et al., "Adverse Reactions to Antiarrhythmic Drugs during Therapy for Ventricular Arrhythmias," *JAMA* 256 (July 4, 1986).
54. Janice B. Schwartz et al., "Adverse Effects of Antiarrhythmic Drugs," *Drugs* 21 (1981): 23–45.
55. See note 53 above.
56. American Heart Association, "Cholesterol and your Heart," 1989.
57. Beatrice Trum Hunter, *Consumer Beware!* (New York: Simon & Schuster, 1971): 18, 286.
58. Donald R. Davis, "Nutrition in the United States: Much Room for Improvement," *Journal of Applied Nutrition,* vol. 35, no. 1 (1983).
59. Roger J. Williams, *The Wonderful World within You* (New York: Bantam Books, 1977).
60. See note 12 above.
61. Ross Hume Hall, *Food for Naught* (New York: Random House, 1976).
62. Weston Price, *Nutrition and Physical Degeneration* (New York: P. B. Hoeber, 1939).
63. Richard A. Kunin, *Meganutrition* (New York: Mc-Graw Hill, 1980).
64. Wilifred Shute, "Vitamin E," *Let's Live,* Jan. 1983.
65. Donald O. Rudin, *The Omega-3 Phenomenon* (New York: Rawson Associates, 1987).
66. Stephen Szanto and John Yudkin, "The Effect of Dietary Sucrose on Blood Lipids, Serum Insulin, Platelet Adhesiveness and Body Weight in Human Volunteers," *Postgraduate Medical Journal* 45 (Sept. 1969): 602–7.
67. See note 12 above.
68. "Dietary Cholesterol Still a Lively Discussion Topic," *JAMA* 259 (March 11, 1988).
69. M. K. Navidi and F. A. Kummerow, "The Nutritive Value of Egg Beaters Compared with Farm Fresh Eggs," *Pediatrics* 53 (April 1974): 565–6.
70. Fred H. Mattson and Scott M. Grundy, "Comparison of Effects of Dietary Saturated, Monounsaturated, and Polyunsaturated Fatty Acids on Plasma Lipids and Lipoproteins in Man," *Journal of Lipid Research* 26 (1985): 194–202.

71. Mary G. Enig, "Status Report Trans Fatty Acid Research," Lipids Biochemistry Group, Department of Chemistry and Biochemistry, University of Maryland, College Park, MD 20742, Dec. 1987.

72. R. A. L. Sturdevant and M. L. Pearce, "Increased Prevalence of Cholelithiasis in Men Ingesting a Serum-Cholesterol-Lowering Diet," *New England Journal of Medicine* 288 (1973): 24–27.

73. *American Journal of Clinical Nutrition* 31 (Nov. 1978): 2005–16.

74. "Alive Talks to Udo Erasmus," *Alive,* Feb./March, 1989.

75. "Fats and Oils: Understanding the Functions and Properties of Partially Hydrogenated Fats and Oils and Their Relationship to Unhydrogenated Fats and Oils," Mary G. Enig, Enig Associates, Inc., Silver Spring, MD, 1989.

76. See note 71 above.

77. "Fish Oil Takes a Dive?" *Science News,* Nov. 28, 1986.

78. "A Fish Oil Story?" *Science News,* Feb. 7, 1987.

79. Udo Erasmus, *Fats and Oils* (Vancouver, Canada: Alive, 1986), 262.

80. See note 57 above.

81. T. Hanis et al., "Effects of Dietary Trans-fatty Acids on Reproductive Performance of Wistar Rats," *British Journal of Nutrition* 61 (1989): 519–29.

82. "Soluble Fiber and Cholesterol," *Harvard Medical School Health Letter,* Oct. 7, 1988.

83. James W. Anderson et al., "Hypocholesterolemic Effects of Oat-bran or Bean Intake for Hypercholesterolemic Men," *American Journal of Clinical Nutrition* 40 (Dec. 1984): 1146–55.

84. Bonnie Liebman, "Jumping on the Bran Wagon," *Nutrition Action Health Letter,* Jan./Feb. 1989.

85. Janis F. Swain et al., "Comparison of the Effects of Oat Bran and Low Fiber Wheat on Serum Lipoprotein Levels and Blood Pressure," *New England Journal of Medicine* 322 (Jan. 18, 1990).

86. See note 13 above.

87. American Heart Association, Press release about Dr. Dean Ornish's study, Nov. 14, 1988.

88. "Effects of Dietary Guar Gum on Hypercholesterolemic Males," *Nutrition Research Newsletter,* July 1984, 71, 72.

89. Benjamin Lau, "Garlic for Health" (Lotus Light Publications, P.O. Box 2, Wilmot, WI 53192).

90. O. M. Kandil, T. H. Abdellah, and A. Elkadi, "Garlic and the Immune System in Humans: Its Effect on Natural Killer Cells," Federation of American Societies for Experimental Biology, Proceedings of 71st Annual Meeting, March 1, 1987, 441.

91. Benjamin Lau, "Detoxifying, Radioprotective and Phagocyte-Enhancing Effects of Garlic," *International Clinical Nutrition Review,* vol. 9, no. 1 (1989): 27–31.

92. "Effect of Onions on Blood Fibrinolytic Activity," *British Medical Journal* (1968).

93. Jeffrey Bland, *Your Health under Siege: Using Nutrition to Fight Back* (Brattleboro, Vt.: Stephen Greene Press, 1981).

94. J. M. Hoeg et al., "Special Communication: An Approach to the Management of Hyperlipoproteinemia," *JAMA* 255 (Jan. 1986): 512–21.

95. James D. Alderman et al., "Effect of a Modified, Well-Tolerated Niacin Regimen on Serum Total Cholesterol, High Density Lipoprotein Cholesterol and the Cholesterol to High Density Lipoprotein Ratio," *American Journal of Cardiology* (Oct. 1, 1989): 725–29.

96. See note 48 above.

97. See note 12 above.

98. See note 13 above.

99. *HealthFacts,* Dec. 1988. (For *HealthFacts'* address, see p. 278.)

100. Jane E. Brody, "Personal Health," *New York Times,* April 27, 1989.

101. Wilfrid E. Shute with Harold J. Taub, *Vitamin E for Ailing and Healthy Hearts* (New York: Pyramid House, 1969).

102. Melvyn R. Werbach, *Nutritional Influences on Illness* (Third Line Press, 4751 Viviana Drive, Tarzana, CA 91356).

103. Richard A. Passwater and Elmer M. Cranton, *Trace Elements, Hair Analysis and Nutrition* (New Canaan, Conn.: Keats Publishing, 1983).

104. Ibid.

105. J. Raloff, "New Misgivings about Low Magnesium," *Science News,* vol. 133, 356.
106. Mildred S. Seelig, "Hyper-reactivity to Vitamin D," *Medical Counterpoint,* July, 1970.
107. Butler Parkinson and Sellers, *Medical Proceedings,* vol. 5 (1959):487.
108. Lloyd T. Iseri et al., "Magnesium Deficiency and Cardiac Disorders," *American Journal of Medicine* 58 (June 1975).
109. Robert C. Wesley, Jr., et al., "Effect of Intravenous Magnesium Sulfate on Supraventricular Tachycardia," *American Journal of Cardiology* 63 (May 1, 1989).
110. Sidney M. Wolfe et al., *Worst Pills Best Pills* (Washington, D.C.: Public Citizens Health Research Group, 1988).
111. Lloyd T. Iseri and James H. French, "Magnesium: Nature's Physiologic Calcium Blocker," *American Heart Journal* 108 (July 1984): 188–93.
112. Jonathan V. Wright, *Dr. Wright's Guide to Healing with Nutrition* (Emmaus, Pa.: Rodale Press, 1984).
113. Leslie M. Klevay, "Interactions of Copper and Zinc in Cardiovascular Disease," *Annals New York Academy of Sciences* 355 (1980): 140–151.
114. See note 103 above.
115. Frans J. Kok, "Decreased Selenium Levels in Acute Myocardial Infarction," *JAMA* 261 (Feb. 24, 1989).
116. See note 102 above.
117. Ibid.
118. Broda O. Barnes and Lawrence Galton, *Hypothyroidism: The Unsuspected Illness* (New York: Thomas Y. Crowell Co., 1976).
119. Library of Congress Catalog Card Number 74-82883.
120. United Fresh Fruit and Vegetable Association, 727 N. Washington St., Alexandria, VA 22314, personal communication, March 1990.

4. CHELATION THERAPY

1. Elmer Cranton and Arline Brecher, *Bypassing Bypass* (Norfolk, VA: Donning Co., 1989).
2. Efrain Olszewer and James P. Carter, "EDTA Chelation Therapy in Chronic Degenerative Disease," *Medical Hypotheses* 27 (1988): 41–49.
3. See note 1 above.
4. Dawn D. Bennett, "Chelation Therapists: Charlatans or Saviors?" *Science News,* March 2, 1985.
5. "Chelation Therapy: A Second Look," *Harvard Medical School Health Letter,* July 1984.
6. See note 1 above.
7. See note 4 above.
8. See note 1 above.
9. Daniel Steinberg, "Beyond Cholesterol: Modifications of Low-Density Lipoprotein that Increase Its Atherogenicity," *New England Journal of Medicine* 320 (April 6, 1989).
10. Norman E. Clarke and Clarke C. Mosher, "Treatment of Angina Pectoris with Disodium Ethylene Diamine Tetraacetic Acid," *American Journal of Medical Science* (Dec. 1956): 654–6.
11. Norman E. Clarke, "Treatment of Occlusive Vascular Disease with Disodium Ethylene Diamine Tetraacetic Acid (EDTA)," *American Journal of Medical Science* (June 1960): 732–44.
12. Morton Walker, *Chelation Therapy: How to Predict or Reverse Hardening of the Arteries* (New York: M. Evans & Co., 1985), 130.
13. See note 1 above.
14. Alfred Soffer, letter to author, Feb. 20, 1987.
15. H. R. Casdorph, "Chelation Therapy: Efficacy in Brain Disorders," *Journal of Holistic Medicine* 3 (1981): 101–17.
16. Efrain Olszewer and James P. Carter, "EDTA Chelation Therapy in Chronic Degenerative Disease," *Medical Hypotheses* 27 (1988): 41–49.
17. Ibid.

18. "ACAM Update," American College of Advancement in Medicine (800/532–3688), March 21, 1990.
19. Donald R. Crapper McLachlan and U. De Boni, "Aluminum in Human Brain Disease—An overview," *Neurotoxicology* 1 (1980): 3–16.
20. Paul Cutler, "Deferoxamine Therapy in High-Ferritin Diabetes," *Diabetes* 38 (Oct. 1989).
21. L. E. Meltzer, M. E. Ural, and Kitchell Jr., "The Treatment of Coronary Artery Disease with Disodium EDTA," in M. J. Johnson, ed., *Metal Binding in Medicine* (Philadelphia: J.B. Lippincott, 1960), 132–36.

5. ARTHRITIS—TRY NUTRITION FIRST

1. R. S. Panush, "Nutritional Therapy for Rheumatic Diseases," *Annals of Internal Medicine* 106 (April 1987).
2. *New York Times,* Aug. 19, 1985.
3. Food and Drug Administration Press Release, Dec. 27, 1988.
4. "Summary of Label Changes," Food and Drug Administration, Feb. 3, 1989.
5. D. L. Scott et al., "Long-term Outcome of Treating Rheumatoid Arthritis: Results after 20 Years," *The Lancet* (May 16, 1987).
6. Theodore Pincus et al., "Severe Functional Declines, Work Disability, and Increased Mortality in Seventy-Five Rheumatoid Arthritis Patients Studied Over Nine Years," *Arthritis and Rheumatism* 27 (Aug. 1984).
7. Arthritis Foundation, "Arthritis Research: What's New." 1988.
8. Executive Committee, "Position Statements: Clinical Ecology," *Journal of Allergy and Clinical Immunology* 78 (Aug. 1986): 269–77.
9. Doris Rapp, "Environmental Medicine: An Expanded Approach to Allergy," *Buffalo Physician,* Feb. 1986.
10. "Adverse Reactions to Foods" (American Academy of Allergy and Immunology, 611 East Wells St., Milwaukee, WI 53202).
11. See note 9 above.
12. "What is Environmental Medicine?" (American Academy of Environmental Medicine, P.O. Box 16106, Denver, CO 80216).
13. Robert Marshall et al., "Food Challenge Effects on Fasted Rheumatoid Arthritis Patients: A Multicenter Study" (Chicago: Human Ecology Research Foundation), first presented at the Third International Food Allergy Symposium of the American College of Allergists, Boston, October 1980.
14. Michael Zeller, "Rheumatoid Arthritis—Food Allergy as a Factor," *Annals of Allergy* 7 (1949): 200–205.
15. Marshall Mandell, *Dr. Mandell's Lifetime Arthritis Relief System* New York: Coward-McCann, 1983), 84.
16. Theron G. Randolph and Ralph W. Moss, *An Alternative Approach to Allergies* (New York: Bantam Books, 1980), 157.
17. Marshall Mandell and Anthony A. Conte, "The Role of Allergy in Arthritis, Rheumatism and Polysymptomatic Cerebral Visceral and Somatic Disorders: A Double-Blind Study," *Journal of the International Academy of Preventive Medicine* 7 (July 1982).
18. See note 13 above.
19. Richard S. Panush et al., "Diet Therapy for Rheumatoid Arthritis," *Arthritis and Rheumatism* 26 (April 1983).
20. See note 1 above.
21. Arthritis Foundation News Release, June 6, 1986.
22. See note 1 above.
23. A. L. Parke and G. R. V. Hughes, *British Medical Journal* 282 (June 20, 1981).
24. Ronald Williams, *British Medical Journal* 283 (August 22, 1981).

25. "Fish, Fatty Acids, and Human Health," *New England Journal of Medicine* 312 (May 9, 1985).

26. Norman F. Childers, *Arthritis—A Diet to Stop It* (Horticultural Publications, 3906 N.W. 31 Pl., Gainesville, FL 32606, 1986).

27. Tak H. Lee et al., "Effect of Dietary Enrichment with Eicosapentaenoic and Docosahexaenoic Acids on In Vitro Neutrophil and Monocyte Leukotriene Generation and Neutrophil Function," *New England Journal of Medicine* 312 (May 9, 1985).

28. Joel M. Kremer et al., "Effects of Manipulation of Dietary Fatty Acids on Clinical Manifestations of Rheumatoid Arthritis," *The Lancet* (Jan. 26, 1985): 184–7.

29. Joel M. Kremer et al., "Fish-Oil Fatty Acid Supplementation in Active Rheumatoid Arthritis," *Annals of Internal Medicine* 106 (April 1987).

30. "Benefits of Eating Fish," *Tufts University Diet and Nutrition Letter,* July 1985.

31. "The Year of the Fish Oil," *Health Facts,* March 1987.

32. *Worst Pills Best Pills* (Public Citizen Health Research Group, 2000 P Street, N.W., Suite 700, Washington, DC 20036, 1988).

33. Dale Alexander, *Arthritis and Common Sense #2* (West Hartford, Conn.: Witkower Press, 1984).

34. Charles A. Brusch and Edward T. Johnson, "A New Dietary Regimen for Arthritis, Value of Cod Liver Oil on a Fasting Stomach," *Journal of the National Medical Association* (July 1959).

35. Michael E. Rosenbaum and Dominick Bosco, *Super Fitness Beyond Vitamins* (New York: New American Library, 1987).

36. D. Ansell et al., "The Effects of Efamol and Efamol Marine on Patients with Rheumatoid Arthritis: A Double Blind, Placebo-Controlled Study" (Paper delivered at the 6th International Congress on Prostaglandins, Florence, Italy, June 1986).

37. Mark A. Stahmann, "The Potential for Alfalfa Protein Concentrates in Animal and Human Nutrition" (Paper delivered at the Fourteenth Farm Seed Conference, 1968, University of Wisconsin, Madison).

38. E. C. Barton-Wright and W. A. Elliott, "The Pantothenic Acid Metabolism of Rheumatoid Arthritis, *The Lancet* (Oct. 26, 1963): 862–3.

39. Patricia Hausman, *The Right Dose* (Emmaus, Pa: Rodale Press, 1987).

40. Stuart M. Berger, *How to Be Your Own Nutritionist* (New York: William Morrow 1987).

41. James Braly and Laura Torbet, *Dr. Braly's Optimum Health Program* (New York: Times Books, 1985).

42. John M. Ellis and James Presley, *Vitamin B6: The Doctor's Report* (New York: Harper & Row, 1973).

43. Richard A. Kunin, *Mega-Nutrition* (New York: New American Library, 1981).

44. John R. J. Sorenson, "Copper Chelates as Possible Active Metabolites of the Antiarthritic and Antiepileptic Drugs," *Journal of Applied Nutrition* vol. 32, nos. 1 & 2, 1980.

45. W. R. Walker, "The 'Copper Bracelet' for Arthritis," *Medical Journal of Australia* (June 18, 1977).

46. W. Ray Walker, "The Results of a Copper Bracelet Clinical Trial and Subsequent Studies," *Inflammatory Diseases and Copper,* ed. John R. J. Sorenson (Clifton, N.J.: The Humana Press, 1982).

47. See note 45 above.

48. Roger J. Williams, *Nutrition Against Disease* (New York: Bantam Books, 1978).

49. Carl C. Pfeiffer, *Mental and Elemental Nutrients* (New Canaan, Conn.: Keats Publishing 1975).

50. See note 43 above.

51. Dava Sobel and Arthur Klein, *Arthritis: What Works* (New York: St. Martin's Press, 1989).

6. CONSTIPATION—HOW TO BANISH IT FROM YOUR LIFE

1. Bernard Jensen, *Tissue Cleansing through Bowel Management.* (Escondido, Calif.: Bernard Jensen, 1981).

2. Ibid.
3. David Reuben, *The Save Your Life Diet* (New York: Random House, 1975).
4. Denis Burkitt, *Don't Forget Fiber In Your Diet* (New York: Arco Publishing, 1979).
5. D. P. Burkitt, "Dietary Fiber and Disease," *JAMA* 229 (Aug. 19, 1974).
6. See note 4 above.
7. Joseph E. Pizzorno and Michael T. Murray, *A Textbook of Natural Medicine* (Seattle, Wash.: John Bastyr College Publications, 1985).
8. James D'Adamo, *One Man's Food* (Toronto: Health Thru Herbs, 1980).
9. Jean Carper, *The Food Pharmacy* (New York: Bantam Books, 1988), 91.
10. *Cancer Control Journal*, vol. 6 no. 7–12 (1985).
11. *Intestinal Toxicology*, ed. Carol Schiller (New York: Raven Press, 1984), 231.
12. Nicholas L. Petrakis and Eileen B. King, "Cytological Abnormalities in Nipple Aspirates of Breast Fluid from Women with Severe Constipation," *The Lancet* (Nov. 28, 1981).
13. Martin E. Plaut, *The Doctor's Guide to You and Your Colon* (New York: Harper & Row, 1982).
14. See note 4 above.
15. Mark Bricklin, *The Natural Healing Annual* (Emmaus, Pa.: Rodale Press, 1985).
16. Shahani and Ayebo, "Role of Dietary Lactobacilli in Gastrointestinal Microecology," *American Journal of Clinical Nutrition* 33 (1980): 2448–57.
17. Dennis Nelson, "Food Combining Simplified," P. O. Box 2302, Santa Cruz, CA 95063.
18. See note 7 above.
19. "Drug Store News," *Inside Pharmacy*, July 20, 1987.
20. Linda Berry, *Internal Cleansing: A Practical Guide to Colon Health* (Capitola, Calif.: Botanica Press, 1985).

7. THE THERAPEUTIC DIET

1. John A. McDougall and Mary A. McDougall, *The McDougall Plan for Super Health and Life-Long Weight Loss* (Piscataway, N.J.: New Century Publishers, 1983).
2. Marian Burros, "What Americans Eat: Nutrition Can Wait, Survey Finds," *New York Times,* Jan. 6, 1988, Sec. 3.
3. Pritikin Research Foundation 1987, 1910 Ocean Front Walk, Santa Monica, CA 90405.
4. Corinne H. Robinson, *Basic Nutrition and Diet Therapy* (New York: Macmillan, 1975).
5. Tom Monte with Ilene Pritikin, *Pritikin: The Man Who Healed America's Heart* (Emmaus, Pa.: Rodale Press, 1988).
6. Jon N. Leonard, J. L. Hofer, and N. Pritikin, *Live Longer Now—The First One Hundred Years of Your Life* (New York: Grosset & Dunlap Publishers, 1974).
7. Ibid.
8. See note 5 above.
9. See note 4 above.
10. "Pritikin vs. AHA Diet: No Difference for Peripheral Vascular Disease," *JAMA* (Oct. 23/30, 1981).
11. Robert C. Atkins, *Dr. Atkins' Health Revolution* (Boston: Houghton Mifflin, 1988).
12. "Nathan Pritikin's Heart," Letters to the Editor, *New England Journal of Medicine* (July 4, 1985).
13. Dean Ornish (Paper presented at the 62nd Annual Meeting of the American Heart Association, New Orleans, La., Nov. 13, 1989).
14. See note 1 above.
15. "Position Paper on Food and Nutrition Misinformation on Selected Topics," *ADA Reports* 66 (March 1975).
16. "Position Paper on the Vegetarian Approach to Eating," *ADA Reports* 77 (July 1980).
17. "Position of the American Dietetic Association: Vegetarian Diets," *ADA Reports* 88 (March 1988).
18. Weston A. Price, *Nutrition and Physical Degeneration* (New York: Paul B. Hoeber, 1939).

19. See note 17 above.
20. *Bulletin of the Walter Kempner Foundation,* Durham, N.C., June 1972.
21. David H. Blankenhorn et al., "Beneficial Effects of Combined Colestipol-Niacin Therapy on Coronary Atherosclerosis and Coronary Venous Bypass Grafts," *JAMA* 257 (June 19, 1987).
22. Michio Kushi, *The Book of Macrobiotics: The Universal Way of Health, Happiness, and Peace* (New York: Japan Publications, 1987), 156–57.
23. Ibid., 266.
24. Ibid.
25. Michio Kushi, *The Macrobiotic Approach to Cancer* (Wayne, N.J.: Avery Publishing Group, 1982).
26. Michio Kushi, *The Cancer-Prevention Diet* (New York: St. Martin's Press, 1983).
27. See note 22 above.
28. American Cancer Society, "Unproven Methods of Cancer Management," Professional Education Publication, 1982.
29. Randi Londer, "Cure by Diet?" *Health,* Oct. 1985.
30. See note 26 above.
31. Jane E. Brody, "Personal Health: Vegetarian Diets for Young Children," *New York Times,* March 25, 1987.
32. Paul Sherlock and Edmund O. Rothschild, "Scurvy Produced by a Zen Macrobiotic Diet," *JAMA* 199 (March 13, 1967).
33. "Position Paper on the Vegetarian Approach to Eating," *ADA Reports* 77 (July 1980).
34. Fredrick J. Stare, M.D., Ph.D., and Virginia Aronson, R.D., M.S., *Your Basic Guide to Nutrition* (Philadelphia: George F. Stickley Co., 1983).
35. See note 22 above.
36. Ibid.
37. Annemarie Colbin, *Food and Healing* (New York: Ballantine Books, 1986).

8. TREATING DISEASE WITH VITAMINS AND MINERALS

1. William H. Philpott and Dwight K. Kalita, *Brain Allergies* (New Canaan, Conn.: Keats Publishing, 1980).
2. Ibid.
3. Jack Smith and James S. Turner, "A Perspective on the History and Use of the Recommended Dietary Allowances," *Currents—The Journal of Food, Nutrition & Health* (Institute of Nutrition, University of North Carolina), April 1986.
4. Richard A. Kunin, *Mega-Nutrition* (New York: New American Library, 1980).
5. Richard Haitch, "Followup on the News," *New York Times,* Nov. 9, 1986.
6. Roger J. Williams, *Nutrition Against Disease* (New York: Bantam Books, 1973).
7. Abram Hoffer, *Common Questions on Schizophrenia and Their Answers* (New Canaan, Conn.: Keats Publishing, 1987).
8. Donald O. Rudin, "Medical Monopoly and the Modern Health Disaster: Defensive Eating and Public Policy," submitted to *Harvard Business Review.*
9. Donald O. Rudin, "The Three Pellagras," *Journal of Orthomolecular Psychiatry,* vol. 12, no. 21983.
10. U.S. Department of Health, Education and Welfare, "HANES: Health and Nutrition Examination Survey," Publication No. (HRA) 74-1219-1 (Rockville, Md., 1974).
11. U.S. Department of Agriculture, "Eating Behavior and Associated Nutrient Quality of Diets: A Study of Food Consumption Patterns in the United States," Human Nutrition Center, Science and Education Administration, Oct. 1982.
12. A. Hoffer, H. Osmond, and J. Smythies, "Schizophrenia: A New Approach. Results of a Year's Research," *Journal of Mental Science* 100 (1954).

13. A. Hoffer, "Does Every Schizophrenic Patient Need Tranquilizers?" *Journal of Orthomolecular Medicine* 2 (1987).
14. Linus Pauling, *How to Live Longer and Feel Better* (New York: W. H. Freeman & Co., 1986), p. 19.
15. Linus Pauling, "Orthomolecular Psychiatry," *Science*, April 19, 1968.
16. American Psychiatric Association, "Megavitamin and Orthomolecular Therapy in Psychiatry," *Task Force Report 7,* July 1973.
17. Charles Marshall, "Can Megavitamins Help Mental Health?" *Vitamins and Minerals, Help or Harm* (Los Angeles: George Stickley Co., 1983).
18. "A Top Priority at NIMH," *Science*, Jan. 23, 1987.
19. See note 4 above.
20. Steven H. Zeisel et al., "Use of Choline and Lecithin in the Treatment of Tardive Dyskinesia," in *Long-Term Effects of Neuroleptics,* ed. F. Cattabeni et al., vol. 24 of series Advances in Biochemical Psychopharmacology (New York: Raven Press, 1980), pp. 463–470.
21. Abram Hoffer and Morton Walker, *Orthomolecular Nutrition* (New Canaan, Conn.: Keats Publishing, 1978).
22. See note 4 above.
23. David R. Hawkins, "The Prevention of Tardive Dyskinesia with High Dosage Vitamins: A Study of 58,000 Patients," *Journal of Orthomolecular Medicine* 1(1986):24–26.
24. See note 18 above.
25. National Alliance for the Mentally Ill, 2101 Welson Blvd., Suite 302, Arlington, VA 22201.
26. William Styron, "Why Primo Levi Need Not Have Died," *New York Times*, Dec. 19, 1988.
27. Elizabeth Rasche Gonzalez, "Sperm Swim Singly After Vitamin C Therapy," *JAMA* 249 (May 27, 1983).
28. Michael Schneir et al., "Dietary Ascorbic Acid Normalizes Diabetes-Induced Under-Hydroxylation of Nascent Type I Collagen Molecules," *Collagen Related Research* 5 (1985): 415–22.
29. Mark Levine, "New Concepts in the Biology and Biochemistry of Ascorbic Acid," *New England Journal of Medicine* (April 3, 1986).
30. Derrick Lonsdale, M.D., "Thou Shalt Do No Harm," *International Journal for Biosocial Research* 4(2) (July 6, 1983).
31. Dr. Karl Folkers, Institute for Biomedical Research, University of Texas at Austin, Austin, TX 78712.
32. National Society for Autistic Children, "Could Your Child Be Autistic?" (Albany, N.Y.: The Society).
33. Bernard Rimland et al., "The Effect of High Doses of Vitamin B6 on Autistic Children: A Double-blind Crossover Study," *American Journal of Psychiatry* 135 (April 1978).
34. Karl H. Schutte and John A. Myers, *Metabolic Aspects of Health* (Kentfield, Calif.: Discovery Press, 1979).
35. See note 1 above.
36. Marshall Mandell and Lynne Waller Scanlon, *Dr. Mandell's 5-Day Allergy Relief System* (New York: Pocket Books, 1980).
37. K. Kennakone and S. Wickramanayake, "Aluminum Leaching from Cooking Utensils," *Nature*, Jan. 1987.
38. Eric R. Braverman with Carl C. Pfeiffer, *The Healing Nutrients Within* (New Canaan, Conn.: Keats Publishing, 1987).
39. "Lecithin Can Suppress Tardive Dyskinesia," *New England Journal of Medicine* (May 4, 1978).
40. See note 20 above.
41. "Vitamin Eases Symptoms of a Schizophrenia Drug," *New York Times*, Nov. 3, 1988.
42. Robert O. Becker and Gary Selden, *The Body Electric* (New York: William Morrow, 1985), 334.
43. Jean Lud Cadet and James B. Lohr, "Free Radicals and the Developmental Pathobiology of Schizophrenic Burnout," *Integral Psychiatry* 5 (1987):40–48.
44. See note 12 above.

9. CATARACT SURGERY—ANOTHER UNNECESSARY OPERATION?

1. American Academy of Ophthalmology, "Cataract—Clouding the Lens of Sight" (San Francisco: The Academy, 1984).
2. Gerald D. Faulkner and Carlos A. Omphroy, *About Cataracts,* 4th ed. (Honolulu, Hawaii: 1987).
3. American Academy of Ophthalmology, "Cataract in the Otherwise Healthy Adult Eye," *Preferred Practice Pattern* (San Francisco: The Academy, Sept. 16, 1989).
4. Otto Hockwin, "The Causes and Prevention of Cataract Blindness," *Endeavor, New Series,* vol. 9, no. 3, 1985, Pergamon Press, Great Britain.
5. Julius Shulman, *Cataracts* (New York: Simon & Schuster, 1984).
6. William B. Rathbun, "An Achilles' Heel of the Human Lens," Research to Prevent Blindness, Inc., Science Writers Seminar, Washington, D.C., Sept. 30–Oct. 30, 1984..
7. See note 5 above.
8. S. D. Varma et al., "Mechanism of In Vitro Photodynamic Damage to Lens," *Lens Research* 2 (2) (1984–85): 145–57. (This study is one in a series.)
9. Shambhu D. Varma, "Vitamin C and the Lens of the Eye: Possible Anticataract Effect," Unpublished paper.
10. Roy H. Rengstorff, "Cutaneous Acetone Depresses Aqueous Humor Ascorbate in Guinea Pigs," *Archives of Toxicology* 58 (1985): 64–66.
11. Roy H. Rengstorff, John P. Petrali, and Van M. Sim, "Cataracts Induced in Guinea Pigs by Acetone, Cyclohexanone and Dimethyl Sulfoxide," *American Journal of Optometry and Archives of American Academy of Optometry* 49 (April 1972): 308–19.
12. William B. Rathbun, Ph.D., "Glutathione Synthesis in Evolution: An Achilles' Heel of Human and other Old World Simian Lens," *Opthalmic Research* 18 (1986): 236–242.
13. Paul F. Jacques et al., "Antioxidant Status Persons with and without Senile Cataract," *Archives of Ophthalmology* 106 (March 1988).
14. David A. Newsome et al., "Oral Zinc in Macular Degeneration," *Archives of Ophthalmology* 106 (Feb. 1988).
15. Vilma Yuzbasiyan-Gurkan and George J. Brewer, "The Therapeutic Use of Zinc in Macular Degeneration," Correspondence, *Archives of Ophthalmology* 107 (Dec. 1989).
16. See note 3 above.
17. Health Products Research, Inc., North Branch, N.J.
18. See note 1 above.
19. See note 3 above.
20. Carrier Operations & Policy, Health Care Financing, Chicago, Ill.
21. See note 3 above.
22. The following account is based on Gary Price Todd's *Nutrition, Health and Disease* (Norfolk, Va.: The Donning Co., 1988).
23. I. Wickelgren, "Vitamins C and E May Prevent Cataracts," *Science News* 135, May 20, 1989.

10. ENERGY MEDICINE

1. William A. Tiller, "What Do Electrodermal Diagnostic Acupuncture Instruments Really Measure," *American Journal of Acupuncture* 15 (Jan.–March 1987).
2. Richard Gerber, *Vibrational Medicine: New Choices for Healing Ourselves* (Santa Fe, N.M.: Bear & Co. 1988).
3. Kathleen McAuliffe, "Brain Tuner," *Omni,* Jan. 1983.
4. Larry Sessions, "Testing the Body Magnetic," *East West,* Oct. 1987.
5. Elmer Green, "Biofeedback and Human Potential," in *Energy Medicine around the World,* ed. T. M. Srinivasvan (Phoenix: Gabriel Press, 1988).

6. Herbert Benson, *Beyond the Relaxation Response* (New York: Times Books, 1984).
7. See note 2 above.
8. T. M. Srinivasan, *Energy Medicine Around the World.* (Phoenix: Gabriel Press, 1988).
9. Maury M. Breecher, "Three Cardiologists Report Prayers for their Patients Are 'Answered,'" *Medical News & International Reports,* Feb. 3, 1986.
10. Clifford C. Kuhn, "A Spiritual Inventory of the Medically Ill Patient," *Psychiatric Medicine* 6, 2 (1988).
11. "Dolores Krieger's Therapeutic Touch," *East West,* Aug. 1989.
12. *BEMI Currents,* Newsletter of the Bio-Electro-Magnetics Institute, 2490 W. Moana Lane, Reno, NV 89509, Spring 1989.
13. The following paragraph is based on note 2 above.
14. "Electronic Evidence of Auras, Chakras in UCLA Study," *Brain/Mind Bulletin* March 20, 1978.
15. Harold M. Schmeck, Jr., "Scientists Explore Body's Magnetic Field," *New York Times,* April 29, 1980.
16. Robert O. Becker and Andrew A. Marino, *Electromagneticism and Life* (Albany: State University of New York Press, 1982).
17. For information about BRAGS, contact Mrs. Ethel S. Pollack, executive secretary, BRAGS, P.O. Box 64, Dresher, PA 19025, (215) 659–5180.
18. Richard B. Borgens et al., "Behavioral Recovery Induced by Applied Electric Fields after Spinal Cord Hemisection in Guinea Pig," *Science,* Oct. 16, 1987, 366–69.
19. Gary Taubes, "An Electrifying Possibility," *Discovery,* April, 1986.
20. See note 16 above.
21. Philip H. Abelson, "Effects of Electric and Magnetic Fields," *Science,* July 21, 1989.
22. "Primary Treatment Is Not Enough for Early Stage Breast Cancer," National Cancer Institute, Office of Cancer Communications, May 18, 1988.
23. H. Roy Curtin, "Traditional and Emerging Methods of Electro-Diagnosis," *Journal of the Society of Ultramolecular Medicine,* 3014 Rigel Ave., Las Vegas, NV 89102.
24. William A. Tiller, "What Do Electrodermal Diagnostic Acupuncture Instruments Really Measure," *American Journal of Acupuncture* 15 (Jan.–March 1987).
25. Julian N. Kenyon, *Modern Techniques of Acupuncture,* vol. 3, (New York: Thorsons Publishers, 1985).
26. Peter V. Madill, "First, Doctor to the Whole Body. Electroacupuncture According to Voll and the Cause of Holistic Dentistry," *American Journal of Acupuncture* 8 (Oct.–Dec. 1980).
27. David W. Eggleston et al., "Evoked Electrical Conductivity on the Lung Acupuncture Points in Healthy Individuals and Confirmed Lung Cancer Patients," *American Journal of Acupuncture* 13 (July–Sept. 1985).
28. Julia J. Tsuei et al., "A Food Allergy Study Utilizing the EAV Acupuncture Technique," *American Journal of Acupuncture* 12 (April–June 1984).
29. See note 26 above.
30. "A Conversation about Energy Medicine," *Complementary Medicine,* March/April 1987.
31. Albert E. Nehl, *The American Vegatester,* Nehl Health Center, P.O. Box 129, Kingston, GA 30145, (404) 336–5521.
32. Howard Roy Curtin, "Hololinguistic Technology," *Case Reports,* Dec. 1986.
33. Catherine E. Spears, "Auricular Acupuncture: New Approach to Treatment of Cerebral Palsy," *American Journal of Acupuncture* 1 (Jan.–March 1979).
34. Philip S. Callahan, "Treating the AIDS Virus as an Antenna," *21st Century,* March–April 1989.

Index

Academy of Orthomolecular Medicine, 159
acetone, 238
Achievable Benefit Not Achieved (ABNA)
    Clinical Services, 158–159
Achtenberg, Jeanne, 26
Acupath 1000, 263
acupuncture, 4, 260–262, 264–265, 268,
    271–273
ADA Reports, 193, 203
Adriamycin, 14
Agriculture Department, U.S., 175, 213
Ahrens, E. H., Jr., 82–83
AIDS, 200, 224, 273
Ainsworth, Thomas H., 76
Aldworth, Grace, 47–48
Alexander, Dale, 148, 149
alfalfa, 151–152
Alford, Robert, 158
allergies, 136–142, 191, 205, 230
Alliance for Alternative Medicine, 51–52
alpha blockers, 65
alternative medicine:
    for cancer, 16–54, 251
    for cataracts, 241–245
    for constipation, 166–174
    economics of, 3, 17, 23
    evaluation techniques of, 2; *see also*
        electrodiagnosis; nutritional status,
        assessment of
    for heart disease, 88–117
    for high blood pressure, 62–74
    locating of, 275–277
    medical background of, 3
    orthodox physicians and medicine compared
        with, 2, 17–19, 27, 32, 136–142
    scientific research on, 3, 17, 29, 32, 33–
        34, 40, 45, 63–64, 71–72, 91–98,
        108–109, 110, 112, 113, 115–116,
        121–126, 150–151, 156, 174
    use of term, 2–3
    see also energy medicine; orthomolecular
        medicine; therapeutic diet
aluminum, 128
Alzheimer's disease, 124, 127–128
American Academy of Allergy and
    Immunology, 136, 137
American Academy of Environmental
    Medicine, 141
American Academy of Medical Acupuncture,
    260
American Academy of Ophthalmology, 235,
    240, 241, 245
American Association of Orthomolecular

Medicine (Huxley Institute), 139, 215,
    222, 232–233
American Biologics (A-B) Research Hospital,
    23, 40, 41
American Cancer Society (ACS), 8–11, 13,
    16, 17, 18, 27–28, 31, 45, 199, 205
American College for Advancement in
    Medicine (ACAM), 120, 124, 127
American College of Cardiology, 86
American Dental Association, 129
American Diabetes Association (ADA), 180
American Dietetic Association (ADA), 190,
    193, 203, 204
American Health, 151
American Heart Association (AHA), 80, 83,
    86, 89–90, 93, 94, 95, 100, 148, 175,
    180, 181, 182
American Holistic Medical Association
    (AHMA), 275
American Journal of Cardiology, 104
American Medical Association (AMA), 17, 18,
    32, 36, 91, 112, 121, 260
American Medical News, 32
American Nutritionists Association, 152
American Psychiatric Association (APA), 214–
    215
American Society of Clinical Hypnosis, 72
American Society of Dowsers, 46, 258
American Wholefoods Cuisine (Goldbeck and
    Goldbeck), 91
amino acids, 66, 68, 89, 91, 118–129, 151,
    231
    in glutathione, 237, 238–239
Anatomy of an Illness (Cousins), 250
Anderson, James W., 101
angina, 89, 118, 119–120, 123, 124, 179
angiograms, 183
angioplasty, balloon, 85–86, 118
angiotensin, 60
angiotensin-converting enzyme (ACE
    inhibitors), 61
Anitschkov, N., 80
Annals of Internal Medicine, 141–142
antiarrhythmic drugs, 88
antibiotics, 220
antidepressive drugs, 221, 222
Antineoplaston Therapy, 19
antipsychotic drugs (neuroleptics), 215–216
Applied Psychophysiology and Biofeedback,
    71
Aron, Bernard S., 10
arrhythmias, 109
arthritis, 127, 132–159, 229, 273

297